Clinical topics in child and adolescent psychiatry

Edited by Sarah Huline-Dickens

RCPsych Publications

© The Royal College of Psychiatrists 2014

RCPsych Publications is an imprint of the Royal College of Psychiatrists,
21 Prescot Street, London E1 8BB, UK
http://www.rcpsych.ac.uk

British Library Cataloguing-in-Publication Data.
A catalogue record for this book is available from the British Library.
ISBN 978-1-909726-17-8

Distributed in North America by Publishers Storage and Shipping Company.

The views presented in this book do not necessarily reflect those of the Royal College of
Psychiatrists, and the publishers are not responsible for any error of omission or fact.

The Royal College of Psychiatrists is a charity registered in England and Wales (228636) and in
Scotland (SC038369).

Printed by Bell & Bain Limited, Glasgow, UK.

Clinical topics in child and adolescent psychiatry

For Michael Carter

Contents

List of tables   vii

List of boxes   ix

List of figures   xi

List of contributors   xiii

Preface   xvii

1   Child psychiatry and the people who have shaped it   1
    Sarah Huline-Dickens

2   Fabrication and induction of illness in children   10
    Christopher Bass, Catia Acosta, Gwen Adshead and Gerry Byrne

3   Personality disorders as disorganisation of attachment and
    affect regulation   26
    Jaydip Sarkar and Gwen Adshead

4   Post-traumatic stress disorder and attachment: possible links
    with borderline personality disorder   41
    Felicity de Zulueta

5   Management of antisocial behaviour in childhood   57
    Sujid Humayun and Stephen Scott

6   Pharmacology for attention-deficit hyperactivity disorder,
    Tourette syndrome and autism spectrum disorder   74
    David Coghill and Eugenia Sinita

7   Pharmacology for anxiety and obsessive–compulsive disorders,
    affective disorders and schizophrenia   94
    Eugenia Sinita and David Coghill

8   Pharmacological management of core and comorbid symptoms
    in autism spectrum disorder   112
    Rachel Elvins and Jonathan Green

9   Pharmacological treatment of depression and bipolar disorder   129
    *Bernadka Dubicka, Paul Wilkinson, Raphael G. Kelvin and
    Ian M. Goodyer*

10 Cognitive–behavioural therapy with children, young people
    and families: from individual to systemic therapy   150
    Nicky Dummett and Roger Lakin

11 Anxiety disorders   165
    Aaron K. Vallance and Victoria Fernandez

12 Somatising: clinical presentations and aetiological factors   183
    Olivia Fiertag and Mary Eminson

13 Somatising: management and outcomes   201
    Olivia Fiertag and Mary Eminson

14 Evaluating psychological treatments for children with autism   218
    Patricia Howlin

15 Attention-deficit hyperactivity disorder: assessment and
    treatment   231
    Peter Hill

16 Schizophrenia   246
    Chris Hollis

17 Tourette syndrome   262
    Mary Robertson

18 Sleep disorders   287
    Gregory Stores

19 Self-harm in adolescents   301
    Alison Wood

20 Adolescent substance misuse: an update on behaviours
    and treatments   315
    Paul McArdle and Bisharda Angom

21 Eating disorders   330
    Dasha Nicholls and Elizabeth Barrett

22 Gender dysphoria in young people   349
    Domenico Di Ceglie

23 The psychiatry of children aged 0–4   365
    David Foreman

Index   382

Tables

4.1 Diagnostic features of complex post-traumatic stress disorder compared with DSM-5 borderline personality disorder   43

6.1 Long-acting stimulant preparations licensed for the treatment of attention-deficit hyperactivity disorder in the UK and mainland Europe   77

6.2 The Dundee chart for switching between different methylphenidate preparations   78

7.1 Doses and indications for medications used to treat depression, anxiety and obsessive–compulsive disorder (OCD) in children and adolescents   97

7.2 Doses and indications for antipsychotics in children and adolescents   104

7.3 Adverse effect profiles of haloperidol and second-generation (atypical) antipsychotics in children and adolescents   108

8.1 Selected medication for behavioural domains in autism   114

9.1 Pharmacological treatment for depression in children and adolescents: UK and US guidelines and licensing   133

9.2 Pharmacological treatment for mania/hypomania and bipolar disorder in children and adolescents: UK and US guidelines and licensing   141

11.1 Evolutionary protective roles associated with anxiety-related behaviours   166

11.2 Fear and its typical developmental stages   166

11.3 Epidemiological characteristics of anxiety disorders in children and adolescents   167

11.4 Medical conditions and drugs that can mimic anxiety symptoms, with potential further investigations   170

11.5 A comparison of two meta-analyses of the efficacy of psychological therapies for anxiety disorders   175

15.1 Norms for digit span recall   236

16.1 Physical investigations in child- and adolescent-onset psychoses   252

17.1 The effect of Tourette syndrome on the young person's quality of life (QoL)   263

17.2 Comorbid disorders and coexistent psychopathology in young people with Tourette syndrome   270

17.3 Main strategies of the management of the motor and vocal/phonic tics of Tourette syndrome in young people, showing the current evidence   277

20.1 European Union countries with lowest and highest prevalences of previous-month cocaine use among 15- to 34-year-olds in 2007   317

23.1 Epidemiology of psychiatric disorders in preschool children   368

23.2 Instruments useful in the assessment of children aged 0–4   370

Boxes

2.1	Assessment of a parent/carer under suspicion	19
3.1	Key components of the body's emotion-driven multisystem machinery	27
3.2	The neural systems that govern affect regulation	29
3.3	Affect dysregulation with personality disorder	33
4.1	Associated symptoms of post-traumatic stress disorder	42
4.2	Yalom's therapeutic factors	53
5.1	Conduct disorder behaviours (amalgamated from ICD-10 and DSM-5)	58
5.2	Oppositional defiant behaviours (amalgamated from ICD-10 and DSM-5)	58
5.3	Examples of factors found in the assessment of antisocial behaviour which may need attention	61
5.4	Intervention principles	66
5.5	Examples of good practice	67
8.1	Important considerations when prescribing for autism spectrum disorder	124
9.1	Specialised clinical care in CAMHS	134
9.2	Predictors of poorer outcome with treatment in depression	136
9.3	Comparative summary of key diagnostic criteria for bipolar affective disorder	138
10.1	Core features of cognitive–behavioural therapy	152
10.2	The cognitive–behavioural formulation	152
10.3	The basics of Socratic questioning	156
10.4	Additional criteria for formulation with children	156
11.1	Advantages and disadvantages of delivering CBT online	176
12.1	Definitions	183
12.2	Major diagnostic categories for somatising disorders in children and adolescents, based on ICD-10	185
12.3	DSM-5: somatic symptom and related disorders	186

12.4	Factors affecting the presentation and persistence of somatising disorders in children and adolescents	189
13.1	Key elements of initial management by primary care or paediatric professionals	202
13.2	Principles of managing somatising disorders in children and adolescents	207
13.3	Elements of cognitive–behavioural family treatment	208
13.4	Liaison roles of child and adolescent mental health services in the management of problem families	213
15.1	Attention-deficit hyperactivity disorder items in DSM-5	232
15.2	Dyspraxia screen	235
15.3	Conditions commonly comorbid with attention-deficit hyperactivity disorder	238
16.1	Differential diagnosis of schizophrenia in childhood and adolescence	253
18.1	Taking a routine history for sleep disturbance	292
18.2	Identification of a sleep disorder	293
18.3	Some fundamentals of good sleep hygiene	294
18.4	Key diagnostic features of delayed sleep phase syndrome	296
19.1	Types of self-harm	301
19.2	Risk assessment	305
19.3	Interventions for self-harm in adolescents	308
19.4	Stepwise approach to self-harm in CAMHS	309
20.1	Practice implications	326
21.1	Reasons for admission to hospital	335
21.2	Features of anorexia nervosa	337
21.3	Features of bulimia nervosa	343
22.1	DSM-5 diagnostic criteria for gender dysphoria	351
22.2	Clinical features of atypical gender identity organisation (AGIO)	357
22.3	Primary therapeutic aims	360

Figures

2.1   The spectrum of healthcare seeking by parents for their children   12

2.2   Parents' desire to consult for their child's symptoms   12

2.3   The main components of acknowledgement   20

5.1   Influences on antisocial behaviour seen at home and at school, and how the consequences may perpetuate it   59

6.1   The Dundee Difficult Times of Day Scale   79

10.1   A template for an individual cognitive–behavioural formulation   153

10.2   Sample recent event-analysis for a panic episode   155

10.3   Systemic cognitive–behavioural formulation template for clinical use   158

10.4   The major attachment patterns, expressed in four-systems terms   162

20.1   Chemical structures of cathinone and dexamfetamine   317

20.2   Effect of parental alcohol dependence on standardised disinhibition factor scores in adopted and non-adopted adolescent offspring   319

20.3   Treatment effect differences for milder and more severe substance misuse   323

22.1   Referrals of children and adolescents to the Gender Identity Development Service at London's Tavistock Centre from the start of the service in 1989 to 2013   354

Contributors

Catia Acosta Specialty Trainee in General Adult Psychiatry, Charing Cross Rotation, West London Mental Health Trust, London, UK

Gwen Adshead Forensic Psychiatrist and Consultant Forensic Psychotherapist, Broadmoor Hospital, Crowthorne, UK

Bisharda Angom, Child and Adolescent Psychiatrist, North Essex Partnership NHS Foundation Trust, Severalls Hospital, Colchester, UK

Elizabeth Barrett Consultant in Child and Adolescent Liaison Psychiatry, Temple Street Hospital, Dublin, Ireland

Christopher Bass Consultant in Liaison Psychiatry, John Radcliffe Hospital, Oxford, UK

Gerry Byrne Clinical Lead, Family Assessment and Safeguarding Service & Infant–Parent Perinatal Service, Oxford Health NHS Foundation Trust, UK

David Coghill Reader in Child and Adolescent Psychiatry, Division of Neuroscience, Medical Research Institute, University of Dundee, UK

Felicity de Zulueta, Former Emeritus Consultant Psychiatrist in Psychotherapy, South London and Maudsley NHS Foundation Trust, and Honorary Senior Lecturer in Traumatic Studies at King's College London, London, UK

Domenico Di Ceglie Consultant Child and Adolescent Psychiatrist and Director of Training, Development and Research, Gender Identity Development Service, Tavistock and Portman NHS Foundation Trust, London, and Honorary Senior Lecturer, Department of Clinical, Educational and Health Psychology, University College London, UK

Bernadka Dubicka Consultant Psychiatrist, The Junction Adolescent Unit, Lancashire Care Foundation Trust, and Honorary Senior Lecturer, University of Manchester, UK

Nicky Dummett Consultant Child and Adolescent Psychiatrist, East Leeds Child and Adolescent Mental Health Service, Leeds, UK

Rachel Elvins Consultant Child and Adolescent Psychiatrist, Salford Child and Adolescent Mental Health Service, Central Manchester University Hospitals NHS Foundation Trust , UK

Mary Eminson Retired Consultant Child and Adolescent Psychiatrist, Bolton NHS Foundation Trust, Bolton, UK

Victoria Fernandez Consultant Child and Adolescent Psychiatrist, South West London and St George's Mental Health NHS Trust, and Honorary Teaching Fellow in Child and Adolescent Psychiatry, Imperial College, London, UK

Olivia Fiertag Locum Consultant Child and Adolescent Psychiatrist, Barnet, Enfield and Haringey Mental Health NHS Trust, London, and Honorary Lecturer, Imperial College, London, UK

David Foreman Visiting Senior Lecturer, Department of Child and Adolescent Psychiatry, King's College London, London, UK, and Consultant in Child and Adolescent Psychiatry to the Isle of Man Government

Ian M. Goodyer Professor of Child and Adolescent Psychiatry, University of Cambridge, and Honorary Consultant Child and Adolescent Psychiatrist, Cambridgeshire and Peterborough NHS Foundation Trust, UK

Jonathan Green Professor of Child and Adolescent Psychiatry, University of Manchester, and Honorary Consultant Psychiatrist, Central Manchester University Hospitals NHS Foundation Trust, UK

Peter Hill Professor Emeritus in Child Mental Health, St George's, University of London, and Great Ormond Street Hospital for Children, London, now working in independent practice, Harley Street, London, UK

Chris Hollis Professor of Child and Adolescent Psychiatry, University of Nottingham and Institute of Mental Health, Queen's Medical Centre, Nottingham, UK

Patricia Howlin Professor of Developmental Disorders, University of Sydney, Australia, and Emeritus Professor of Clinical Child Psychology, King's College London, London, UK

Sarah Huline-Dickens Consultant Child and Adolescent Psychiatrist, Plymouth Community Healthcare and Honorary Clinical Senior Lecturer, Peninsula College of Medicine and Dentistry, UK

Sajid Humayun Lecturer in Criminology, School of Law, University of Greenwich, London, UK

Raphael G. Kelvin Consultant Child and Adolescent Psychiatrist, Cambridgeshire and Peterborough NHS Foundation Trust, and Associate Lecturer, University of Cambridge, UK

Roger Lakin Consultant Child and Adolescent Psychiatrist, East Leeds Child and Adolescent Mental Health Service, Leeds, UK

Paul McArdle Consultant Child and Adolescent Psychiatrist, Northumberland, Tyne and Wear NHS Foundation Trust, Newcastle upon Tyne, UK

Dasha Nicholls Honorary Senior Lecturer and Consultant Child and Adolescent Psychiatrist, Great Ormond Street Hospital, London, UK

Mary Robertson Emeritus Professor of Neuropsychiatry, University College London, UK, Honorary Professor, Department of Psychiatry and Mental Health, University of Cape Town, South Africa, and Visiting

Professor and Honorary Consultant, Atkinson Morley Wing, St George's Hospital Medical School, London, UK

Jaydip Sarkar Consultant, Department of General and Forensic Psychiatry, Institute of Mental Health, Singapore

Stephen Scott Professor of Child Health and Behaviour, Institute of Psychiatry, King's College London, London, UK

Eugenia Sinita Head of Research and Development & Consultant in Adult Psychiatry, Department of Research and Development, National Centre of Mental Health, Clinical Psychiatric Hospital, Chisinau, Republic of Moldova

Gregory Stores Emeritus Professor of Developmental Neuropsychiatry, Department of Psychiatry, University of Oxford, UK

Aaron K. Vallance Consultant Child and Adolescent Psychiatrist, Surrey and Borders Partnership NHS Trust, and Clinical Senior Lecturer, Faculty of Medicine, Imperial College London, UK

Paul Wilkinson Honorary Consultant in Child and Adolescent Psychiatry and Lecturer, University of Cambridge, UK

Alison Wood Consultant Child and Adolescent Psychiatrist, Fairfield Hospital, Bury, UK

Preface

Caught up in the drama and conflict of other people's lives, children are often to be found in Paula Rego's art in those sinister, paradoxical or unexpected ways familiar to child psychiatrists. Sometimes they are looking after parents, sometimes they are about to be abused or humiliated, and sometimes they are even performing their own abortions. Her image on the cover of this book features J. M. Barrie's character Peter Pan, or The Boy Who Wouldn't Grow Up. Though apparently playful and mischievous, Peter Pan is in flight, and his escape from parents and family is a means of coping with painful displacement, or something worse.

As described in the introduction to this book (Chapter 1), there has always been a hope that a study of troubled children would produce recorded information of *how mental illness began* (Evans *et al*, 2008: p. 456) (my italics). This aim is an important one, and one that often attracts child psychiatrists to the work in the first place. Unfortunately, for many clinicians it is so often forgotten in the business of endless restructuring of service provision and policy revision.

However much policy material is produced, the real function of most child psychiatrists is to assess and treat mental disorders in childhood and adolescence. This book is aimed at them, to help them keep up to date with clinical topics. The clinical topic can be seen to reflect the medical approach to a clinical problem and embody a certain habit of thought, often involving the application of clinical reasoning and diagnostic decision-making. Most chapters in this book concern discrete clinical disorders, although some are about an aspect of treatment, such as pharmacological management. All are central to the work of practising clinicians in the specialty, and many will be relevant to other doctors, psychologists, child and adolescent mental health professionals, social workers, teachers and students, and trainees in all of these fields.

The selection of topics has largely been guided by what has appeared in the journal *Advances of Psychiatric Treatment* in the form of educational articles published since 1994. These chapters therefore represent a scholarly trend of practice over the past two decades. Many of the chapter authors have made contributions to the specialty: maybe not always in the shape of new knowledge (although this is true for some), but in the conceptualisation of their topics for purposes of medical education and the development of good practice.

The following four contemporary themes – continuity into adult life, the integration of biological and social aetiology, the influence of neuroscience, and the increasing use of research and evidence – have been discernible from conference material, editorials and journal articles over the past few years. These themes have formed the axes for the revision of all of the chapters in this volume since the time of original publication and for the chapters that have been newly commissioned.

Continuity into adult life

The continuity of mental disorder from childhood into adult life has, of course, been recognised for a long time. In the case of schizophrenia, for example, in a series of 1054 individuals with dementia praecox, Kraepelin found that 57% met this diagnosis before the age of 25, with 3.5% aged 10 or under and a further 2.7% between 10 and 15 years old. Indeed, he reminds us that it was this 'predisposition of youth' that led Hecker to coin the term hebephrenia, which means insanity of youth (Kraepelin, 1919). We also have more information now on the long-term nature of many other neurodevelopmental disorders, such as autism spectrum disorder (ASD), attention-deficit hyperactivity disorder (ADHD) and Tourette syndrome, which are seen very widely in clinical practice. It is surely time to place continuity at the centre of service design and research. Within the paradigm of continuity throughout the lifespan, there have also been calls for some time for more attention to be paid to disorders of infants and young children (see below).

Integration of biological and social aetiology

As more sophisticated techniques emerge for investigating gene–environment interactions, we understand that certain children with genetic susceptibilities may be more influenced by negative environments; children who are exposed to multiple family adversities are more likely to demonstrate disturbance; and stressful environments can affect all levels of the emotional system, including the hypothalamic–pituitary–adrenal axis, neurotransmitter systems and brain architecture (Jenkins, 2008).

In a paper on vulnerability to mental disorders, Goldberg (2009) discussed 'the interaction between our genetic constitution and social environments that either allow genes to manifest themselves in the phenotype, or suppress them altogether. It is now possible to describe the biology of secure attachment, and describe the physiological changes that accompany [it]'. Children who are raised in families in which a parent has a mental illness find themselves in a situation where the risks are both genetic and environmental. The many ways in which this might affect children are well described (e.g. see Stallard et al, 2004). Advances in understanding are likely to occur in investigating the early developmental origins of mental disorder, and mechanisms of adaptation and resilience need to be better understood.

Findings from neuroscience

A consensus is emerging that developmental and biological disruptions in early life often lead to adult psychiatric disorder. This might happen through cumulative damage or as a result of an event occurring during a sensitive period. As well as the genetic and cellular events leading to brain formation, evidence is accumulating that the uterine and postnatal environments, together with early relations in life, can affect childhood brain development and behaviour (Leckman & March, 2011). Furthermore, it seems likely that not all children will be affected equally, so that susceptibility to these processes may be genetically determined and various areas of the brain may mature at different rates in different children. These findings, together with technological advances such as in brain imaging, give us a more sophisticated understanding of the relationship between genetics and the environment.

Research and evidence

Finally, it is important to acknowledge that there has been a growth in the academic aspect of our specialty. The conspicuous increase in the volume of literature about neurodevelopmental psychiatry over the past two decades in, for example, ASD, ADHD and Tourette syndrome, has been accompanied by an increase in publications about their treatment. Since 2005, there has been a proliferation of guidance from the National Institute for Health and Care Excellence (NICE), so that treatments can now be based on published work. At the time of writing there are specific NICE guidelines for children and adolescents who present with eating disorders, self-harm, post-traumatic stress disorder (PTSD), depressive disorder, obsessive–compulsive disorder (OCD), ADHD, autism, conduct disorder, psychosis and schizophrenia, and the list continues to grow. The Faculty of Child and Adolescent Psychiatry is the only faculty of the Royal College of Psychiatrists currently to insist on research training as a mandatory part of the higher training curriculum and this will be crucial to the development of the discipline.

An outline of this book

The three newly commissioned chapters for this volume serve to illustrate these themes particularly well. David Foreman, in marshalling a wealth of research evidence, describes the epidemiology of disorders of young children (aged 0–4 years) in terms of disorders across the rest of the lifespan, and in so doing he not only creates a paradigm shift, but also draws attention to the paradox that this group is increasingly neglected by child psychiatry even though cost-effective treatments are available. Changes in service configuration, however, will be required.

Mary Robertson draws on her extensive career in research and treatment of Tourette syndrome to richly describe the familiar phenomenology of a disorder that straddles psychiatry and neurology, and also to provide us with new material on psychosocial impact, aggression and neuroscience.

The third new chapter, by Aaron Vallance & Victoria Fernandez, serves to summarise the central topic of anxiety: a common disorder whose impact is easily underestimated, especially when comorbid with other disorders. The chapter comprehensively describes the aetiological factors and reviews evidence-based treatment.

The remaining chapters have been revised or updated since their publication in *Advances in Psychiatric Treatment*. At a time when child abuse and neglect is a major public health problem, the chapter by Christopher Bass and colleagues provides clinicians with a review of fabricated illness (formerly known as Munchausen syndrome by proxy). This chapter emphasises the need for adult and child psychiatrists to work together and orders the clinical reasoning processes associated with such cases, in addition to informing us about new findings about the perpetrators.

Spanning the worlds of developmental psychopathology and neuroscience, with many implications for the continuity of disorders into adult life, the chapter by Jaydip Sarkar & Gwen Adshead exemplifies how there has been a transformation of approach to the topic of personality disorders. This chapter, strong in theoretical orientation, describes how disorganisation of the capacity for affect regulation has come to be understood as central to the origin of personality development and disorder. These cases form the bulk of work for child psychiatrists and become the future patients of adult psychiatry. It is time that those leading services recognised this and adapted interventions accordingly. Associated with this topic is the chapter by Felicity de Zulueta, who discusses the aetiology of complex PTSD in terms of attachment theory, and examines the similarities between complex PTSD and borderline personality disorder. This chapter is important for providing a more international perspective to the practice of the specialty.

Although child psychiatry developed to deal with antisocial behaviour in troubled or maladjusted children, as described in Chapter 1, there has since been much debate about whether these children should still be centrally the business of the specialty. The chapter on antisocial behaviour in childhood by Sajid Humayun & Stephen Scott summarises new information about treatment studies and includes children with so-called callous-unemotional traits, who appear to be an aetiologically distinct group with low empathy and high fearlessness. The evidence is presented that there may be higher genetic heritability for these traits than for ordinary conduct disorder and that there may also be a different pattern of neurocognitive deficits.

Several chapters reflect the growing evidence base and increasingly widespread practice of using psychopharmacological treatment in children and adolescents. In a pair of chapters, David Coghill & Eugenia Sinita survey the psychopharmacological treatments of the major disorders seen in child and adolescent mental health services (CAMHS), with particular emphasis on one on evidence-based practice and ensuring safety in the use of medications for ADHD. Rachel Elvins & Jonathan Green focus on the pharmacological management of core symptoms and comorbidity in ASD. With increasing recognition of this disorder and accumulation of empirical evidence, this is likely to be an area of developing demand for services from child psychiatrists. The chapter by Bernadka Dubicka and colleagues summarises the significance of the data on the treatment of mood disorders, and investigates the matter of suicidality, which is a term variously defined, and its relation to the use of antidepressants in young people. As one would expect, the answers are not simple.

The chapter by Nicky Dummett & Roger Lakin provides some very practical strategies for clinicians in the application of cognitive–behavioural therapy (CBT), but accompanied by rigorous formulation of the child's presenting problems. Refreshingly, these authors make connections between the worlds of CBT and other therapeutic approaches and draw attention to the importance of continuing to conceptualise problems systemically. Mary Eminson's lucid descriptions of the practice of paediatric liaison in her two articles of 2001 have been updated into two chapters jointly written with Olivia Fiertag. The first reminds us of the clinical presentations of the somatising disorders and the second deals with management and outcomes. These chapters remind us of the important role that child psychiatry has within paediatrics.

Patricia Howlin also focuses on psychological management by taking an overview of what counts as effective interventions for children and young people with ASD. Although not a clinical topic, and therefore not in the style of the other contributions, this chapter reviews the recent evidence base for psychosocial treatments of ASD. Child psychiatrists are increasingly confronted with children with these complex disorders, which are far more widespread than previously recognised, and the despair these children can cause their families. Howlin concludes that many psychosocial interventions have yet to be shown to be definitively helpful in these conditions and emphasises the problem of lack of services for individuals with ASD after they graduate from CAMHS.

Continuing the neurodevelopmental thread, and crystallising all the themes of the book, Peter Hill provides us with a masterclass and comprehensive revision of the topic of ADHD. This chapter is dedicated to the memory of his late coauthor, Mary Cameron, who wrote the original version with him in 1996. Chris Hollis, in his chapter on adolescent schizophrenia, summarises new research as well as the core features, course and outcome of this disorder, and investigates its neurobiology as well as continuity into adult life. He concludes, in conformity with other conclusions in this book, that adult-based diagnostic criteria have validity in adolescents. Sadly, however, the disorder has a poorer outcome when first occurring in youth.

Other chapters give the clinician updated guidance by experts on the assessment and treatment of sleep disorders (Gregory Stores), self-harm (Alison Wood) and substance misuse (Paul McArdle & Bisharda Angom), including the use of more contemporary substances in the modern age. The fields of both eating disorders, written about here by Dasha Nicholls and Elizabeth Barrett, and gender dysphoria, by Domenico di Cegli, have been under some recent transformation. Research activity on the range of eating problems in younger children has advanced considerably, as has the trend for increasingly individualised treatments. As for the fascinating and complex world of gender identity and dysphoria, di Cegli's chapter reminds us that nowhere is psychiatry or its patients free from harmful cultural, social and often religious attitudes. In the case of these problems, their social and legal recognition in recent years in the UK at least has transformed the experience of those of transgender, who are now protected by equality legislation. This then is an area of optimistic and progressive social change.

References

Evans B, Rahman S, Jones E (2008) Managing the unmanageable: interwar child psychiatry at the Maudsley Hospital, London. *History of Psychiatry*, **19**, 454–475.

Goldberg D (2009) The interplay between biological and psychological factors in determining vulnerability to mental disorders. *Psychoanalytic Psychotherapy*, **23**, 236–247.

Jenkins J (2008) Psychosocial adversity and resilience. In *Rutter's Child and Adolescent Psychiatry* (5th edn) (eds M Rutter, D Bishop, D Pine, *et al*), pp. 377–391. Wiley-Blackwell.

Kraepelin E (1919) *Dementia Praecox and Paraphrenia* (trans RM Barclay, ed GM Robertson). Krieger/Chicago Medical Book Company.

Leckman J, March J (2011) Developmental neuroscience comes of age. *Journal of Child Psychology and Psychiatry*, **52**, 333–338.

Stallard P, Norman P, Huline-Dickens S, *et al* (2004) The effects of parental mental illness upon children: a descriptive study of the views of parents and children. *Clinical Child Psychology and Psychiatry*, **9**, 39–52.

Sarah Huline-Dickens
BSc MA MSc BMBCh MRCPsych FAcadMed
Consultant Child and Adolescent Psychiatrist
Honorary Clinical Senior Lecturer

CHAPTER 1

Child psychiatry and the people who have shaped it

Sarah Huline-Dickens

'The greatest terror a child can have is that he is not loved, and rejection is the hell he fears. And with rejection comes anger, and with anger some kind of crime in revenge for the rejection, and with the crime guilt – and there is the story of mankind.'

John Steinbeck, *East of Eden*, 1952

John Steinbeck was centrally concerned with social exclusion, and the story of child and adolescent psychiatry has also shared this focus. It begins with the delinquent child and only later includes children with other behavioural and emotional problems. Often depending on private charity and voluntary organisations, marginalised children and young people in Britain had little to help them, and services were scattered before the establishment of the National Health Service (NHS) in 1947. In the USA, the specialty grew from a turbulent period of mass migration and social change in the 20th century, but it was aided by important European influences.

The origins of child psychiatry derive from a convergence of theories and practice from public health and paediatrics, asylum psychiatry, psychoanalysis, psychology, social work, education and criminology. This has led to richness from one point of view but confusion from another (Parry-Jones, 1994). It has also resulted in problems in defining the work of child psychiatry and what child psychiatrists do. Some 20 years ago, Parry-Jones commented 'Many questions bear on the future of the subspecialty, concerning its scope, its place in psychiatry and medicine, and issues about staff roles and organization' (Parry-Jones, 1994: p. 794), and these matters are just as pressing for the professional today. Often it can seem that child psychiatrists, just like Dr Martin Dysart in Peter Shaffer's 1973 play *Equus*, are struggling with their own sense of purpose while trying to understand the complex or perplexing patients they are trying to help.

When child guidance clinics were founded in the UK, the aim was to prevent delinquency and antisocial behaviour. There may well have been a deficiency of theoretical orientation behind this desire: the team-working approach encouraged diplomacy and integration but, in the words of Evans *et al*, it 'brought about a marked loss in terms of maintaining theoretical coherence and accuracy' (Evans *et al*, 2008: p. 469). There was, however, a hope, expressed by the Maudsley's first superintendent Edward Mapother in 1932, that a study of these children would produce recorded information of *how mental illness began* (Evans *et al*, 2008: p. 456) (my italics).

There is evidence now of increasing interest in child and adolescent psychiatry and its history. The public health importance of emerging disorders, the need for special education in many circumstances, public attitudes towards delinquency, crime and disability, and a social history involving significant developments in the interwar period are all reasons for this. And there is the abiding conflict between nature and nurture which makes many of the clinical cases child psychiatrists deal with so richly interesting.

Some of the seminal changes that have occurred in psychiatry in general, and in child psychiatry in particular, are still within the lifetimes of psychiatrists working today, so that 'There is a zone in history where the past merges with the present' (Crammer, 1990: p. 175). The formation of the Royal College of Psychiatrists in 1971 and the NHS reorganisation of 1974, which effectively led to the closure of the asylums, number among these changes. As this book goes to press, the ramifications of another large change, the Health and Social Care Act 2012, will be beginning to be felt.

In almost every decade there has been at least one useful historical review by a clinician, and sometimes several. Examples of these are the excellent guide by Barton Hall (1947), and those by Rosen (1968: pp. 285–300), Warren (1971), Hersov (1986) and Wardle (1991), the latter containing many serviceable chronological tables. Parry-Jones's (1994) scholarly review is both tightly structured and comprehensive. Black & Gowers (2005) provide a briefer overview, and Cottrell & Kraam (2005) an understanding of more contemporary developments in service organisation.

More recent studies by non-clinicians such as Evans *et al* (2008) make interesting additions to this body of work and introduce new questions. By examining patients' notes, management accounts and types of treatments available, this study is unusual in describing how practice influenced the growth of the specialty, rather than adopting a primarily critical approach emphasising medicalisation, accidental discoveries and the inherent weaknesses of classification systems so prominent in other historical and political accounts.

Developmental history

So the beginning of this story will be in the 1850s, when the term paediatrics was first used to describe the study of infant and child health in Europe, perhaps reflecting a concern with national efficiency and strength in that period. For example, the context of the military losses of the Franco-Prussian war (1870–1871) may have been instrumental in the emergence of infant welfare clinics in France (Levene, 2011). Indeed, war came to play a significant part in the history of the development of the discipline in Europe.

In the 1850s in Britain most kinds of insanity were still confined to the asylum. At a time when literature about children in English life (*Jane Eyre* and *Wuthering Heights* were published in 1847 and *David Copperfield* in 1850) was beginning to emerge, some children were incarcerated as a matter of course. Although it is not widely recognised, children as young as 5 were admitted to asylums (Parry-Jones, 1990). Of 46 young people under the age of 16 admitted to Oxfordshire County Asylum between 1846 and 1866, 25 were recorded as having epilepsy, 19 were classed as idiots, 2 were hallucinating, 4 had delusional ideas, 2 were paranoid, 1 was thought to be manic and several were suicidal.

The development of child and adolescent psychiatry through child guidance to what is now known as child and adolescent mental health followed slightly different paths in the USA and Britain. In the USA, according to several authors (Barton Hall, 1947; Rosen, 1968: pp. 285–300), maladjustment appeared to be a growing topic of public interest in the early part of the 20th century. The reasons for this are probably complex but two factors stand out: this was a time of extraordinary migration to America, with total immigration soaring to more than 8 million individuals in 1901–1910, most of whom settled in the cities. During this period too, children were still labouring in industrial workplaces, which no doubt required their full contribution to the labour force. In the powerful photographs of the social reformer Lewis Hine, such as *Little Spinner in Globe Cotton Mill*, 1909, or *Noon Hour in the Ewen Breaker*, 1911, we see images of children working in filthy and perilous conditions.

In this context we find reference to an early psychiatric clinical study of delinquent youth begun in 1909 and culminating in *The Individual Delinquent* (1915), by William Healy (1869–1963) (cited by Barton Hall, 1947), and it appears that at this time a psychiatric lens was beginning to be applied to delinquency elsewhere as well. Rosen (1968: pp. 285–300) reports that by 1932, 50 cities in the USA had established clinics for such children.

Along the way, certain publications can be seen to have shaped developments. In 1914, for example, the Children's Bureau recommended the need for establishing good, regular habits early, and to this end in 1921 the Baby Hygiene Association of Boston joined forces with the psychiatrist Douglas Thom to form a Habit Clinic. Children between the ages of 2 and 5 with undesirable habits were managed with the combined force of professionals from psychiatry, psychology and social work (Rosen, 1968: pp. 285–300).

The child guidance clinic

So it was that we arrive at a pivotal period in the story of our specialty's development. During the decade 1920–1930 the child guidance clinic emerged in the USA, focused on problem children and with the objective of treatment and rehabilitation. A team approach was used and the systemic paradigm adopted that the child's problem was symptomatic of a troubled family and social situation.

In Britain meanwhile, and in a somewhat parallel development, in 1923, the year of its opening, London's Maudsley Hospital had only a small department for the treatment of children, run by Dr W. S. Dawson with the help of the hospital almoner. The strategic goals of the institution set out in 1907 made no reference to the treatment of children, so the provision of children's services had not been planned. However, from its small beginnings the children's department at the Maudsley expanded rapidly in the late 1920s, with referrals rising from 90 in 1924 to 432 in 1931 (Evans *et al*, 2008).

Training of staff for clinical work with children in other centres in Britain also began in the 1920s. The staff at the Tavistock Clinic for Functional Nerve Cases in London, some of whom had experienced the effects of the First World War, established services for civilian adults, but soon also found themselves treating children and publishing related works. Among the latter is *The New Psychology and the Parent* by H. Crichton Miller, the clinic's first director (Barton Hall, 1947).

At this time, Leo Kanner (1894–1981), a psychiatrist born in a small village in what is now Ukraine, left his early career in Berlin in 1924 to establish himself in the USA, founding the children's psychiatric service at Johns Hopkins Hospital in 1930. Recognised as the first 'child psychiatrist', he published *Child Psychiatry*, the first English-language textbook on the subject, in 1935. Known principally for his work on autism, his paper 'Autistic disturbances of affective contact' (Kanner, 1943) was highly influential in the study of this disorder.

The first child guidance clinic in Europe was the East London Child Guidance Clinic, established in 1927 by the Jewish Health Organization and directed by Emmanuel Miller. Miller (1893–1970) is credited with the introduction of the child guidance movement from the USA to the UK, and in 1968 he edited *Foundations of Child Psychiatry*. He helped to establish the Institute for the Study and Treatment of Delinquency and also founded what later became the Association for Child and Adolescent Mental Health. During a demonstration of the work of the East London Child Guidance Clinic reported by *The British Medical Journal* (1936), a Lady Cynthia Colville gave a brief talk on the work of the clinic and how 'Thieving, spiteful, and backward children became transformed after a few sessions at the clinic into normal and happy youngsters, ready to take up life and meet it on its own terms'. Clearly, there was a great deal of optimism in the air.

Similar clinics began to be established elsewhere in the UK as a result of the Commonwealth Fund of 1927, which had been formed by an act of philanthropy. One such was the London Child Guidance Clinic, to which John Bowlby was appointed in 1936. Work at the clinic provided the source for his classic paper 'Forty-four juvenile thieves, their characters and home life' (Bowlby, 1944). Bowlby (1907–1990) was born in London and trained as a psychiatrist as well as a psychoanalyst. His early interest in childhood delinquency later extended to children who were affectionless, hospitalised or institutionalised. Most known for his work on attachment theory, which was based on a theory of evolutionary adaptation and inspired by the ethological approaches of Lorenz and Tinbergen, his work has been profoundly influential.

The Hampstead War Nurseries

The Second World War is the next milestone, heralding another era of mass movement and social change. In this period in Britain, the many city children who came to be wartime evacuees in the 1940s were found to be in poor health. This was also a time of traumatic loss and separation from family, and this was the context for the establishment of the Hampstead War Nurseries in the winter of 1940–1941 by a group of engaged and energetic colleagues in Anna Freud's circle. Young-Bruehl (1989) gives an account of the nurseries, which were intended to care for children whose families had been broken up in one way or another. The creation of the nurseries also, of course, afforded opportunities for observation and research into children in institutional settings. One of the members of this group, the social worker and film-maker James Robertson, made the classic film *A Child Goes to Hospital,* which did a great deal to challenge restrictive hospital visiting policies.

Wartime research also afforded other discoveries. The tragedy of the famine – known as the hunger winter – in war-time Holland in 1944–1945 led to findings about the influence of starvation on the fetus (although these were not published until much later). The most exposed cohort of individuals conceived at the height of the famine had a two-fold increase in risk of schizophrenia (Susser *et al*, 1996) and it now seems likely that this kind of critical assault on fetal growth is associated with other neurodevelopmental disorders.

The postwar period

After the war, trends in the development of the specialty have included the influence of psychoanalytic ideas, the establishment of in-patient units for adolescents, increasing professionalism of disciplines allied to child psychiatry, teaching and research, an increase in the number of child psychiatrists and a proliferation in treatment approaches. These are all comprehensively discussed elsewhere (e.g. Warren, 1971; Hersov, 1986; Wardle, 1991; Rutter & Stevenson, 2008) and only the first two of these themes will be mentioned here as they are of more importance to the narrative.

Although the role of psychoanalytical thinking and its influence on child psychiatry has been controversial and has attracted vociferous criticism, Adler and Freud, and colleagues who followed them, contributed theoretical concepts and frameworks which led to many developments in practice. For example, Alfred Adler (1870–1937), who fled anti-Semitism in Europe in 1935 to migrate to America, made a particular contribution in considering the effect of obstacles to the shaping of the individual child's self-esteem. Karl Abraham (1877–1925) wrote on infantile trauma and manic–depressive insanity; Sigmund Freud (1856–1939), whose many ideas were influential generally in the culture (the significance of the emotional life on the generation of symptoms, the importance of repression and symbolism, the dynamic model of the unconscious, trauma and memory, transference and countertransference, and so on), also extended his work to the realm of childhood. Melanie Klein (1882–1960) elaborated a theory of defences to deal with anxiety and also analysed in great detail the mother–child relationship. Anna Freud (1895–1982), as well as being director of the Hampstead War Nurseries and a training programme for psychoanalytic work with children, wrote on defence mechanisms and the ego. The paper by Rous & Clark (2009) gives a brief overview of the history of the psychoanalytical movement in the NHS and the Freud/Klein controversy, and outlines the contemporary situation of psychotherapy provision in a public service.

In service development, the emergence of adolescent psychiatry as a subspecialty occurred only with the establishment of the first modern in-patient units after the Second World War. These were opened at the Maudsley Hospital in 1947 and St Ebba's Hospital (Epsom, Surrey) in 1949 (later moving to Long Grove in Epsom). The emergence of adolescents as a group recognised as having particular needs and concerns is very recent, and only in the past decade have services been obliged to provide specifically for young people aged between 16 and 18. The opening of these two units marked a shift in thinking at that time. It occurred soon after two other major changes: the birth of the NHS and the reforms recommended by C. P. Blacker in a report commissioned by the Ministry of Health, *Neurosis and the Mental Health Services*, in 1946. In this, he suggested the separation of the child guidance clinics led by psychologists and run by local authorities from the child psychiatry departments led by child psychiatrists and run by health authorities. The conflict over where the specialty belongs is therefore a well-rehearsed one, and child psychiatrists may find it salutary to remind themselves that their path has never been easy and there was no golden age.

The reformation: community services

Entering a more modern era in the narrative, critics of the child guidance movement were always plentiful and early included those from within the ranks. So, for example, Kanner considered that help provided by child guidance clinics encouraged rigidity and inhibited inventiveness (Warren, 1971) and the Association for the University Teachers of Psychiatry called for their abolition in 1961. Later, the number of critics multiplied and the child guidance approach was seen by many (including Rutter & Stevenson, 2008) to foster professional isolationism as well as lead to lengthy open-ended treatment. Naturally, the team approach has come under opprobrium too and it is interesting to speculate, as Hersov (1986) does, what would have been the outcome had the team clustered around a prototypical child with neurosis rather than one who was delinquent. An outright critic of more recent times, the historian John Stewart, has blamed child guidance clinics for pathologising childhood, medicalising a whole generation of children and emphasising that problems result from emotional and psychological rather than material causes (such as poverty) (e.g. see Stewart, 2013).

There thus has followed a period of reformation, beginning with the merging of local authority child guidance clinics and in-patient services in 1974 to form community services. Ultimately, we have arrived at the widely misunderstood but much quoted model of a four-tiered provision of services, which began in the 1990s. More recently, a baffling number of policy initiatives have been steadily produced, concisely and helpfully summarised by Cottrell & Kraam (2005) and also by Richardson & Wyatt (2010). It is always to be hoped that social policy can in some way improve the national well-being of children, and the UNICEF report on 21 of the most industrialised nations in 2007 certainly demonstrates that it needs to (UNICEF, 2007). The UK scored particularly poorly at the bottom of a composite chart of indices and was among the nations in which child poverty was above the 15% level. But it has been understood for a long time that the relationship between socioeconomic status and child psychiatric disorder is steeply positive (with a prevalence of disorder of 5% among the children of the professional classes, 15% among those of unskilled workers and 20% among those whose parents have never worked (Melzer *et al*, 2000). It is clearly unfair that children should be so differentially afflicted; unfair that they should be exposed to so little that is nurturing; and frankly often unfair that they are conceived in the first place.

The tension continues over whether child and adolescent mental health services (CAMHS) are part of children's services or part of the health service. Partridge & Richardson (2010) usefully distinguish between the need for society to care for the well-being of its population (universalism, if you like) and the responsibility of CAMHS to attend to mental disorder (which is, after all, a specialty). Professionals in CAMHS cannot be expected to improve the emotional well-being of every child, but child psychiatrists have played and continue to play an important role in their professional lives with this generally disadvantaged group.

The child psychiatrists of the future

What do we know of the explicitly stated theoretical models that were being used historically? W. S. Dawson, who established the children's department at the Maudsley, had the view that insanity was essentially a disorder of conduct shown by a failure to adjust the self to surroundings. He based this belief on a dynamic model in which the instinctive urges are controlled in accordance with social demands (Dawson, 1944). Although interested in an evolutionary perspective and also in Freud, the work he encouraged also had a strong empirical basis. There was systematic recording of information on admission to the Maudsley in the 1930s and children were given full medical, including neurological, examinations (Evans *et al*, 2008). In his view, 'Intensive study of the child is undertaken in the hope that not only may such nervous manifestations and other behaviour difficulties be handled successfully, but that *the development of neurosis and even of psychosis at a later age may be prevented*' (my italics) (Dawson, 1944: p. 298).

With the rise of scientific approaches over the past 50 years (e.g. as reviewed by Rutter & Stevenson, 2008), the problem of lack of theory may now be beginning to be resolved. Michael Rutter (b. 1933) – the first Professor of Child Psychiatry in England and head of the first academic department for the specialty at the Maudsley in 1972 (Black & Gowers, 2005) – has done much to establish the specialty on a more rigorous scientific basis. Notable for his interest in epidemiology, Rutter's comprehensive population surveys in London and the Isle of White published in 1970 are still regarded as classic studies in the field.

The child psychiatrists who shape the future will be specialist doctors who will have a sound grasp of biomedical, neurodevelopmental, psychological and social medicine. They will be informed in behavioural and cognitive approaches, and family and psychoanalytic theories. They will be familiar with the continuity of childhood mental disorder into adult life, and thus the whole range of psychopathology in their patients and in those patients' families. They will be able to appreciate the influence of the interaction of genes and environment on the developing brain, be confident in psychopharmacology, appreciate how research and evidence can inform practice and remain alert to how findings from neuroscience might shape the specialty. *Clinical Topics in Child and Adolescent Psychiatry* has been edited with them in mind, with the aim of contributing to a developmental understanding of our specialty as well as of our patients.

> TYRONE: Mary! For God's sake, forget the past!
> MARY (with strange objective calm): Why? How can I? The past is the present, isn't it? It's the future, too. We all try to lie out of that but life won't let us.
>
> Eugene O'Neill, *Long Day's Journey into Night*, 1956

References

Barton Hall, M (1947) *Psychiatric Examination of the School Child*. Edward Arnold.

Black D, Gowers SG (2005) A brief history of child and adolescent psychiatry. In *Seminars in Child and Adolescent Psychiatry* (2nd edn) (ed S Gowers), pp. 1–6. Gaskell.

Bowlby J (1944) Forty-four juvenile thieves, their characters and home life. *International Journal of Psychoanalysis*, **25**, 19–52.

Cottrell D, Kraam A (2005) Growing up? A History of CAMHS (1987–2005). *Child and Adolescent Mental Health*, **10**, 111–117.

Crammer J (1990) *Asylum History: Buckinghamshire County Pauper Lunatic Asylum – St John's*. Gaskell.

Dawson WS (1944) *Aids to Psychiatry* (5th edn). Baillière, Tindall & Cox.

Evans B, Rahman S, Jones E (2008) Managing the unmanageable: interwar child psychiatry at the Maudsley Hospital, London. *History of Psychiatry*, **19**, 454–475.

Hersov L (1986) Child psychiatry in Britain – the last 30 years. *Journal of Child Psychology and Psychiatry*, **27**, 781–801.

Kanner L (1943) Autistic disturbances of affective contact. *Nervous Child*, **2**, 217–250.

Levene A (2011) Childhood and adolescence. In *The Oxford Handbook of the History of Medicine* (ed M Jackson), pp. 321–337. Oxford University Press.

Melzer D, Gatward R, Goodman R, *et al* (2000) *The Mental Health of Children and Adolescents in Great Britain*. Office for National Statistics.

Parry-Jones W (1990) Juveniles in 19th century Oxfordshire asylums. *British Journal of Clinical and Social Psychiatry*, **7**, 51–58.

Parry-Jones W (1994) History of child and adolescent psychiatry. In *Child and Adolescent Psychiatry: Modern Approaches* (3rd edn) (eds M Rutter, E Taylor, L Hersov), pp. 794–812. Blackwell.

Partridge I, Richardson G (2010) Introduction. In *Child and Adolescent Mental Health Services: An Operational Handbook* (2nd edn) (eds G Richardson, I Partridge, J Barrett), pp. 1–8. RCPsych Publications.

Richardson G, Wyatt A (2010) CAMHS in context. In *Child and Adolescent Mental Health Services: An Operational Handbook* (2nd edn) (eds G Richardson, I Partridge, J Barrett), pp. 9–20. RCPsych Publications.

Rosen G (1968) *Madness in Society: Chapters in the Historical Sociology of Mental Illness*. Routledge & Kegan Paul.

Rous E, Clark A (2009) Child psychoanalytic psychotherapy in the UK National Health Service: an historical analysis. *History of Psychiatry*, **20**, 442–456.

Rutter M, Stevenson J (2008) Developments in child and adolescent psychiatry over the last 50 years. In *Rutter's Child and Adolescent Psychiatry* (5th edn) (eds M Rutter, D Bishop, D Pine, *et al*), pp. 3–17. Wiley-Blackwell.

Susser E, Neugebauer R, Hoek HW, *et al* (1996) Schizophrenia after prenatal famine: further evidence. *Archives of General Psychiatry*, **53**, 25–31.

Stewart J (2013) *From Child Guidance in Britain, 1918–1955: The Dangerous Age of Childhood*. Pickering & Chatto

The British Medical Journal (1936) East London Child Guidance Clinic. *British Medical Journal*, (30 May), 1123.

UNICEF (2007) *Child Poverty in Perspective: An Overview of Child Well-Being in Rich Countries: A Comparative Review (Innocenti Report Card 7)*. UNICEF.

Wardle CJ (1991) Twentieth-century influences on the development in Britain of services for child and adolescent psychiatry. *British Journal of Psychiatry*, **159**, 53–68.

Warren W (1971) You can never plan the future by the past. *Journal of Child Psychology and Psychiatry*, **11**, 241–257.

Young-Bruehl E (1989) *Anna Freud*. Macmillan.

CHAPTER 2

Fabrication and induction of illness in children

Christopher Bass, Catia Acosta, Gwen Adshead
and Gerry Byrne

In the fabrication or induction of illness in children, an adult – characteristically a parent and usually the mother – presents a child to healthcare professionals as ill when in fact the symptoms of the illness are falsified, fabricated or actively induced by the adult. There have been many changes in nomenclature since Meadow first described this manifestation of disturbed parenting and caregiving as 'Munchausen syndrome by proxy' (Meadow, 1977). Other terms have since been introduced, including 'factitious disorder by proxy' (DSM-IV: American Psychiatric Association, 1994), 'factitious disorder imposed by another' (DSM-5: American Psychiatric Association, 2013), 'paediatric condition falsification' (Ayoub et al, 2002) and, in the UK, 'factitious or induced illness' (Department of Health, 2002). The term 'medical child abuse' has also been used in the USA (Roesler & Jenny, 2009), to reflect the role of the doctor in ordering interventions and procedures that are invasive and unnecessary, which (inadvertently) maintain the abuse. In this chapter, we will use the term 'fabricated or induced illness by carers' (FII), which has also been adopted by the Royal College of Paediatricians in the UK (Royal College of Paediatrics and Child Health, 2009). In practice, however, the majority of perpetrators (85%) are parents.

All of these definitions have limitations because they attempt to describe a spectrum of abnormal illness behaviour involving a perpetrator and how this behaviour affects a child. Abnormal healthcare seeking behaviour in the perpetrator can range from hypervigilant preoccupation with a child's symptoms at one end of the spectrum through to intentional induction of illness or poisoning of the child at the other. However conceptualised, FII is a form of child abuse that involves an abnormal form of care-eliciting behaviour in the caregiver, usually manifested as an abnormal relationship with healthcare professionals that has an adverse effect on the child.

Epidemiology

The incidence of FII is unknown, but the behaviour is widely believed to be underreported. In 1996, the combined annual incidence of identified FII, non-accidental poisoning and non-accidental suffocation in the UK and Ireland among children 5–16 years of age was 0.5 per 100 000; among those 1–4 years old it was 1.2 per 100 000; among those 0–11 months old it was 2.8 per 100 000; 8 deaths were recorded (McClure *et al*, 1996). Watson *et al* (1999) studied children who had experienced 'parental abnormal illness behaviour' and reported an incidence of FII, non-accidental poisoning and non-accidental suffocation of 89 per 100 000 under-16-year-olds over a 2-year period in the Manchester health district, but no mortality. Denny *et al* (2001) in New Zealand reported an incidence of FII of 2.0 per 100 000 children under the age of 16 and of 1.2 per 100 000 using the same criteria as McClure *et al*, but found no deaths.

These figures are likely to be an underestimate of the true incidence. Detection can be difficult, especially in cases that involve false accounts of symptoms or fabricated symptoms (such as tampering with a child's specimens). Induced illness, which results in greater morbidity or even death, may be more easily detected, although there remain concerns that some types of sudden death in children may be the result of this form of child abuse (Craft & Hall, 2004; Galvin *et al*, 2005).

Fabricated or induced illness is most often seen in children under 5 years of age who are unable to verbalise their own problems. Older children are also affected, and they may actively collude with their parents in the sick role. Boys and girls are equally affected, and FII is perpetrated by all social classes. The average age at which FII is diagnosed is 48.6 months (range 0–204 months), with an average interval between the onset of symptoms and diagnosis of 21.8 months (range 0–195 months) (Sheridan, 2003).

Manifestations of abnormal caregiving behaviour

The complex ways in which a parent can respond to a child's symptoms is shown Figures 2.1 and 2.2. It is clear that a range of behaviours involve healthcare professionals and result in a variety of outcomes for the child. These include:

- overconsultation with healthcare professionals (compared with normative rates), refusal to accept a diagnosis or comply with suggested treatments and persistent antagonism towards healthcare professionals
- exaggeration of existing symptoms
- providing false accounts of non-existent symptoms (e.g. 'he keeps having fits', 'she suddenly stops breathing)
- fabrication of symptoms (e.g. contaminating body fluids used for medical investigation by putting substances in a child's urine sample to simulate illness)
- actively inducing symptoms, which involves either direct or indirect behaviour that causes physical harm (e.g. administering medications inappropriately, smothering to simulate apnoeic attacks, tampering with hospital equipment).

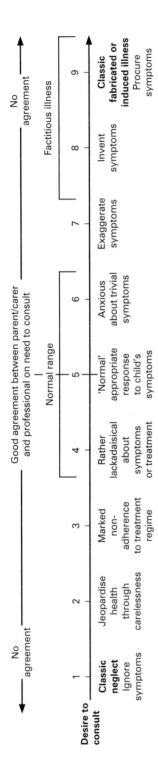

Fig. 2.1 The spectrum of healthcare seeking by parents for their children. After Eminson (2000), with permission.

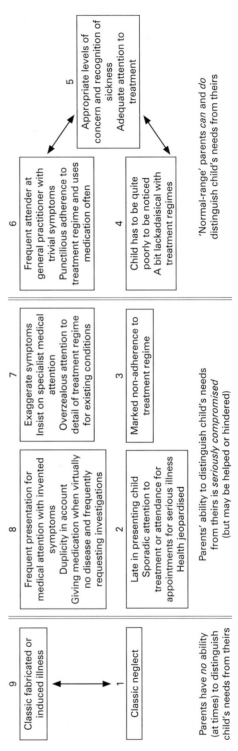

Fig. 2.2 Parents' desire to consult for their child's symptoms. After Eminson (2000), with permission.

It is not known whether there is an escalation from milder to more severe forms of behaviour. It is known, however, that mild forms may coexist with more severe forms.

Although it is the induction of illness that usually carries the greatest risk of serious physical harm to the child, children can also suffer harm as a result of the repeated inappropriate investigations (such as lumbar punctures), unnecessary medical interventions (such as oesophageal reflux surgery) or the administration of medication that the false accounts or fabricated signs or symptoms bring about.

One of the most problematic aspects of this behaviour is that general practitioners, accident and emergency (A&E) staff and paediatricians may unwittingly be involved in causing potentially dangerous iatrogenic complications (Roesler & Jenny, 2009).

Impact on children

In her literature review of 451 cases of FII, Sheridan (2003) reported that 27 (6%) of the children died and 33 (7%) suffered long-term or permanent injury. Over half of children subjected to FII suffer indirect psychological harm, including emotional abuse or neglect, which can be manifested in behavioural problems, school non-attendance and major concentration difficulties. Furthermore, affected children live in a fabricated sick role and may eventually simulate illness in themselves, sometimes continuing the behaviour into adulthood (Sanders, 1995). Some suffer persistent consequences into adolescence, even in the absence of the original perpetrating parent (Shapiro & Nguyen, 2011). Three-quarters of index children are affected by other forms of maltreatment, physical abuse, neglect, further fabrications or inappropriate medicating (Bools et al, 1992).

Social and demographic characteristics of perpetrators

People who fabricate or induce illness in children are nearly always female. Sheridan's review (2003) reported that 76% of the perpetrators were the biological mother and 7% the father. Between 14 and 30% had ties to the healthcare profession. Some professional carers have been reported to abuse those dependent on them, which again suggests that the reciprocal role relationships may be important for this type of abuse (Adshead & Bluglass, 2004). Unlike other types of child abuse, FII seems to be perpetrated by all social classes, is not always associated with other types of family violence or crime, young, inexperienced parents or socioeconomic deprivation. In one series of 41 children from 37 families there were high rates of privation, childhood abuse and significant loss or bereavement in the 34 mothers who were responsible for the fabrication or induction of illness. Only 4 (11%)

of these parents (including 2 fathers) were employed (Gray & Bentovim, 1996). Furthermore, a later case series, of 28 women (Bass & Jones, 2011), reported that a majority of perpetrators were either unemployed (53%, or 15 individuals) or in receipt of long-term disability living allowance (25%, or 7 individuals), and had a mean age of 31; 39% (11 individuals) had spent time in foster care.

Potentially relevant psychosocial factors include the following.

Childhood sexual and physical abuse

In the Bass & Jones (2011) case series, 15 (54%) of the 28 women had had severe abusive experiences in childhood. Childhood sexual abuse was reported by 12 (43%) participants and severe physical abuse by 7 (25%). Of note was the fact that from an early age some participants began to feign symptoms in order to avoid beatings or to prevent visits with abusive parents/carers.

In the 37 sets of parents studied by Gray & Bentovim (1996), 8% had experienced physical abuse and 35% emotional deprivation. None had a history of sexual abuse – perhaps because the series began in 1984, when sexual abuse was less discussed.

Marital and family difficulties

In Gray & Bentovim's sample, 40% reported serious marital problems, often of long duration, on admission or in subsequent therapy sessions. Of note is that these problems had previously been denied or minimised. One quarter of the mothers seemed to use the child's illness concerns as a way of re-engaging the fathers, who in 70% of cases were either absent or peripheral to the family system.

Bereavement

The Gray & Bentovim study reported that 14% of mothers had experienced a loss or bereavement involving children in the perinatal period (difficulties in conception, miscarriage, stillbirth or death); 11% of these mothers had experienced at least one bereavement of a significant adult (parents or supportive family member) and 32% had experienced the loss of a partner through either separation or divorce. One-third to a quarter of these mothers had suffered two or more of these types of difficulty. A study of attachment in 67 mothers who had demonstrated FII found that a high number had experienced unresolved distress and bereavement (Adshead & Bluglass, 2005).

Other factors

Other parental factors associated with abnormal illness behaviour in children include somatoform disorder, factitious disorder, being in receipt of disability living allowance, keeping children home from school, frequent visits to doctors with unexplained symptoms and failure to attend appointments (Bass & Jones, 2011).

Assessors should also note any frequent house moves, registration with new general practitioners and attempts to register for disability living allowance for the child. It is important to note that the parents of children who are victims of serious and substantiated physical abuse and neglect change their child's primary care provider more frequently than those of non-abused children (Friedlaender et al, 2005). It is essential therefore that full copies of the child's medical and general practitioner records are made available when interviewing a suspected perpetrator of FII.

Psychopathology of the fabricators

It may be helpful to consider the psychopathology of child abusers more generally, and then to focus on mechanisms that may give rise to this particular form. Fabricated or induced illness by carers of children is exploitation of the vulnerable, and potentially criminal behaviour. Child abuse is not associated with any specific psychiatric diagnosis, and it can occur in the absence of diagnosis. Most studies of child abuse by parents emphasise abnormalities in the parent–child relationship which are usually present from birth. Child abuse is more common among younger parents who have insecure backgrounds, are ambivalent about parenthood, and who have unplanned babies who are unwell or disabled (Paz et al, 2005).

Perpetrators of FII have been diagnosed with a range of psychiatric diagnoses, the most common of which are discussed here.

Somatoform and factitious disorders

Some researchers have noted the role of somatising behaviour in perpetrators, i.e. the tendency to express their anxiety physically, and have suggested that the mothers were treating their children as an extension of their own bodies. Bools et al (1994) found a high prevalence of somatising and factitious disorders in their sample, and Gray & Bentovim (1996) reported that 38% of mothers described medical problems of various degrees of severity. In 3% there was evidence of hypochondriasis and in 16% there was evidence of chronic factitious disorder. Bass & Jones (2011) reported 57% with somatisation disorder, 65% with fabricated or factitious disorder and 39% with both.

These findings are not unexpected, as there is evidence that somatising behaviour in adulthood is associated with adverse experiences of care and illness in early childhood (Craig et al, 2002). The distinction between somatising disorders and factitious disorders is chiefly one of perceived and conscious motive (Bass & Jones, 2011). In somatising disorder, the adult is not consciously or deliberately fabricating but is gripped by a conviction that they have a serious physical disorder. In factitious disorders, it is thought that an individual who fabricates, induces or even exaggerates is consciously

15

choosing this behaviour or at least consciously aware of the deception and possible gains involved. In practice, this distinction of motivation may be hard to detect.

Of the medically unexplained symptoms reported by somatising mothers, a high proportion are 'pseudoneurological' (faints and pseudoseizures), gastroenterological (abdominal pain and nausea), and obstetric and gynaecological (Bass & Jones, 2011). It is of interest that the symptoms most commonly fabricated in children by carers are epilepsy and syncope (Barber & Davis, 2002).

Affective and psychotic illnesses

Gray & Bentovim (1996) reported that 43% of their sample had a history of depression. Only 5% had been treated for psychotic illness, namely schizophrenia and bipolar affective disorder.

Personality disorder

Personality disorder is reported as highly prevalent in child abusers generally (Dinwiddie & Bucholz, 1993). However, there is a danger of circularity of argument, because the diagnosis of personality disorder is based on the abusive behaviour. It is likely that some types of personality disorder (for example, antisocial personality disorder) are a risk factor for child abuse generally, but the diagnosis alone provides little information.

This point is of particular relevance in cases of FII. More than one study found high rates of emotionally unstable personality disorder, borderline type, in fabricators, at times also associated with other types of personality disorder (Bools et al, 1994; Bass & Jones, 2011). However, it would be misleading to suggest that borderline personality disorder causes the behaviour, since so many mothers with borderline personality disorder do not abuse their children in this way. Nevertheless, borderline personality disorder is associated with a variety of parenting problems (Hobson et al, 2005), almost certainly mediated through the attachment style of affected parents (see below).

Motivation and triggers

The issue of motive has been a major cause of debate among workers in this field. Meadow's original contention was that the mothers carried out this behaviour to draw attention to their own needs and distress. Authors such as Schreier & Libow (1994) have suggested that the mothers form disturbed relationships with healthcare professionals that replicate past disturbed relationships with carers. Of relevance here may be that some case series have revealed that many of these mothers themselves experienced childhood abuse (Bools et al, 1994; Gray & Bentovim, 1996; Adshead & Bluglass, 2005). However, a history of childhood abuse is neither necessary nor sufficient to explain FII, since most adult survivors of abuse do not abuse their children.

Gray & Bentovim (1996) suggested that early stressful and traumatic events experienced by parents contribute to an ambivalent attitude and grievance towards the child and a perception that the child is ill. The seeking of medical assistance in the belief that the child is ill is then seen as a way of receiving help themselves.

It has also been suggested that FII represents an abnormality in the attachment system between mother and child, which regulates caregiving and care-eliciting behaviours (George & Solomon, 1996). Attachment insecurity is overrepresented in maltreating parents, including those who perpetrate FII, compared with non-clinical samples (Adshead & Bluglass, 2004, 2005) and is associated with hostile and helpless states of mind (Lyons-Ruth *et al*, 2006). An attachment perspective may also be relevant because of the known influence of insecurity of attachment on medically unexplained symptoms and abnormal illness behaviour. Ciechanowski *et al* (2002) found that patients with preoccupied and fearful attachment reported significantly more physical symptoms compared with secure patients. Controlling for age, income and recent experience of violence by an intimate partner, Waldinger *et al* (2006) showed that fearful attachment fully mediated the link between childhood trauma and somatisation among women.

Some believe that FII is a form of complex deceptive behaviour. Scrutiny of Social Services records or discussions with relatives or other informants, such as the general practitioner, may reveal a history of lying. Pseudologia fantastica is a dramatic form of pathological lying in which grandiose stories are constructed, often built on a matrix of truth (Dike *et al*, 2005). Unlike a person with delusional psychosis, someone with pseudologia fantastica will abandon the story or change it if confronted with contradictory evidence or sufficient disbelief. Bass & Jones (2011) reported that 61% of their sample exhibited lying or fabrication of stories.

The role of the psychiatrist

Investigation

Strictly speaking, the psychiatrist has no role to play until FII has been identified and confirmed. However, because it may be difficult for child protection services to gather actual evidence, professionals may put pressure on psychiatrists to state whether or not FII has taken place. This should be resisted, because of the risk that the psychiatrist might step outside their legal area of expertise. Ideally, psychiatric assessment will not take place until the paediatric review has confirmed that there is no organic cause for the child's illness or presentation and/or until there has been a legal fact-finding hearing. If the alleged perpetrator is denying the behaviour, then the assessing psychiatrist should prepare two opinions: one based on a perpetrator being found to have carried out the behaviour; one based on a situation where there is no perpetrator identified. Psychiatrists who state their opinion about the guilt of an alleged perpetrator may find that they interfere with any criminal justice proceedings, and risk being referred to the General Medical Council.

The assessment process relies heavily on paediatric assessment and investigation, and the exclusion of other causes for the child's 'symptoms'. However, psychiatrists (either from liaison or child psychiatry) may be called in to assess parents who have a history of psychiatric disorder, usually in the context of risk assessment. In such circumstances, it is important for the psychiatrist to remind colleagues that a psychiatric history does not automatically make a parent more likely to abuse their child, nor does it mean that all of their concerns about their child will be abnormal. Specifically, it is important to state that a history of borderline personality disorder, factitious disorder or a somatoform disorder does not necessarily help to identify FII.

Psychiatrists should be especially wary of accepting instructions in legal proceedings (either family or criminal) where FII is suspected, but has not been confirmed as legal fact. Psychiatrists may come under enormous pressure to provide an opinion as to whether a parent 'has FII' and therefore, by inference, has carried out the behaviour in question (Adshead, 2005). Since there is no evidence base that supports a link between any psychiatric diagnosis and either past or future abusive behaviour, it would be highly misleading for psychiatrists to offer any opinion until the facts about the identity of the perpetrator have been established. It must be remembered that there is no adult diagnosis of 'FII in children' (or of Munchausen syndrome by proxy), so it is not possible to say that a mother 'has' this, especially not on the basis of a single interview conducted in an out-patient department.

Assessment

Both adult and child psychiatrists have important roles to play in the management of identified cases in which illness has been fabricated or induced in a child. When decisions are being taken about the care of children involved, adult psychiatrists may be asked to assess the risk posed by both the abusing and the non-abusing parent.

Assessment of the child

Child psychiatrists may be asked to provide assessments of family dynamics and parenting skills, opinions about the possibilities of family interventions and support, assessments of the effects of the behaviour on the child, and treatment for both the child and the other family members.

Sanders & Bursch (2002) offer useful guidelines for conducting assessments of possible FII at the request of the courts. In all but the mildest of cases, the child is separated from the potentially fabricating adult until the risk and prognosis are fully established. The domains assessed are: child, parent, parent–child, family, social and professional; and in all these domains there are factors with better and worse outcome prognosis (Jones & Bools, 1999). The criteria for evaluation of whether change has occurred and interventions have been successful or not should also be established at the assessment stage (Jones *et al*, 2000).

Assessment of the adult(s)

The assessment of the perpetrating parent is a complex process that requires the collection of information from a wide variety of sources, with the parent's consent. It is essential to read the medical records of the parent (both hospital and primary care) and also, if possible, of the abused child or children. Specifically, it may be useful to look at hospital attendance rates and put these in context of the other events in the parent's life. Relevant Social Services records should be accessed and, if possible, any criminal record. The amount and type of information available will depend to some extent on the context in which the assessment is taking place: most commonly, it will be in the context of care proceedings, where the parent's solicitor may have to be approached to gain access to both health and criminal records.

Both adult and child psychiatrists may find themselves in situations where they are interviewing a parent who is only suspected of having fabricated or induced illness in their child, i.e. it has not yet been proven. If this is the case, then the process of preparation before interviewing the parent is especially important and complex (Box 2.1).

Box 2.1 Assessment of a parent/carer under suspicion

Preparation for the assessment of a parent/carer suspected of inducing or fabricating illness in a child should ideally include:

- the parent/carer's medical records (hospital and general practitioner records, both paper and electronic)
- the child's medical records
- social work records/reports
- police records/videos
- legal documents (mother's and father's statements; reports written by the child's guardian *ad litem*)
- interview with the parent and partner (audiotaped, with consent)
- interview with the grandparents (audiotaped, with consent)
- telephone interview with general practitioner, social workers, paediatrician and guardian.

Information gathering will also include interviews with key informants such as social workers and the child's grandparents. Evidence of inconsistencies in the medical history, comments from medical practitioners and social workers about parenting skills, episodes of antisocial behaviour and dissimulation or frank lying might be revealed. It is also important to establish whether the parent acknowledges any of the concerns and is willing to commit to therapeutic work to change their behaviour. This will have a major impact on outcome (Fig. 2.3) in the long term (Bools, 2007).

Psychiatrists are often asked to provide opinions about the parenting capacity of a parent suspected of this type of abuse or of the non-abusing parent. It is important that psychiatrists who do this have expertise in the field. This usually means that they are child psychiatrists. Adult psychiatrists should not offer expert opinions about parenting capacity unless they: (a) have the skills to carry out a thorough parenting assessment; and (b) can demonstrate to the courts exactly how they have done so. Parenting capacity or its absence cannot be established by an ordinary psychiatric interview of the adult alone: it usually includes assessment of the parent with the child, and information from foster carers or those who supervise contact.

Some screening tools may be of assistance. The Relationship Scales Questionnaire (RSQ; Griffin & Bartholomew, 1994) and the Parental Bonding Instrument (PBI; Parker et al, 1987) may provide an indication of the parent's attachment security. It may be useful to assess for any disorder of personality either using the Structured Clinical Interview for

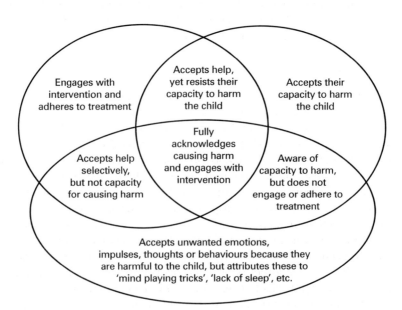

Fig. 2.3 The main components of acknowledgement. Adapted by D. Jones from David (1990), with permission.

DSM-IV Axis II Personality Disorders (SCID-II; First *et al*, 1997) or the International Personality Disorder Examination (IPDE) screening versions (Loranger, 1999). It is important to make clear in any report that these are not diagnostic tools and that they cannot provide confirmatory or refutatory evidence where the facts are disputed.

Management

Detection of FII usually results in care proceedings to determine whether the abusing parent should continue to care for the child. In most cases, courts will place the child in the care of the non-abusing parent (if separated), grandparents or the local authority. Abusing parents may or may not have contact or access, depending on individual circumstances.

For parents who are found by the court to have harmed their children, there are usually two issues at stake. First, they may need an assessment of parenting capacity in relation to their other children, and this may require admission to a residential family unit. Then there is the issue of whether reunification of the family is possible. This will depend on the assessment of risk to the child, and the attitudes of the parent to working with professionals, including therapists.

Treatment for parents

When parent and child are permanently separated

There are a very few specialist services that can provide treatment for both perpetrator and child where there has been severe parenting breakdown. Often, the parent will be rejected by regular psychological therapy services as being too disturbed, but is not disturbed enough to reach criteria for the intervention of forensic services.

Most parents will need treatment for both mood disorders and personality disorders, usually of the emotionally unstable, borderline type. There has been considerable expansion of treatment services for personality disorders, and there is ample evidence that personality pathology responds to treatments that address affect and arousal regulation, such as dialectical behaviour therapy (DBT) and mentalisation-based therapy (MBT) (National Collaborating Centre for Mental Health, 2009). Studies of the treatment of patients with emotionally unstable personality disorder have demonstrated that, although many patients report substantial reductions in symptom severity, improved social and vocational function are more difficult to achieve (National Collaborating Centre for Mental Health, 2009; Gunderson *et al*, 2011; Bateman, 2012).

In addition to treatment for the underlying condition, perpetrators need therapy to address the impact of harming a child, as well as the effect of the loss of that relationship. Therapy needs to address feelings of guilt, shame and sometimes associated suicidal thoughts. It is worth noting that where feelings of guilt and shame are wholly absent, the perpetrator's capacity to mentalise the effect of the harm on the child needs to be questioned and explored. It is also fundamental to consider the child's protection from future harm, protecting other children (decision-making regarding risk to siblings and/or the public) and ensuring that the parent is supported and/ or treated to help them deal with the public consequences of having their child or children taken from them.

As for all psychological therapies, successful treatment requires both engagement with and commitment to therapy. Personality pathology is treatable (National Collaborating Centre for Mental Health, 2009), but psychological therapies are not indicated for individuals who are so deceptive that they cannot establish a therapeutic alliance. In addition, individuals who cannot admit their behaviour present almost insurmountable obstacles to psychological therapy. However, if the individual is willing to engage in psychological treatment, the initial focus of therapy must include their acknowledgement of their behaviour.

Where reunification of parent and child is planned

Where reunification is to be considered, assessment and treatment of the parent–child relationship is essential. The courts seek psychiatric advice on whether the abusing parent can be sufficiently rehabilitated to be reunited with their child and the rest of the family. As suggested above, where there is frank denial of the behaviour or other evidence of antisocial attitudes or cruelty, this is not likely to be possible. In about 20% of cases, the abuse recurs if the child remains with the parent who abused them (Bools et al, 1993). Other siblings are also at risk.

However, there is evidence that reunification of families is sometimes possible and successful. A study by Berg & Jones (1999) followed all 17 children from 16 families selected for admission to a specialist residential family unit between 1992 and 1996. There was one recurrence of FII, leading to mild harm to the child. A favourable outcome was associated with: acknowledgement of fabrication and the psychosocial context within which it occurred; less severe abuse; improvements in the parent's psychological functioning and empathy for the child; and improved parent–child relationships and child attachment behaviour towards the parents. A better outcome was seen where changes in the family system and a therapeutic alliance with the fabricator's partner and extended family could be established. For more delineation of prognostic factors see Jones & Bools (1999) and Jones et al (2005).

Careful assessment is needed before selecting families for possible intervention. The initial assessment (Jones et al, 2000) should determine the degree and quality of the acknowledgement of abuse by the perpetrator, their partner and the wider family, and an assessment of their willingness and individual capacities to engage in a programme of risk management and treatment. Further factors that influence selection include the potential for working in partnership and the existence of better prognostic features.

Conclusion

Fabricated or induced illness by carers is a rare but serious disorder that has adverse effects on a child's health and development, and can be fatal. It usually involves abnormal illness behaviour in the perpetrator (most often the mother, but rarely a professional carer) and there is evidence of high rates not only of somatoform and factitious disorders, but also of coexisting personality disorders in the perpetrators. The symptoms that are fabricated or induced in the children can on occasion resemble the somatic complaints reported by the mother, and early identification is key if harm to the child is to be avoided. The recently updated guideline on identifying child maltreatment provides helpful information (National Institute for Health and Clinical Excellence, 2013: paras 1.2.11–1.2.12).

Assessment in suspected cases is labour intensive, and professionals should expect to spend considerable time collating material and collaborating with other parties. An attempt should be made to assess the degree to which the perpetrator acknowledges the abusive behaviour, as without this any chance of reuniting the perpetrator and child is negligible. Assessments of parenting capacity and parent–child interaction may be needed to determine whether reunification is viable, but this must take into consideration the timescales for the child. Close collaboration between professions is essential, not only between different medical disciplines but also social services and schools. Collation of material from a variety of different sources is required before reports to the court can be prepared.

References

Adshead G (2005) Evidence-based medicine and medicine-based evidence: the expert witness in cases of factitious disorder by proxy. *Journal of the American Academy of Psychiatry and Law*, **33**, 99–105.

Adshead G, Bluglass K (2004) Attachment representations and factitious illness by proxy: relevance for assessment of parenting capacity in child maltreatment. In *A Matter of Security: The Application of Attachment Theory to Forensic Psychiatry and Psychotherapy* (eds F Pfäfflin, G Adshead), pp. 211–224. Jessica Kingsley.

Adshead G, Bluglass K (2005) Attachment representations in mothers with abnormal illness behaviour by proxy. *British Journal of Psychiatry*, **187**, 328–333.

American Psychiatric Association (1994) *Diagnostic and Statistical Manual of Mental Disorders (4th edn) (DSM-IV)*. APA.

American Psychiatric Association (2013) *Diagnostic and Statistical Manual of Mental Disorders (5th edn) (DSM-5)*. APA.

Ayoub CC, Alexander R, Beck D, *et al* (2002) Position paper: definitional issues in Munchausen by proxy. *Child Maltreatment*, **7**, 105–111.

Barber M, Davis P (2002) Fits, faints, or fatal fantasy? Fabricated seizures and child abuse. *Archives of Disease in Childhood*, **86**, 230–233.

Bass C, Jones D (2011) Psychopathology of perpetrators of fabricated or induced illness in children: case series. *British Journal of Psychiatry*, **199**, 113–118.

Bateman, A (2012) Treating borderline personality disorder in clinical practice. *American Journal of Psychiatry*, **165**, 560–564.

Berg B, Jones D (1999) Outcome of psychiatric intervention in factitious illness by proxy (Munchausen syndrome by proxy). *Archives of Disease in Childhood*, **81**, 465–472.

Bools C (2007) *Fabricated or Induced Illness in a Child by a Carer*. Radcliffe Publishing.

Bools CN, Neale BA, Meadow SR (1992) Co-morbidity associated with fabricated illness (Munchausen syndrome by proxy). *Archives of Disease in Childhood*, **67**, 77–79.

Bools C, Neale B, Meadow R (1993) Follow up of victims of fabricated illness (Munchausen syndrome by proxy). *Archives of Disease in Childhood*, **69**, 625–630.

Bools C, Neale B, Meadow R (1994) Munchausen syndrome by proxy: a study of psychopathology. *Child Abuse and Neglect*, **18**, 773–788.

Ciechanowski P, Walker E, Katon W, *et al* (2002) Attachment theory: a model for health care utilisation and somatisation. *Psychosomatic Medicine*, **64**, 660–667.

Craft AW, Hall DM (2004) Munchausen syndrome by proxy and sudden infant death. *BMJ*, **328**, 1309–1312.

Craig T, Cox A, Klein K (2002) Intergenerational transmission of somatisation behaviour: a study of chronic somatisers and their children. *Psychological Medicine*, **32**, 805–816.

David A (1990) Insight and psychosis. *British Journal of Psychiatry*, **156**, 798–808.

Denny SJ, Grant CC, Pinnock R (2001) Epidemiology of Munchausen syndrome by proxy in New Zealand. *Journal of Paediatrics and Child Health*, **37**, 240–243.

Department of Health (2002) *Safeguarding Children in Whom Illness is Fabricated or Induced*. Department of Health Publications.

Dike C, Baranowski M, Griffith E (2005) Pathological lying revisited. *Journal of the American Academy of Psychiatry and Law*, **33**, 342–349.

Dinwiddie SH, Bucholz KK (1993) Psychiatric diagnoses in self-reported child abusers. *Child Abuse and Neglect*, **17**, 465–476.

Eminson MD (2000) Background. In *Munchausen Syndrome by Proxy Abuse: A Practical Approach* (eds MD Eminson, RJ Postlethwaite), pp. 24–25. Butterworth-Heinemann.

First M, Gibbon M, Spitzer R, *et al* (1997) *User's Guide for the Structured Clinical Interview for DSM-IV Axis II Personality Disorders: SCID-II*. American Psychiatric Association.

Friedlaender E, Rubin D, Alpern E, *et al* (2005) Patterns of health care use that may identify young children who are at risk of maltreatment. *Paediatrics*, **116**, 1303–1308.

Galvin HK, Newton AW, Vandeven AM (2005) Update on Munchausen syndrome by proxy. *Current Opinion in Pediatrics*, **17**, 252–257.

George C, Solomon J (1996) Representational models of attachment: links between caregiving and attachment. *Infant Mental Health Journal*, **17**, 198–216.

Gray, J, Bentovim, A (1996) Illness induction syndrome: paper I – a series of 41 children from 37 families identified at the Great Ormond Street Hospital for Children NHS trust. *Child Abuse and Neglect*, **20**, 655–673.

Griffin D, Bartholomew K (1994) The metaphysics of measurement: the case of adult attachment. *Advances in Personal Relations*, **5**, 17–52.

Gunderson J, Stout J, McGlashan T, *et al* (2011) Ten year course of borderline personality disorder. *Archives of General Psychiatry*, **68**, 827–837.

Hobson R, Patrick M, Crandell L, *et al* (2005) Personal relatedness and attachment in infants of mothers with borderline personality disorder. *Developmental Psychopathology*, **17**, 329–347.

Jones D, Bools,C (1999) Factitious illness by proxy. In *Recent Advances in Paediatrics* (vol. 1) (ed TJ David), pp. 57–71. Churchill Livingstone.

Jones D, Byrne G, Newbold C (2000) Management, treatment and outcomes. In *Munchausen Syndrome by Proxy Abuse: A Practical Approach* (eds MD Eminson, RJ Postlethwaite), pp. 276–294. Butterworth-Heinemann.

Jones DPH, Hindley N, Ramchandani P (2005) Making plans: assessment, intervention and evaluating outcomes. In *The Developing World of the Child* (eds W Rose, J Aldgate, D Jones). Jessica Kingsley.

Loranger A (1999) *International Personality Disorder Examination (IPDE): DSM-IV and ICD-10 Interviews*. Psychological Assessment Resources.

Lyons-Ruth K, Dutra L, Schuder M, *et al* (2006) From infant attachment disorganisation to adult dissociation: relational adaptation or traumatic experiences? *Psychiatric Clinics of North America*, **29**, 63–86.

McClure RJ, Davis PM, Meadow SR, *et al* (1996) Epidemiology of Munchausen syndrome by proxy, non-accidental poisoning, and non-accidental suffocation. *Archives of Disease in Childhood*, **75**, 57–61.

Meadow R (1977) Munchausen syndrome by proxy: the hinterland of child abuse. *Lancet*, **2**, 343–345.

National Collaborating Centre for Mental Health (2009) *Borderline Personality Disorder: The NICE Guideline on Treatment and Management* (National Clinical Practice Guideline Number 78). British Psychological Society & Royal College of Psychiatrists.

National Institute for Health and Clinical Excellence (2013) *When to Suspect Child Maltreatment (Issued: July 2009; Last Modified: March 2013)* (NICE Clinical Guideline 89). NICE.

Parker G, Kiloh L, Hayward L (1987) Parental representation of neurotic and endogenous depressives. *Journal of Affective Disorders*, **13**, 75–82.

Paz I, Jones D, Byrne G (2005) Child maltreatment, child protection and mental health. *Current Opinion in Psychiatry*, **18**, 411–421.

Roesler T, Jenny C (2009) *Medical Child Abuse: Beyond Munchausen Syndrome by Proxy.* American Academy of Pediatrics.

Royal College of Paediatrics and Child Health (2009) *Fabricated or Induced Illness by Carers (FII): A Practical Guide for Paediatricians.* Royal College of Paediatrics and Child Health.

Sanders M (1995) Symptom coaching: factitious disorder by proxy with older children. *Clinical Psychology Review*, **15**, 423–442.

Sanders M, Bursch B (2002) Forensic assessment of illness falsification, Munchausen by proxy, and factitious disorder, NOS. *Child Maltreatment*, **2**, 112–124.

Schreier H, Libow JA (1994) Munchausen by proxy syndrome: a modern pediatric challenge. *Journal of Pediatrics*, **125** (issue 6 suppl.), S110–S115.

Shapiro M, Nguyen M (2011) Psychological sequelae of Munchausen's syndrome by proxy. *Child Abuse and Neglect*, **35**, 87–88.

Sheridan MS (2003) The deceit continues: an updated literature review of Munchausen syndrome by proxy. *Child Abuse and Neglect*, **27**, 431–451.

Waldinger R, Schulz M, Barsky A, *et al* (2006) Mapping the road from childhood trauma to adult somatization: the role of attachment. *Psychosomatic Medicine*, **68**, 129–135.

Watson S, Eminson DM, Coupe W (1999) quoted in: Eminson, M (2000) Background. In *Munchausen Syndrome by Proxy Abuse: A Practical Approach* (eds M Eminson, RJ Postlethwaite), pp. 31–32. Butterworth-Heinemann.

CHAPTER 3

Personality disorders as disorganisation of attachment and affect regulation

Jaydip Sarkar and Gwen Adshead

Personality disorders are common psychiatric disorders that carry significant costs for healthcare services. People with personality disorders present a problem in psychiatry because they demonstrate both symptoms of psychological distress and social rule-breaking behaviour. They therefore invite punitive as well as therapeutic responses, which can lead to confusion and negativity among service providers (Watts & Morgan, 1994).

Personality disorders are developmental conditions that begin in childhood and adolescence. Research into gene–environment interactions indicates that the caregiving environment influences the expression of genetic neuropharmacological vulnerability. For example, a hostile care-giving environment makes antisocial behaviour much more likely in boys with variations in allele length for serotonergic proteins compared with those without this mutation (Livesley *et al*, 1993; Caspi *et al*, 2002; Kim *et al*, 2009).

In this chapter, we suggest that the major feature of personality disorders is a failure of affect regulation. We present evidence on the neurobiology of affect regulation and on its development within attachment relationships in a heuristic model that explains both the symptoms of and effective treatment strategies for personality disorders. Being heuristic in nature, this model will, we hope, form the basis of further empirical research. Emotions and affects are essentially similar terms and we use them interchangeably.

Affects

What are they and where are they formed?

Emotion indicates a departure from a basic state of calm (Freeman, 1999: p. 124). Damasio's (1994) view is that emotions are bodily experiences (somatosensory states) in response to external and internal influences. Several areas of the somatosensory cortex are associated with the

26

recall of emotional experiences, especially the insula, cingulate cortex, hypothalamus and several nuclei of the brain-stem tegmentum (Damasio, 2003). The bodily states created include autonomic, neuroendocrine and somatomotor responses that are subjectively experienced as feelings and are expressed through a range of somatomotor responses, including facial, gestural, vocal and behavioural reactions. Thus, behaviour is merely one expression of an affective state; individuals also use words (written and spoken) and facial expression to communicate them.

What are their functions?

Affects act as a driving force or catalyst to assist humans in pursuit of goal-directed behaviours that help us find sources of energy, fend off external noxious agents, and make and maintain social relationships to support a life-sustaining homeostasis (Panksepp, 1998). This is achieved by the complex interplay of multiple systems and events within the body that leads to an automated regulation of life. The 'machinery' involved includes a number of systems (Box 3.1), nested within each other, that are ultimately driven by emotions. No one system acts in isolation: simple systems are regulated by more complex ones (Damasio, 2003). Affect regulation is one aspect of the more complex systems required for optimal homeostasis. This nested principle, with the emotions governing the motivational machinery of the body, includes, but goes beyond, the reductionist view of affects simply as states elicited by rewards and punishments (Rolls, 2000).

Humans are unique among animals in their long period of total dependence on others for survival after birth. Like other non-human primates that live in social groups, people instinctively make and maintain different types of social relationship for survival. These relationships are a function of time, complexity and interpersonal attachments. To be effective, interpersonal affective responses need to be both regulated and organised. In particular, the most favourable management of relationships requires the capacity to regulate negative affects such as anger and anxiety. This is especially true of relationships characterised by discrepancies of power and

---

Box 3.1 Key components of the body's emotion-driven multisystem machinery

- The endocrine system
- Simple reflexes (e.g. the startle reflex, which is protective in nature and has survival value)
- The immune system
- Drives and motivations (e.g. hunger, thirst and curiosity)
- Approach and avoidance behaviours that lead to appetites and desires

those that involve dependency and neediness, for example relationships with partners, children, family members and professional carers.

We suggest that the need and the ability to coexist with others in order to survive optimally are fundamental to the development and maintenance of affect regulation. In other words, the affects fine-tune the organism's struggle for survival, but affect regulation can improve the quality of that survival.

Affect production and regulation

Regulation in any homeostatic system (including that of affect) means not only initiating a response to a stimulus, but also modulating it appropriately and turning it off when no longer required. Regulation also implies that the response itself is organised and effective. Phillips *et al* (2003) suggest that affective experience involves:

- identification of the emotional significance of a stimulus
- production of an affective state in response
- regulation of the affective state.

Identification of emotional significance

Two areas of the brain – the amygdala and the insula – are involved in the identification of the emotional significance of a stimulus. The amygdala is responsible for modulation of vigilance and attention to emotionally salient information. The insula conveys aversive sensory information to the amygdala, and the two areas act in concert to detect and respond to threatening and aversive stimuli. They can be conceptualised as a defence radar alerting the organism to the presence of threat in its environment and stimulating a fight or flight self-preservative response (see Phillips *et al*, 2003).

Regulation of the affective state

Affect regulation is largely dependent on the functioning of two neural systems: a ventral and a dorsal system (Phillips *et al*, 2003).

The ventral system includes the amygdala, insula, ventral striatum and ventral (affective) regions of the anterior cingulate gyrus and prefrontal cortex. It is important for rapid appraisal of emotional material, and automatic affective regulation in response to social interactions, including the capacity for interpersonal empathy.

The dorsal system includes the hippocampus and dorsal (cognitive) regions of the anterior cingulate gyrus and prefrontal cortex. It supports selective and sustained attention, planning and effortful (rather than automatic) regulation of affective states, and autonomic responses to those states. Here affect regulation involves cognitive appraisals: using logic and rational evaluations based on past experience and anticipated outcomes.

These contributions of the two systems might be summarised as insight and foresight respectively (Freeman, 1999: p. 124) (Box 3.2).

The role of attachment relationships in affect regulation

Schore (2002, 2003) has set out an explanatory framework for affect dysregulation, based on research into the neural development of the infant brain. He reviews the evidence that the rearing environment (in the form of the infant's relationship with the mother or other primary carer) has a direct effect on the development of brain structures and pathways involved in affect regulation. Animal research by Suomi (1999, 2003) has also demonstrated the importance of the interaction between the genetic basis of neural and synaptic development (temperament) and the developing infant's socioemotional environment (nurture) in the development of neurotransmitter systems and cytoarchitecture.

Secure attachment

In humans, attachment operates through the interaction of two behavioural systems: caregiving and care-eliciting (George & Solomon, 1996). These foster identification of affects, the response to them and the regulation of the affective system. It is useful to conceptualise the interaction between a caregiver and care-elicitor as one that regulates the experience of emotions through a crescendo–decrescendo process (Schore, 2002). A distressed infant responds to threats in its environment by experiencing a high degree of arousal, mediated by the sympathetic division of the autonomic nervous system. This is a catabolic system, making available large amounts of energy to prepare the infant for a self-preservative action repertoire of a fight/flight mode. The infant experiences the peripheral and central effects of noradrenaline (norepinephrine) (e.g. more rapid heart and pulse rate, increased blood pressure, dilated pupils),

---

Box 3.2 The neural systems that govern affect regulation

Insight is mediated by the ventral system:

- amygdala
- insula
- ventral striatum
- ventral (affective) regions of the anterior cingulate gyrus and prefrontal cortex.

Foresight is mediated by the dorsal system:

- hippocampus
- dorsal (cognitive) regions of the anterior cingulate gyrus and prefrontal cortex.

which are uncomfortable. By soothing the infant, the caregiver helps in recruiting the child's parasympathetic system, which has opposite effects and restores homeostasis. There is a return to normal rate and rhythm of the autonomic system. The sympathetic system supports an action-consuming state, whereas the parasympathetic system supports a withdrawal–conservation state.

The earliest attachment figure conceivably acts as a primary affect regulator, one that ameliorates and terminates the infant's distress, augments within reasonable limits its experience of happiness and pleasure, and offers predictable and replicable affect regulation. The basic language of attachment relationships thus consists of episodes of interactive signals produced by the autonomic nervous system in both infant and caregiver. These episodes emerge at about 2 months of age, and they are highly arousing, affect-laden and short interpersonal events that expose the infant to high levels of cognitive and social information (Feldman et al, 1999). As the infant grows, it is the relationship, rather than a particular caregiver, that becomes the (accessory) affect regulator.

Right prefrontal cortex regulation of the autonomic nervous system lies at the heart of the development of affect regulation in an infant. The right hemisphere is also centrally involved in corporeal self-identity and its relation to the environment, distinguishing self from non-self (Devinsky, 2000). Infant–maternal attachment behaviour is almost exclusively body to body, and it is now accepted that the right hemisphere is involved in the social and biological functions of the attachment system in the infant (Wang, 1997). Furthermore, this hemisphere is crucial in the receptive and expressive empathic processes (Adolphs et al, 2000), which are processed unconsciously using extensive reciprocal connections with both limbic systems.

A good-quality affect regulatory system, based on secure attachment, leads to optimal right hemispheric maturation at a critical period during the first 2–3 years of life (Schore, 2002). Any experience that disturbs the development of secure attachment at a time of heightened dependence (e.g. abuse, neglect or inconsistent caring) can lead to impaired development of neural pathways that subserve emotional behaviours, such that impaired emotional regulation is likely to persist throughout the individual's lifetime.

The final task in terms of emotion processing involves the internalisation of affect-regulating capacity. Up to about 5 years of age, children locate both affects and their stimuli outside of the self. Any adverse emotional experience is therefore ascribed to the object (including humans) causing it: an externalisation of affects. Later, children locate emotions internally and still later they can identify mixed and conflicting emotions (Levine et al, 1997). Thus, emotion is initially perceived as being caused, and is in reality regulated, by others, but over the course of early life it becomes increasingly self-regulated as a result of neurophysiological development (Thompson, 1990: p. 371).

Insecure attachment

The successful outcome of secure attachment is the development of the basic machinery to self-regulate affects later in life (Fonagy *et al*, 2002). Insecure attachment can prevent the development of a proper affect regulatory capacity. The individual is left with either an inability to balance sympathetic hyperarousal in response to threat, or the production of an untimely or inadequate parasympathetic response. Dysregulation of this nature leads to prolonged persistence of a catabolic state of fight/flight hyperarousal, or a sudden and inappropriate shift into an anabolic withdrawal–conservation state of 'freezing'. The latter occurs when a situation is perceived to be hopeless and one's own agency inadequate, leading to inhibition and avoidance in order to become 'unseen' (a state of dissociation) as a defensive strategy of last resort. Alternatively, there could be rapid cycling between states of hyperarousal and withdrawal, resulting in gross disorganisation of both affects and associated behaviours.

Affect dysregulation and symptoms of personality disorder

Individuals who have experienced insecure attachment are at risk of developing dysregulated and disorganised affective systems. Both small-scale (Patrick *et al*, 1994; Fonagy *et al*, 1997) and larger studies (Johnson *et al*, 1999) have found that early childhood adversity, especially neglect, is a risk factor for the development of personality disorders. Childhood sexual abuse is also a risk factor for the development of self-harming and suicidal behaviour in adulthood (Andrews *et al*, 2003) – behaviour commonly seen in people with personality disorders.

One major outcome of this is that people with personality disorders have significant difficulty in establishing and maintaining interpersonal relationships that require good affect regulation. They seem to withdraw from and alienate others and/or engage in confusing and disorganised relationships. This characteristic is observed particularly within dependency relationships during adulthood (e.g. relationships with peers, partners, children and professional carers), which may be experienced as disparities of power and vulnerability, giving rise to a sense of threat and fear. Inability to regulate negative affects within dependency relationships increases the chance of responding with unregulated hostility or anger. This puts these individuals at a double disadvantage: not only do they tend to alienate caregivers, but they are likely to do it at times of greatest need.

In exhibiting this behaviour, individuals with personality disorders are moving away from the recently (in evolutionary terms) evolved adaptive species-preservative behaviour seen in mammals towards a more ancient self-preservative behaviour. As the name suggests, species-preservative behaviour has evolved to improve the chances of survival of a species, and it is based on parental care, nursing, social interaction, pair-bonding and mutual defence (Henry & Wang, 1998). If trauma results in a stressful loss of control, the self-preservative fight/flight catecholamine coping response takes priority. Problems arise when this style becomes the default coping response to a wide range of events, people and circumstances. It is then maladaptive and inappropriately accessed.

Regulation of negative affect

The problem is not that people with personality disorders are 'affectless' but that they have too much or too little affect, depending on the perceived social stimulation, i.e. the affective system is dysregulated and the responses disorganised. Affect dysregulation also implies an unpredictability that goes beyond either an excessive or diminished response.

Heightened perception of threat seems to be a major problem for people with personality disorders, one that emphasises a lack of safety with and an essential untrustworthiness of others. This is compounded by an inability to repair the emotional states stimulated by threat or fear. They seem to lack the capacity to soothe themselves after fearful experiences (van der Kolk & Fisler, 1994), becoming and remaining hyperaroused in an uncontrollable, dysregulated manner. Their difficulty in providing an internal discourse for themselves to manage negative affects leads to the expectation or requirement of an external solution when they feel bad – preferably from another person whom they identify as having a caring role.

In people with personality disorders there appears to be a deficit, if not an absence, of the shift in locus from external to internal affect regulation. They appear to continue to believe that emotions are almost always an outcome of external developments caused by other people. This is a problem of excessive externalisation of experience of negative affects, a task that should have been resolved around 5 years of age. Such responses are therefore age inappropriate and immature.

Regulation and specific personality disorders

In its *Diagnostic and Statistical Manual of Mental Disorders* (DSM), the American Psychiatric Association (2013) groups personality disorders into three clusters (Box 3.3). The World Health Organization's (1992) *International Classification of Diseases and Health Related Problems* (ICD) does not use this clustering, but describes similar types of disorder.

Cluster A

Cluster A personality disorders (paranoid, schizoid, schizotypal) are characterised by increased paranoia and suspiciousness of others. People with paranoid personality disorders have increased suspiciousness and arousal based on the excessive fear that arises from their heightened perception of threat, underregulation of fear and a fight/flight response

Box 3.3   Affect dysregulation with personality disorder

Cluster A

Prototype: paranoid personality disorder

- Consistent underregulation of the affects of fear and terror
- Overregulation of positive affects – narrow range of affective expression
- Overregulation (muting) of all affects in schizoid personality disorder

Cluster B

Prototype: borderline personality disorder

- Dysregulation (under- or over-) of both positive and negative affects, but predominantly demonstrated with fear, anger, sadness and anxiety
- Underregulation of fear, arousal and anger, and overregulation of feelings of empathy, remorse and guilt in antisocial and narcissistic personality disorders
- Underregulation of most affects in histrionic personality disorder

Cluster C

Prototype: anxious/avoidant personality disorder

- Underregulation of social emotions, e.g. shame and guilt
- Underregulation of anxiety and sadness
- Positive affects usually experienced only when with others

pattern. Those with schizoid and schizotypal personality disorders also have a predominantly constricted affect. Individuals with schizoid personality disorder also experience lack of pleasure and an affective indifference towards others, suggesting perhaps a muting of all affective responses on account of overregulation of affects. Schizotypal personality disorder is characterised by inappropriate affect and heightened social anxiety, secondary to paranoia, and lacking in habituation.

Cluster B

Cluster B personality disorders (borderline, antisocial, histrionic and narcissistic) are the classic example of dysregulation, and borderline personality disorder is the prototype. In this cluster there is clinical evidence of dysregulation of all negative affects, primarily involving fear and anger, but including depression and anxiety.

People with borderline personality disorder alternate between having either no trust in others or a highly risky tendency to fail to see threat when it is present. They also experience predominantly depressive mood disorders and poorly controlled anger, and form underregulated, intense attachments that are often a source of further affective distress and arousal.

Histrionic personality disorder is characterised by shallow or labile affect, excitement-seeking and an exaggerated emotional expression.

Individuals with antisocial personality disorder show an excessive capacity for blaming others (externalisation of affect) and have little or no regard for the feelings of others, as exemplified by impairment in empathy, remorse and guilt. They share certain characteristics with those with narcissistic personality disorder, who also show little empathy but also excessive envy and jealousy. People with either disorder seem to see others as highly risky and unstable sources of aggression or threat, and their own aggression, paranoia and cruelty to others are likely to be due to underregulation of arousal in response to threat. They seem to have difficulty in regulating emotions that have a social valence, suggesting a dysfunction based in the prefrontal cortex. Not surprisingly, people with these particular disorders have the greatest difficulty in adapting to social norms and customs.

Cluster C

The avoidance behaviour so characteristic of Cluster C personality disorders (avoidant, dependent and obsessive–compulsive) may be seen as avoidance of situations, people and thoughts that provoke unmodulated affect, usually severe anxiety and panic, in a classic behavioural style.

People with obsessive–compulsive (anankastic in ICD-10) personality disorder show excessive doubt and caution, avoiding risks altogether, whereas those with avoidant personality disorders have a heightened fear of criticism and disapproval, with a possible heightened sense of shame and ridicule. People with dependent personality disorder have exaggerated fears of their own ability to care for themselves and therefore avoid being alone, depending on others to validate their existence.

Substance misuse

Substance misuse is a common feature of personality disorders. It often starts in adolescence. Ethanol, in particular, may be neurotoxic to processes such as synaptogenesis or dendritisation, making the adolescent brain increasingly vulnerable to environmental challenges, which in turn may make adult psychiatric disturbance more likely (Olney *et al*, 2000).

It is likely that the pathways that mediate the euphoric properties of psychostimulants evolved as neural systems for social attachment. There is evidence that brain activation patterns in adults responding to attachment figures (partners or children) are similar to neural responses to cocaine-induced euphoria (Bartels & Zeki, 2000). The brain structures involved include bilateral activation in the anterior cingulate gyrus, medial insula and ventral striatum. These findings suggest that the explanation for the high rates of substance misuse among people with personality disorders may therefore lie, in part at least, in their dysfunctional or absent social attachments. Substance use (and misuse) acts as a social integrator, both externally with peers and internally through the induction of a pleasurable state. This state replaces the very basic human quality of gregariousness.

Furthermore, substances are used as external regulators of negative affects because the individual perceives these affects to be externally, not internally, caused.

Violence

Only two of the personality disorders are associated with high rates of violence and rule-breaking: antisocial personality disorder and psychopathy. The Cluster A and Cluster C diagnoses are not associated with violence to others; and borderline personality disorder is associated with self-harm, rather than violence to others. However, forensic services frequently admit patients where there is a link between their personality disorder and violence.

Blair (2001) suggests that violence can take one of two forms: reactive violence, which is elicited in response to frustration or threat, and instrumental violence, which is goal-directed, purposeful and apparently unprovoked.

Reactive violence has been conceptualised as a response to perceived threat, mediated by the hypothalamus–periaqueductal grey matter system. The amygdala feeds information into the periaqueductal grey matter system on the current state of threat, thus determining whether the response is fight or flight. The orbitofrontal cortex has extensive projections to autonomic control centres in the medial hypothalamus and periaqueductal grey matter, and it is damage specifically to this part of the frontal lobe that leads to greatest risk of reactive violence (Grafman *et al*, 1996). Thus, reactive violence is a consequence of inadequate regulation of threat-based affects, largely by the dorsal prefrontal cortex.

Instrumental violence is a function of cruelty and lack of empathy (Hare *et al*, 1991), which in turn has been linked to muted autonomic responses to sad and fearful facial expressions. In this type of violence, it has been speculated that the affect-regulating system of the prefrontal cortex remains intact, but there is a fundamental problem within the amygdala, the area concerned with properly identifying fearful and sad emotions (Blair, 2001).

Implications for treatment

Essentially, all therapeutic interventions in psychiatry seek to regulate affects by various means (Bradley, 2000: p. 146). Cognitive psychotherapies are likely to engage the dorsal prefrontal system, which is involved in the use of reason, logic and foresight, to influence affect regulation. Relationship-based therapies (including individual and group psychodynamic therapies), which are based on emotional experiences, are likely to be processed in the ventral prefrontal cortices. This is consistent with evidence that mild to moderate degrees of personality disorder can be treated using a combination of psychotherapies (Bateman & Tyrer, 2004).

An affect-regulation model of personality disorder also helps to explain the use of polypharmacy to treat it. This includes all classes of psychotropic drugs, which are often used on a trial and error basis (Tyrer & Bateman, 2004). It has been proposed that, although most psychotropics have some specificity for psychiatric disorders, most have a generic affect-regulating (anxiety-regulating) function. Antipsychotic medications are most effective for the most intense and disorganising anxiety (psychotic reactions), whereas antidepressants and sedatives have an anxiolytic effect in the less disorganising types (LeDoux, 1996). This may explain the efficacy of mood-stabilising agents in the management of personality disorders. Given the prevalence of substance misuse in personality disorder, it is hardly surprising that any prescribed drugs that reduce arousal or regulate affect will be as effective (or ineffective) as illicit drugs; nor is it surprising that people with personality disorders may misuse prescribed drugs.

Affect regulation is also relevant in group processes such as therapeutic communities, which are clearly effective for mild to moderate personality disorder (Lees & Manning, 1999). Community members report feeling more confident in dealing with their own (insight) and others' negative feelings (empathy), especially hostility and rage. The therapeutic benefit of such communities for people with personality disorders may arise from the secure attachment to the community that they can make, which allows them to develop a greater capacity to manage negative affect internally.

Management of adolescent personality disorder

Affect regulation forms an integral part of the management of adolescent personality disorder. The three essential components of such an approach are:

(a) enhancing the carer's capacity to provide better quality socioemotional interactions with the young person
(b) the young person's acquisition and use of skills to regulate their emotions
(c) for the young person to use what is learnt in (a) and (b) to improve their relationships with others.

These general principles are reflected in the systemic approaches used to work with young people. An especially significant difference from adult services is the need to work with the young person's school/college, family members and the social network.

The National Institute for Health and Care Excellence (NICE) guidelines for borderline personality disorder note that there has been only one published randomised controlled trial of interventions for adolescents with the disorder – perhaps because clinicians are reluctant to diagnose personality disorders in young people (National Institute for Health and Clinical Excellence, 2009). Similarly, there is no mention of any evidence relating to the treatment of comorbid personality disorders in young people with depression or eating disorders, even though these are common comorbidities in adulthood. Such a lack of evidence makes treatment complex, especially since the transition between adolescence and adulthood may be a critical period for intervention in the adolescent-onset group.

Treatments for emotional disorder

Dialectical behaviour therapy

Dialectical behaviour therapy (DBT) has been adapted for a wide range of clinical settings and groups, including adolescents (Adshead et al, 2012). There is preliminary evidence to support an adapted version of DBT for adolescents who meet criteria for borderline personality disorder (Rathus & Miller, 2002). Adolescent DBT differs from adult DBT in that it is designed to be delivered over fewer sessions (24 sessions over 12 weeks), includes parents in the treatment, places a greater emphasis on the family, and focuses on teaching a smaller number of skills. Teaching these skills to other family members can enable them to act as coaches so that skills can be generalised in the young person's everyday environment.

Rathus & Miller (2002) found that adolescents engaging in DBT had fewer hospital admissions, higher rates of treatment completion, reduction in suicidal ideation and fewer symptoms of borderline personality disorder than those who received treatment as usual. An adolescent in-patient unit that used DBT recorded a significant reduction in behavioural incidents compared with a unit run on psychodynamically oriented principles (Katz et al, 2004). James et al (2011) offered DBT to a group of adolescents in local authority care. They found a significant reduction in self-reported depression scores (Beck Depression Inventory), hopelessness (Beck Hopelessness Scale) and episodes of self-harm. Dialectical behaviour therapy has also been shown to have some positive effects in female juvenile rehabilitation centres (Trupin et al, 2002). This study highlighted both the impact of DBT on the young people and changes in the staff's reactions to them. Staff who had completed in-depth training in DBT showed a reduction in the use of punitive responses.

STEPPS

Systems Training for Emotional Predictability and Problem Solving (STEPPS; Blum et al 2009) is an emotion regulation therapy (ERT) developed for adolescents with symptoms of borderline personality disorder and emotion dysregulation. The effectiveness of an adaptation of STEPPS was examined in a randomised controlled pilot study involving 43 young people (aged 14–19) in five mental health centres in The Netherlands (Schuppert et al, 2009). Participants were randomly assigned to ERT plus treatment as usual or to treatment as usual alone. Both groups showed equal reductions in symptoms of borderline personality disorder over time. The group receiving ERT reported more sense of control over their mood swings and attributed mood swings not only to external factors.

Multisystemic therapy

Multisystemic therapy is a package of interventions for young people at risk of antisocial behaviour. A number of treatment trials have shown it to be effective with selected groups of young people and their families. Families have reported increased family cohesion, and young people have fewer arrests and self-reported offences (Adshead *et al*, 2012).

Although psychological interventions can improve problem behaviour, it is not yet clear whether they effect change in underlying personality structures. Given the role of insecure attachment in the development of disordered personalities, it seems important to provide a secure base for therapy and to promote young people's curiosity and learning of new cognitions and appraisals of both themselves and others (Adshead *et al*, 2012).

Conclusion

Affect regulation is only one aspect of personality disorder, but it is arguably the most critical. Given its developmental origins, it is a key foundation on which other aspects of personality – thoughts, perceptions and behaviour – are built.

This chapter is purposely limited in scope and does not discuss neuroendocrine regulation or the involvement and interaction of various neurotransmitters and neuromodulators. Neither does it deal with the problem of comorbid mental illness and the fact that personality disorders rarely occur singly. Finally, the chapter has not covered all subtypes of personality disorder, especially psychopathy and schizotypy. We suggest that there are fundamental differences in the brain mechanisms underlying these two subtypes, which may be the result of altered patterns of neural connectivity and responses that are largely genetically based rather than a product of gene–environment interaction.

Our key conclusion is that a personality disorder is like many other complex medical conditions. It has degrees of severity and can manifest with varying levels of behavioural dysfunction and symptomatic distress. Mild degrees of personality disorder are probably compatible with reasonable mental health and functioning; more severe disorder or comorbid psychiatric conditions will cause more dysfunction and result in referral to mental health services. Given the continuity of morbidity from childhood to adulthood, it would seem sensible that services for emerging personality disorder are developed, and a workforce trained to meet the needs of people with personality disorders.

References

Adolphs R, Damasio H, Tranel D, *et al* (2000) A role for somatosensory cortices in the visual recognition of emotion as revealed by three-dimensional lesion mapping. *Journal of Neuroscience*, **20**, 2683–2690.

Adshead G, Brodrick P, Preston J, *et al* (2012) Personality disorder in adolescence. *Advances in Psychiatric Treatment*, **18**, 109–118.

American Psychiatric Association (2013) *Diagnostic and Statistical Manual of Mental Disorders (5th edn) (DSM-5)*. APA.

Andrews G, Corry J, Slade T, *et al* (2003) Child sexual abuse. In *Comparative Quantification of Health Risks: Global and Regional Burden of Disease Attributable to Selected Major Risk Factors* (eds M Ezzati, AD Lopez, A Rodgers, *et al*), pp. 1851–1940. World Health Organization.

Bartels A, Zeki S. (2000) The neural basis of romantic love. *NeuroReport*, **11**, 3829–3834.

Bateman AW, Tyrer P (2004) Psychological treatment for personality disorders. *Advances in Psychiatric Treatment*, **10**, 378–388.

Blair RJR (2001) Neurocognitive models of aggression, the antisocial personality disorders, and psychopathy. *Journal of Neurology, Neurosurgery and Psychiatry*, **71**, 727–731.

Blum N S, Bartels NE, St John D, *et al* (2009) *Systems Training for Emotional Predictability and Problem Solving (STEPPS-UK version) (CD-ROM)*. Level One Publishing.

Bradley SJ (2000) *Affect Regulation and the Development of Psychopathology*. Guilford Press.

Caspi A, McClay J, Moffitt T, *et al* (2002) The role of the genotype in the cycle of violence in maltreated children. *Science*, **297**, 851–854.

Damasio AR (1994) *Descartes' Error: Emotion, Reason and the Human Brain*. Penguin Putnam.

Damasio AR (2003) *Looking for Spinoza: Joy, Sorrow and the Feeling Brain*. Heinemann.

Devinsky O (2000) Right cerebral hemisphere dominance for a sense of corporeal and emotional self. *Epilepsy and Behaviour*, **1**, 60–73.

Feldman R, Greenbaum CW, Yirmiya N (1999) Mother–infant affect synchrony as an antecedent of the emergence of self-control. *Developmental Psychology*, **35**, 223–231.

Fonagy P, Target M, Steele M, *et al* (1997) Morality, disruptive behavior, borderline personality disorder, crime, and their relationship to security of attachment. In *Attachment and Psychopathology* (eds L Atkinson, KJ Zucker), pp. 233–274. Guilford Press.

Fonagy P, Gergely G, Jurist EL, *et al* (2002) *Affect Regulation, Mentalisation and the Development of the Self*. Other Press.

Freeman WJ (1999) *How Brains Make up Their Minds*. Orion Books.

George C, Solomon J (1996) Representational models of attachment: links between caregiving and attachment. *Infant Mental Health Journal*, **17**, 198–216.

Grafman J, Schwab K, Warden D, *et al* (1996) Frontal lobe injuries, violence, and aggression: A report of the Vietnam head injury study. *Neurology*, **46**, 1231–1238.

Hare RD, Hart SD, Harpur TJ (1991) Psychopathy and the DSM–IV criteria for antisocial personality disorder. *Journal of Abnormal Psychology*, **100**, 391–398.

Henry JP, Wang S (1998) Effects of early stress on adult affiliative behaviour. *Psychoneuroendocrinology*, **23**, 863–875.

James A, Winmill L, Anderson C, *et al* (2011) A preliminary study of an extension of a community dialectic behaviour therapy (DBT) programme to adolescents in the looked after care system. *Child and Adolescent Mental Health*, **16**, 9–13.

Johnson JG, Cohen P, Brown J, *et al* (1999) Childhood maltreatment increases risk of personality disorder during early adulthood. *Archives of General Psychiatry*, **56**, 600–606.

Katz L, Cox B, Gunasekara S, *et al* (2004) Feasibility of DBT for suicidal adolescent inpatients. *Journal of the American Academy of Child and Adolescent Psychiatry*, **43**, 276–282.

Kim J, Cicchetti D, Rogosch F, *et al* (2009) Child maltreatment and trajectories of personality and behaviour functioning: implications for development of personality disorder. *Development and Psychopathology*, **21**, 889–912.

LeDoux J (1996) *The Emotional Brain: The Mysterious Underpinnings of Emotional Life*. Simon & Shuster.

Lees J, Manning N (1999) *Therapeutic Community Effectiveness: A Systematic International Review of Therapeutic Communities for People with Personality Disorder and Mentally Disordered Offenders* (CRD Report 17). NHS Centre for Research and Dissemination, University of York.

Levine D, Marziali E, Hood J (1997) Emotion processing in borderline personality disorders. *Journal of Nervous and Mental Disease*, **185**, 240–246.

Livesley WJ, Jang KL, Jackson DN, *et al* (1993) Genetic and environmental contributions to dimensions of personality disorder. *American Journal of Psychiatry*, **150**, 1826–1831.

National Institute for Health and Clinical Excellence (2009) *Borderline Personality Disorder: Treatment and Management (NICE Clinical Guideline 78)*. NICE.

Olney, J, Farber, N. B, Wozniak, D. F, *et al* (2000) Environmental agents that have the potential to trigger massive apopototic neurodegeneration in the developing brain. *Environmental Health Perspective*, **108** (suppl. 3), 383–388.

Panksepp J (1998) *Affective Neuroscience*. Oxford University Press.

Patrick M, Hobson RP, Castle P, *et al* (1994) Personality disorder and the mental representation of early social experience. *Developmental Psychopathology*, **94**, 375–388.

Phillips ML, Drevets WC, Rauch SL, *et al* (2003) Neurobiology of emotion perception. I: The neural basis of normal emotion perception. *Biological Psychiatry*, **54**, 504–514.

Rathus JH, Miller AL (2002) Dialectical behaviour therapy adapted for suicidal adolescents. *Suicide and Life-Threatening Behavior*, **32**, 146–157.

Rolls ET (2000) Précis of brain and emotion. *Behavioral and Brain Sciences*, **23**, 177–234.

Schore AN (2002) Dysregulation of the right brain: a fundamental mechanism of traumatic attachment and the psychopathogenesis of posttraumatic stress disorder. *Australian and New Zealand Journal of Psychiatry*, **36**, 9–30.

Schore AN (2003) The human unconscious: the development of the right brain and its role in early emotional life. In *Emotional Development in Psychoanalysis, Attachment Theory and Neuroscience: Creating Connections* (ed V Green), pp. 23–54. Brunner–Routledge.

Schuppert HM, Giesen-Boo J, van Gemert TG, *et al* (2009) Effectiveness of an emotion regulation group training for adolescents: a randomised controlled pilot study. *Clinical Psychology and Psychotherapy*, **16**, 467–47.

Suomi S (1999) Attachment in rhesus monkeys. In *Handbook of Attachment* (eds J Cassidy, P Shaver), pp. 181–197. Guilford Press.

Suomi SJ (2003) Gene–environment interactions and the neurobiology of social conflict. *Annals of the New York Academy of Sciences*, **1008**, 132–139.

Thompson RA (1990) Emotion and self-regulation. In *Nebraska Symposium on Motivation, 1990. Vol. 38: Perspectives on Motivation* (ed. R. A. Dienstbier), p. 371. University of Nebraska Press.

Trupin E, Stewart DE, Beach B, *et al* (2002) Effectiveness of a dialectical behaviour therapy program for incarcerated female juvenile offenders. *Child and Adolescent Mental Health*, **7**, 121–127.

Tyrer P, Bateman AW (2004) Drug treatment for personality disorders. *Advances in Psychiatric Treatment*, **10**, 389–398.

van der Kolk BA, Fisler R (1994) Child abuse and neglect and loss of self-regulation. *Bulletin of the Menninger Clinic*, **58**, 145–168.

Wang S (1997) Traumatic stress and attachment. *Acta Physiologica Scandinavica*, **161** (suppl. 640), 164–169.

Watts D, Morgan G (1994) Malignant alienation: dangers for patients who are hard to like. *British Journal of Psychiatry*, **164**, 11–15.

World Health Organization (1992) *The ICD-10 Classification of Mental and Behavioural Disorders: Clinical Descriptions and Diagnostic Guidelines*. WHO.

CHAPTER 4

Post-traumatic stress disorder and attachment: possible links with borderline personality disorder

Felicity de Zulueta

This chapter principally concerns the relationship between trauma, attachment and the emergence of personality disorder. Clearly, whether or not young people should be given a diagnosis of personality disorder is an area of controversy. As explained by Sarkar & Adshead in Chapter 3, personality disorders can be viewed as developmental conditions that begin in childhood and adolescence. Some clinicians prefer to use diagnoses that emphasise trauma rather than challenging behaviours, and in this chapter I will use the term complex post-traumatic stress disorder (complex PTSD) instead of the possible alternative of emerging borderline personality disorder.

Owing to the reluctance of clinicians to diagnose personality disorders in young people, there is little established research evidence on effective treatments for that age group. Consequently, much of this chapter relates to adults. However, it gives an understanding of how abuse in childhood can lead to this complex condition, and it may be of relevance to older adolescents and indeed to the parents (especially mothers) of children presenting to child and adolescent mental health services.

In both ICD-10 (World Health Organization, 1992) and DSM-5 (American Psychiatric Association, 2013), the diagnostic criteria for PTSD require that the individual has been exposed to 'a stressful event or situation of exceptionally threatening or catastrophic nature' (according to ICD-10) which may elicit 'fear-based re-experiencing, emotional, and behavioural symptoms' (according to DSM-5). Research shows that the events resulting in most diagnoses of PTSD are actually quite common and that none of these traumas is so powerful that exposure typically leads to PTSD (Kessler *et al*, 1999: p. 55). The disorder is more frequent and severe in victims of man-made rather than natural disasters because of the meaning that can be attributed to the former (Lifton & Olson, 1976: pp. 10–14), and is less likely to occur in well-integrated communities than in fragmented ones (Quarantelli, 1985: p. 192). These findings tie in with the main conclusion of treatment guidelines published by the National Institute for Health and Care Excellence (NICE), which singles out the lack of social support as the most important risk factor for PTSD (National Collaborating Centre for Mental Health, 2005: p. 94).

Social support is a vague term, but there is little doubt that it includes the attachments that individuals develop with each other, in both family and community life. It is through the study of attachment research that we can begin to make sense of findings that show strong links between the pathophysiology of PTSD and that of attachment disorders (Van der Kolk, 1996; Henry, 1997; Wang, 1997; Schore, 2001).

An understanding of the development of attachment and its disorders is therefore helpful to our understanding of PTSD, and particularly of complex PTSD (Herman, 1992*a,b*). Attachment research can also guide the development of therapeutic approaches for complex PTSD (de Zulueta, 2006*a,b*), an important area that is not addressed by the NICE guidelines (National Collaborating Centre for Mental Health, 2005).

DSM-5 expands on the criteria for PTSD by including dissociative reactions, negative alteration of cognitions and mood, and insecure relationships with others. In addition to the key diagnostic symptoms, DSM-5 acknowledges that 'the disorder may be especially severe or long-lasting when the stressor is interpersonal and intentional (eg. torture, sexual violence)'. This combination (Box 4.1) has been variously referred to as complex PTSD (Herman, 1992*a*) and 'disorders of extreme stress not otherwise specified' (Pelcovitz *et al*, 1997). The list closely resembles the symptoms of DSM-5 borderline personality disorder except for the last item, referred to as 'a change from previous personality characteristics', which is probably best covered by the ICD-10 diagnosis of 'enduring personality change'.

Box 4.1 Associated symptoms of post-traumatic stress disorder

- Impaired affect modulation, self-destructive and impulsive behaviour
- Dissociative symptoms
- Somatic complaints
- Feelings of ineffectiveness, shame, despair, hopelessness, guilt; feeling permanently damaged; loss of previously sustained beliefs
- Hostility, social withdrawal, feeling constantly threatened, impaired relationships with others
- Change from previous personality characteristics

(Van der Kolk, 2005)

Table 4.1 Diagnostic features of complex post-traumatic stress disorder (PTSD) compared with DSM-5 borderline personality disorder

Complex PTSD	Borderline personality disorder[a]
Impaired affect modulation	Impulsivity in at least two potentially self-damaging areas; recurrent suicidal or self-damaging behaviour; affective instability; inappropriate, intense anger or difficulty in controlling anger
Dissociative symptoms	Transient, stress-related paranoid ideation or severe dissociation; identity disturbance such as a markedly and persistently unstable self-image of sense of self; chronic feeling of emptiness
Impaired, insecure relationships with others	Frantic efforts to avoid real or imagined abandonment; a pattern of unstable and intense interpersonal relationships

a. American Psychiatric Association, 2013.

Complex PTSD and borderline personality disorder

The distinction between the diagnosis of complex PTSD and that of borderline personality disorder (Table 4.1) remains controversial. Both can be seen to result from damage to the attachment system (Fonagy & Target, 1997; de Zulueta, 2006*b*). However, borderline personality disorder is often thought of as a stigmatising diagnosis that elicits a negative response from healthcare workers.

There is some debate about renaming borderline personality disorder. One suggestion is that it should be called an 'emotional regulation disorder'. This term is favoured by Linehan, the creator of dialectical behaviour therapy, a useful approach in treating the symptoms of some of these patients (Koerner & Linehan, 2000).

The development of attachment behaviour and PTSD

Like all mammals, human infants are genetically predisposed to seek contact with an attachment figure, usually their caregiver, a behaviour that is essentially triggered by fear. The same fear and sense of helplessness are inherent to the experience of psychological trauma. Bowlby describes it as follows:

> 'Man, like other animals, responds with fear to certain situations, not because they carry a *high* of pain and danger, but because they signal an *increase* of risk. Thus, just as animals of many species, including man, are disposed to respond with fear to sudden movement or a marked change in level of sound or light because to do so has survival value, so are many species, including man, disposed to respond to separation from a potentially caregiving figure and for the same reasons' (Bowlby, 1988: p. 30. Italics as in original).

Attachment behaviour involves the limbic and paralimbic areas of the right hemisphere and the supraorbital area of the brain. With deep connections to the autonomic system, the supraorbital area is critical to the modulation of emotional and social behaviour, the affect-regulating functions involved in attachment behaviour (Schore, 2001).

It is through the process of attunement that takes place between infant and caregiver that infants become able to modulate their emotions. The different types of attachment behaviour that develop between infants and their various caregivers were originally identified by Ainsworth and her team (Ainsworth et al, 1978). Using the 'strange situation', a structured separation test carried out on 1-year-old infants, they described three types of attachment: secure; insecure avoidant; and insecure anxious – ambivalent or resistant.

Secure attachment

From their interactions with their caregivers, infants are thought to develop a mental representation or, as Bowlby defined it, a 'working model' (1988: pp. 129–133) of how the caregiver is likely to respond in times of trouble. The secure child has a mental representation of the caregiver as responsive at such times. This type of attachment becomes a primary defence against trauma-induced psychopathology (Schore, 2001). In addition, if the caregiver or another important attachment figure in the child's life is able to give meaning to the child's experiences and share and predict their behaviour, the child can internalise this capacity. Such a developmental acquisition, described by Fonagy & Target (1997) as 'reflective functioning' or 'mentalisation', enables people to understand the mental states of others and thereby foster successful social interactions. Its development in a child provides them with further protection against future re-traumatisation.

The development of the child's representation of self is closely inter-twined with their internal representation of their attachment figures. Hence, securely attached children will tend to feel loved and valuable and feel confident and capable of forming good attachments.

Insecure attachment

Insecure attachments develop when infants do not have a mental representation of a responsive caregiver in times of need: they develop various strategies to gain access to their caregiver in order to survive (Ainsworth et al, 1978). The most insecurely attached are infants with a disorganised/disoriented attachment due to their caregivers' abusive or neglectful behaviour (Main & Hesse, 1992). They show an unpredictable response to their caregiver in the strange situation and are seen to freeze in a state of fear without solution. In some cases, the infant can trigger PTSD in the caregiver (Main & Hesse, 1992).

Vignette 1

A Kurdish woman from Turkey with a diagnosis of complex PTSD presented with her small son, who had been referred to social services for failure to thrive. The mother had been severely beaten by the child's father and, unfortunately for this little boy, when he became distressed, his eyes resembled his father's. This triggered in his mother a reliving of her past experience of domestic violence, with all the anger and fear that this involved. Thus, the mother not only induced traumatic states in her child, but she was also unable to comfort him because, owing to her PTSD, she had lost the capacity to empathise with him.

The result of such a situation is very damaging, both to the child's future capacity to regulate emotions and because it can lead to the development of early structural dissociation. This process involves three stages in the infant's psychobiological response to feeling threatened by their caregiver (Perry *et al*, 1995).

The first is the fight-or-flight response, mediated by the sympathetic nervous system. This bypasses the cortical centres and their capacity for symbolic processing, with the result that traumatic experiences are stored in somatic, behavioural and affective systems.

If the fight-or-flight response is not possible, as is usually the case with a very small child, the parasympathetic state takes over and the child 'freezes', which in nature fosters survival. Vocalisation is inhibited and the child, like a young animal, loses the capacity to speak. This trauma-induced mutism is due to the release of endogenous opiates and the shutting down of Broca's speech area (as observed in positron emission tomography scans of adults with PTSD) (Rauch *et al*, 1996).

If the caregiver's threat or rejection continues, the infant enters a state of 'fear without solution', in which both responses are activated, leading to an inward flight or dissociative response (Main & Hesse, 1992): sexually abused girls often describe themselves as being on the ceiling looking down at their abuser doing things to them. Although in fear of their caregiver, these children must maintain their vital attachment to them. This can only be achieved by resorting to dissociation, i.e. 'forgetting' their traumatic interaction in order to preserve an idealised attachment to their caregiver. This results in the creation of different self-states, or representations of themselves in relation to their caregiver, and a lack of self-continuity in relation to the 'other' such as can be seen in people with borderline personality disorder (Fonagy & Target, 1997; Ogawa *et al*, 1997; Ryle, 1997; de Zulueta, 2006c), complex PTSD (Herman, 1992b) and other dissociative disorders.

At a cognitive level, this means that these survivors will tend to feel guilty and blame themselves rather than their caregiver for what happens to them. By taking the blame, being 'bad' and keeping the caregiver as an idealised figure in their mind, they retain a sense of control in the face of otherwise unbearable helplessness. They can also preserve the hope that in the future, if they behave well, they will finally attain the love and care

45

they never had. This cognitive defence, aptly called the 'moral defence' by Fairbairn (1952), is ferociously maintained to avoid the unbearable realisation, and its accompanying grief and anger, that there is no such idealised caregiver.

The cost of maintaining a 'traumatic attachment' to an abusing or neglectful caregiver can be a heavy one. In seeking the parental care they never had, these survivors tend to destroy their intimate relationships and sabotage their achievements and progress in order to continue their search for the idealised parent they still yearn for, albeit unconsciously (de Zulueta, 2006c). Addressing the traumatic attachment and its cognitive distortions may be central to the treatment of patients with a history of childhood abuse or severe neglect (de Zulueta, 2006c).

Henry (1997) noted that many people with complex PTSD arising from childhood abuse and neglect also suffer from alexithymia, finding it difficult to speak about their emotions and thereby to share and cope with disturbing feelings. Consequently, they tend to re-enact their traumatic experience rather than think about it, thus experiencing re-traumatisation (Van der Kolk, 1989). Alexithymia also appears to be associated with an interhemispheric transfer deficit and is more likely to occur if the trauma is repeated, as in sexual abuse (Zeitlin et al, 1993).

The psychobiology of neglect and abuse

Evidence suggests that traumatisation in early life can result in damage to the cortical and subcortical limbic systems of the right hemisphere, leaving the child with a reduced capacity to play, to empathise and to form sustaining relationships (Schore, 2001). Their inability to modulate emotions is central to an understanding of these patients: they cannot deal with sympathetic-dominant affects such as terror, rage and elation, nor can they deal with parasympathetic-dominant affects such as disgust and, in particular, shame.

Shame is an emotion that is often ignored. People who have been neglected or abused in childhood can grow up into adults whose sense of self is extremely fragile. When exposed to further shame or 'disrespect', they may attempt to destroy the 'other' in order to ward off an unbearable sense of total annihilation. As one patient with a history of homicide said to his therapist, 'Better be bad than not be at all' (Gilligan, 1996). Our prisons are full of such individuals.

The inability to modulate emotions often causes survivors of trauma to self-medicate using alcohol or drugs or to resort to immediate violence when feeling out of control or threatened.

The reliving of traumatic experiences can result in release of natural opiates and accompanying analgesia: this effect can fuel acts of re-traumatisation, self-harm or violence as a form of relief from unbearable emotional states.

Understanding PTSD as a 'sensitisation disorder' of the attachment system

Post-traumatic stress disorder is classified in ICD-10 as a stress-related disorder and in DSM-5 as a trauma- and stressor-related disorder. In 1997 Yehuda reported that 'contrary to all initial expectations and hypotheses, the neuroendocrinology of PTSD does not resemble the neuroendocrine alterations observed in stress'. High cortisol levels have traditionally been associated with stress but, among her sample of victims of road traffic accidents, only those who showed a lower than normal release of cortisol developed PTSD. She commented, 'It may be that PTSD reflects a biologic sensitisation following stress due to pre-existing risk factors. If so, perhaps it might be more appropriate to consider the symptoms and neurobiologic changes following trauma as reflecting a posttraumatic *sensitisation* disorder rather than a posttraumatic stress disorder' (Yehuda, 1997: p. 69; italics as in original).

This hypothesis is supported by evidence showing correlations between maltreatment and suppressed cortisol levels in children (Hart *et al*, 1995). Yehuda's view that PTSD is a 'sensitisation disorder' that may be attributed to a priming of the hypothalamic–pituitary axis seems very likely. It could be the result of either trauma-induced damage to the attachment system during early development or repeated or chronic traumatisation in later life (Wang, 1997; Cichetti & Rogosch, 2001). In adults, low urinary cortisol levels have been found in Holocaust survivors with PTSD and in Vietnam veterans. The levels were strongly negatively correlated with degrees of emotional numbing (Yehuda, 1997: pp. 58–62).

There also appears to be evidence of transmission of this sensitisation to PTSD down the generations. Yehuda *et al* (2002) noted low cortisol levels in both Holocaust survivors and their adult offspring, together with an increased risk of PTSD in both parents and offspring. Similarly, the 1-year-old infants of women who developed PTSD after direct exposure to the destruction of New York's World Trade Center when they were pregnant showed reduced cortisol levels, as did the mothers (Yehuda *et al*, 2005). These findings support Yehuda's earlier contention (Yehuda, 1997) that the children of mothers who suffer from PTSD and associated low cortisol levels also have low cortisol levels, which is likely to predispose them to developing PTSD in later life.

The important aspect of the 2005 study by Yehuda *et al* is that transmission of vulnerability to PTSD happened to infants still in the womb when their mothers developed PTSD. This finding ties in with research in the field of epigenetics by Meaney & Szyf (2005), which has shown that maternal behaviour can affect the stress responses of offspring via modulation of DNA methylation of critical genes. Thus, PTSD in a pregnant woman can alter the cortisol levels of her infant (Yehuda *et al*, 2005).

The evidence of transmission of low cortisol levels and its significance in terms of predisposing individuals to PTSD highlights the role of the transgenerational transmission of vulnerability to PTSD. It further confirms Schore's (2001) view that a secure attachment is a primary defence against trauma-induced psychopathology. This possibility is even more likely if we take into account Van Ijzendoorn & Bakermans-Kranenberg's (1997) review of the research in the field of attachment, which shows a 75% correspondence between a mother's attachment and that of her offspring. These findings have to be taken into account when analysing possible genetic transmission of PTSD.

The conceptual basis of the treatment of complex PTSD

In guidance that covers adults and children, NICE recommends trauma-focused cognitive–behavioural therapy (CBT) or eye movement desensitisation and reprocessing (EMDR) as the first-line treatments for simple PTSD (National Collaborating Centre for Mental Health, 2005). For older children and young people specifically, it stipulates that trauma-focused CBT should be offered to those with severe post-traumatic symptoms or with severe PTSD in the first month after the traumatic event; and that children and young people with PTSD, including those who have been sexually abused, should be offered trauma-focused CBT adapted to suit their age, circumstances and level of development. There is also a research recommendation to assess absolute and relative efficacy and cost-effectiveness of EMDR and trauma-focused CBT in children. Drug treatments should not be routinely prescribed for children and young people with PTSD.

There are currently no national guidelines regarding the treatment of complex (or 'developmental') PTSD. This is in part due to the confusion surrounding its diagnosis and the lack of randomised controlled therapeutic trials in this field. In adults, an evidence-based guide that reviews the research on the treatment of complex PTSD provides useful guidelines for the treatment of these disorders (Courtois & Ford, 2009). The same authors have recently published a text describing the differing therapeutic strategies available for children (Courtois & Ford, 2013).

There are also an increasing number of outcome studies reporting on different therapeutic modalities for the treatment of borderline personality disorder (Bateman & Fonagy, 2001; Beecham et al, 2006), which, as discussed above, is very similar to complex PTSD. Both Bateman and Fonagy use an attachment-based model in their therapeutic work. It therefore makes sense to extend attachment theory and research to the treatment of people with complex PTSD, many of whom have borderline personality traits or borderline personality disorder with PTSD symptoms. The latter are often not given the appropriate treatment in specialist treatment centres for borderline personality disorder because of the failure to acknowledge the importance of emotional dysregulation and dissociation.

Such an integrative, attachment-based approach to the treatment of people with complex PTSD allows for the inclusion of psychoanalytically derived treatments such as cognitive analytic therapy (CAT) (Ryle, 1997) and affect-focused therapies such as dialectical behaviour therapy (Koerner & Linehan, 2000), as well as new therapeutic modalities mentioned in the section 'Treatment of complex PTSD' below. In this volume (Chapter 3), Sarkar and Adshead have reviewed the use of dialectical behaviour therapy, Systems Training for Emotional Predictability and Problem Solving (STEPPS) and multisystemic therapy for adolescents with personality disorder. The use of EMDR is worthy of mention in this context too, as it is included in treatment guidelines for many countries, including the UK, Holland and Australia. A strong evidence base supports EMDR for the treatment of PTSD (Foa *et al*, 2009), and a meta-analysis by Bisson & Andrew (2007) revealed no statistically significant difference in efficacy between EMDR and trauma-focused CBT.

Eye movement desensitisation and reprocessing

In EMDR, the processing of traumatic memories is achieved by evoking the memory and applying bilateral stimulation in accordance with a clearly outlined protocol (Shapiro, 1995). The stimulation can involve eye movements, sounds or tapping the patient above the knees, depending on the client's preference and with their full consent. Henry (1997) pointed out that, since PTSD can produce a functional dissociation of emotional processing across the two hemispheres of the brain, the therapeutic role of EMDR may be that of enabling this processing to be restored across the corpus callosum – a region that can be reduced in volume in survivors of child abuse, for instance (McCrory *et al*, 2010).

It is not necessary for the patient to give a detailed account of their traumatic experiences during EMDR: they only have to give the therapist a rough idea of what they are processing.

It is the bilateral stimulation in EMDR that essentially distinguishes it from trauma-focused CBT (Ehlers & Clark, 2000) and may also be why it is so effective in the treatment of somatic symptoms. Such symptoms often predominate in the presentation of patients with complex PTSD from the Middle East, Africa and the Far East (Al Krenawi, 2005). The additional fact that these individuals often do not speak much English and that they feel so much shame in relation to their experiences of rape and torture makes the use of EMDR a very useful tool in their therapy.

It is very important to follow Shapiro's protocol when using EMDR for complex PTSD in patients with high levels of dissociation on the Dissociative Experiences Scale (Bernstein & Putnam, 1986). In such cases in particular, this powerful approach can cause the patient to feel overwhelmed by horrific traumatic and fragmented memories that they cannot process.

Assessment of adult patients with complex PTSD

The assessment of adult patients with complex PTSD can extend to two or even three sessions. The primary purpose of the assessment is threefold:

- to establish whether the patient has the resources, both internal and external, to be treated for their PTSD symptoms
- to establish whether it is safe to proceed with therapy without risk of re-traumatising the patient
- to determine how complex the treatment is likely to be, bearing in mind the attachment history and current levels of support.

Substance and alcohol addiction are contraindicated and the patient should be referred to addiction services before any PTSD treatment can be contemplated.

Self-destructive behaviour and suicide risk tend to increase in the early phase of treatment. It is therefore important to assess these and put in place support systems if necessary, involving community mental health teams or general practitioners. Risk assessment should take into account the patient's potential for violence to self and others and their levels of dissociation in relation to their behaviour towards other members of the family. Usually, such information can be obtained only by meeting with the partner or another close relation or friend, who can also provide essential information about changes in the patient's behaviour and personality over time. A family meeting is often useful to further establish levels of risk and need in the family, as well as giving them an opportunity to understand what complex PTSD is all about using an attachment model. This usually reduces the patient's fear of being seen as 'mad' and empowers both patient and family in working with the therapeutic process.

If the patient is from a minority ethnic group, cultural issues must be addressed. The first is to use an appropriate interpreter if the patient does not speak English – it is not appropriate to use a member of the family. Some, however, choose to speak English despite obvious difficulties. This may be to protect them from distressing associations and memories linked to early life (de Zulueta, 1995) or because they do not trust the interpreter for political reasons or because of their feelings of shame, a particular problem if the interpreter is from the same community.

Specific cultural differences often need to be addressed. For example, in certain Middle Eastern and African communities a woman who has been raped becomes a social outcast. This means that the rape cannot be acknowledged, sometimes even by her husband, because of the fear of rejection or 'honour killing'. Working with the terrible shame these women feel requires a very sensitive approach if the patient is to remain in treatment. Similarly, young men and women from most non-Western cultures often have to show far more respect in relation to their parents than is usual in a White British community.

In the case of mothers whose children are the victims of rape, a careful assessment may be particularly important.

Vignette 2

> A refugee was referred to us for the treatment of PTSD following her rape during a civil war in her country. She had become pregnant as a result of this abuse and, after arrival in the UK, had given birth to a male infant. She disclosed that sometimes the eyes of her baby triggered in her terrifyingly vivid memories of her past abuser, such that she would find herself identifying her infant with the man who had repeatedly raped her in captivity. As a result she feared she might do harm to the baby in one of her dissociative states. Her fear was well founded and had to be addressed by providing her with extra psychiatric and child care support before any trauma-focused therapy could take place.

Treatment of complex PTSD

Treatment must be carried out from what Bowlby (1988) called a 'secure base' (further discussed below). This can lead to increasing violence or even homicide. In cases of child abuse, victims who are still living with their family, be it with either the abuser or the caregiver who allowed the abuse to happen, may need to move out of the family home before engaging in therapy addressing their traumatic experiences, and the family should be seen for a family assessment and therapy. Unfortunately, clinical experience is often that hard-pressed social services ignore the need to protect the child, justifying abuse and neglect as culturally appropriate.

The need for phase-oriented treatment

The conceptual infrastructure underpinning the therapeutic work in the Traumatic Stress Service at London's Maudsley Hospital follows the guidelines set up in the USA by Herman (1992*b*) and Bloom (1997). It is based on an attachment model within a systemic framework in which PTSD symptoms are understood as the psychobiological manifestation of a disrupted attachment system requiring an approach that addresses both the internal world of the individual and their social attachment network (de Zulueta, 2006*b*).

Once the patient has been assessed by a team member, the findings are discussed in a team meeting and the treatment best suited to the patient's individual and social needs is decided. Therapists offer a range of therapeutic orientations, including psychodynamic, systemic and attachment-based psychotherapy, CBT and EMDR. Within these different individual approaches, however, narrative exposure therapy (Schauer *et al*, 2005), CBT techniques (Ehlers & Clark, 2000) and particularly EMDR (Shapiro, 1995) are often used to process the traumatic memories at the appropriate stage in treatment.

Phase 1: Stabilisation

The focus here is on providing safety – a secure base – and helping the patient achieve some degree of affect modulation to enable them to cope with the traumatic work that will follow without dissociating or being re-traumatised. With severely traumatised or unstable patients, this can take a relatively long time. It is achieved through psychoeducation, the establishment of a cohesive support network and techniques focusing on affect modulation. The last is provided not only by the use of the 'safe place' in EMDR, but by a host of new therapeutic modalities. These include mindfulness and meditation techniques that use vagus innervation to the supraorbital area of the brain, and more somatically oriented approaches for the treatment of PTSD such as sensorimotor therapy (Ogden & Pain, 2006).

With asylum seekers, it is often important to attend to housing and immigration problems first. Medication can play an important role in treating concomitant severe depression, and overwhelmingly high levels of arousal and flashbacks can be reduced by prescribing very low levels of an antipsychotic medication such as olanzapine, as outlined in the NICE guidelines (National Collaborating Centre for Mental Health, 2005).

Phase 2: Remembering, processing and grieving

Avoidance and fear of the traumatic memory are central to post-traumatic psychopathology. Therefore a paced and modulated approach to this material is essential.

Techniques from CBT and EMDR can be used to process traumatic memories, often in combination with another therapeutic approach such as narrative exposure therapy (Schauer *et al*, 2005), which is particularly effective with refugees.

In many patients suffering from complex PTSD, often with borderline personality traits if not a diagnosis of borderline personality disorder, resolution of their intense traumatic attachments to their internal abusive or neglectful caregiver usually needs to be addressed during this phase. This allows the patient to let go of their still infantile need for their parent and the resulting sabotage of their therapeutic gains (de Zulueta, 2006c). Some patients may not feel ready to go through this stage of grieving and loss, which is equivalent to the Kleinian depressive position; they should not be forced to do so because of the risk of re-traumatisation.

Phase 3: Personality integration and rehabilitation

Personality integration and rehabilitation can be ongoing throughout the therapy. However, it becomes increasingly important towards the end of treatment, when patients begin to reconnect with life in the 'here and now' and are encouraged to engage in gratifying activities such as sports, dance, art or other right-hemisphere based activities, as well as their life in their community. They examine with their therapist the changes they have made and, by reconnecting with others, facilitate the process of ending the

---

Box 4.2 Yalom's therapeutic factors

- Instillation of hope
- Universality
- Imparting information
- Altruism
- The corrective recapitulation of the primary family group
- Development of socialising techniques
- Imitative behaviour
- Interpersonal learning
- Group cohesiveness
- Catharsis
- Existential factors

(Yalom, 1995)

---

therapy. Termination of therapy is often painful, as it does bring back the feelings of separation and loss related to their past, but for this reason it is extremely important.

Group therapy

By its very nature group therapy is, as Yalom (1995) has outlined in his 11 curative factors (Box 4.2), an excellent treatment mode for adults with PTSD: the possibility of sharing and helping others to make sense of what has happened to them while working together towards recovery and rehabilitation gives patients hope and dispels their overriding sense of loneliness. In the early phase of stabilisation, the group model can be used to teach and practise general psychoeducation techniques. Subsequently, therapy can continue with specific groups of individuals who have suffered a common trauma.

Conclusion

When Lindemann in 1944 defined psychological trauma as 'the sudden cessation of human interaction', he was addressing its essential feature, the sudden disruption of an individual's attachment system and all its manifestations, particularly at the level of attunement – which I believe is the core injury in PTSD. Attachment research provides a comprehensive understanding of the psychobiological symptoms of both simple and complex ('developmental') PTSD (Van der Kolk, 2005) and supports Yehuda's view that PTSD is in fact a sensitisation disorder of the hypothalamic–pituitary axis. It also accounts for the fact that many people with complex PTSD, usually those with an earlier experience of attachment failure, do not respond to CBT or EMDR alone, requiring the other interventions outlined above, focusing particularly on the different manifestations of emotional dysregulation and dissociation.

If we understand PTSD as resulting from the disruption of the attachment system, we can also understand why the lack of social support – more specifically the lack of empathic and attuned relationships – is the most important risk factor for this disorder. This finding makes sense of the fact, for instance, that an asylum seeker with a history of severe political abuse can remain free of symptoms of PTSD while living within his own community in London, only to present with severe symptoms when removed from those to whom he is attached and attuned. It also explains why many people with a history of childhood abuse can remain free of symptoms of complex PTSD until they experience the loss of an important attachment figure in adulthood.

Finally, an attachment perspective may contribute to the resolution of the diagnostic impasse between complex PTSD and borderline personality disorder.

References

Ainsworth MDS, Blehar MC, Waters E, *et al* (1978) *Patterns of Attachment: A Psychological Study of the Strange Situation*. Lawrence Erlbaum.

Al Krenawi A (2005) Mental health practice in Arab countries. *Current Opinion in Psychiatry*, **18**, 560–564.

American Psychiatric Association (2013) *Diagnostic and Statistical Manual of Mental Disorders (5th edn) (DSM-5)*. APA.

Bateman A, Fonagy P (2001) Treatment of borderline personality disorder with psychoanalytically oriented partial hospitalization: an 18-month follow-up. *American Journal of Psychiatry*, **158**, 36–42.

Beecham J, Sleed M, Knapp M, *et al* (2006) The costs and effectiveness of two psychosocial treatment programmes for personality disorder. *European Psychiatry*, **21**, 102–109.

Bernstein EM, Putnam FW (1986) Development, reliability and validity of a dissociation scale. *Journal of Nervous and Mental Disease*, **174**, 727–735.

Bisson J, Andrew M (2007) Psychological treatment of post-traumatic stress disorder (PTSD). *Cochrane Database of Systematic Reviews*, issue 3, CD003388.

Bloom S (1997) *Creating Sanctuary: Toward the Evolution of Sane Societies*. Routledge.

Bowlby J (1988) *A Secure Base: Clinical Applications of Attachment Theory*. Routledge.

Cichetti D, Rogosch FA (2001) Diverse patterns of neuroendocrine activity in maltreated children. *Development and Psychopathology*, **13**, 677–693.

Courtois CA, Ford JD (eds) (2009) *Treating Complex Traumatic Stress Disorders: An Evidence-Based Guide*. Guilford Press.

Ford JD, Courtois CA (eds) (2013) *Treating Complex Traumatic Stress Disorders in Children and Adolescents: Scientific Foundations and Therapeutic Models*. Guilford Press.

de Zulueta F (1995) Bilingualism, culture and identity. *Group Analysis*, **28**, 179–190.

de Zulueta F (2006a) *From Pain to Violence: The Roots of Human Destructiveness*. John Wiley & Sons.

de Zulueta F (2006b) The treatment of PTSD from an attachment perspective. *Journal of Family Therapy*, **28**, 334–351.

de Zulueta F (2006c) Inducing traumatic attachment in adults with a history of childhood abuse: forensic applications. *British Journal of Forensic Practice*, **8** (3), 4–15.

Ehlers A, Clark DM (2000) A cognitive model of post traumatic stress disorder. *Behaviour Research and Therapy*, **38**, 334–351.

Fairbairn WRD (1952) *Psychoanalytic Studies of the Personality*. Routledge & Kegan Paul.

Foa EB, Keane TM, Friedman MJ (2009) *Effective Treatments for PTST: Practice Guidelines of the International Society for Traumatic Stress Studies*. Guilford Press.

Fonagy P, Target M (1997) Attachment and reflective function: their role in self-organization. *Development and Psychopathology*, **9**, 679–700.

Ford JD, Courtois CA (eds) (2013) *Treating Complex Traumatic Stress Disorders in Children and Adolescents: Scientific Foundations and Therapeutic Models*. Guilford Press.

Gilligan J (1996) *Violence: Our Deadly Epidemic and Its Causes*. G. P. Putnam & Sons.

Hart H, Rubia K (2012) Neuroimaging of child abuse: a critical review. *Frontiers in Human Neuroscience*, **6**, 52.

Hart J, Gunnar M, Cicchetti D (1995) Salivary cortisol in maltreated children: evidence of relations between neuroendocrine activity and social competence. *Development and Psychopathology*, **7**, 11–26.

Henry J (1997) Psychological and physiological responses to stress: the right hemisphere and the hypothalamic–pituitary–adrenal axis. An inquiry into problems of human bonding. *Acta Physiologica Scandinavica*, **161**, 164–169.

Herman JL (1992a) Complex PTSD: a syndrome in survivors of prolonged and repeated trauma. *Journal of Traumatic Stress*, **5**, 377–391.

Herman J (1992b) *Trauma and Recovery: The Aftermath of Violence from Domestic Abuse to Political Terror*. Basic Books.

Kessler RC, Sonnega A, Bromet E, et al (1999) Epidemiological risk factors for trauma and PTSD. In *Risk Factors for Posttraumatic Stress Disorder* (ed R Yehuda), pp. 23–59. American Psychiatric Press.

Koerner K, Linehan M (2000) Research and dialectical behaviour therapy for patients with borderline personality disorder. *Psychiatric Clinics of North America*, **23**, 151–167.

Lifton RJ, Olson E (1976) The human meaning of total disaster: The Buffalo Creek experience. *Psychiatry*, **39**, 1–18.

Lindemann E (1944) Symptomatology and management of acute grief. *American Journal of Psychiatry*, **101**, 141–148.

Main M, Hesse E (1992) Disorganized/disoriented infant behavior in the Strange Situation, lapses in the monitoring of reasoning and discourse during the parent's Adult Attachment Interview, and dissociative states. In *Attachment and Psychoanalysis* (eds M Ammaniti, D Stern), pp. 86–140. Gius Laterza e Figli.

McCrory E, De Brito SA, Viding E (2010) Research review: the neurobiology and genetics of maltreatment and adversity. *Journal of Child Psychology and Psychiatry*, **51**, 1079–1095.

Meaney, MJ, Szyf M (2005) Environmental programming of stress responses through DNA methylation: life at the interface between a dynamic environment and a fixed genome. *Dialogues in Clinical Neuroscience*, **7**, 103–123.

National Collaborating Centre for Mental Health (2005) *Post-Traumatic Stress Disorder (PTSD): The Management of PTSD in Adults and Children in Primary and Secondary Care* (Clinical Guideline 26). National Institute for Clinical Excellence.

Ogawa JR, Sroufe LA, Weinfield NS, et al (1997) Development of the fragmented self: longitudinal study of dissociative symptomatology in a nonclinical sample. *Development and Psychopathology*, **9**, 855–879.

Ogden P, Pain C (2006) A sensorimotor approach to the treatment of trauma and dissociation. *Psychiatric Clinics of North America*, **29**, 263–279.

Pelcovitz D, Van der Kolk BA, Roth SH, et al (1997) Development of a criteria set and a Structured Interview for Disorders of Extreme Stress (SIDES). *Journal of Traumatic Stress*, **10**, 3–16.

Perry BD, Pollard RA, Blakeley TL, et al (1995) Childhood trauma, the neurobiology of adaptation, and 'use-dependent' development of the brain: how 'states' become 'traits'. *Infant Mental Health Journal*, **16**, 271–291.

Quarantelli EL (1985) An assessment of conflicting views on mental health: the consequences of traumatic events. In *Trauma and its Wake: Vol. I The Study and Treatment of Post-Traumatic Stress Disorder* (ed CR Figley), pp. 182–220. Brunner/Mazel.

Rauch SL, Van der Kolk BA, Fisler RE, *et al* (1996) A symptom provocation study of post traumatic stress disorder using positron emission tomography and script driven imagery. *Archives of General Psychiatry*, **53**, 380–7.

Ryle A (1997) The structure and development of borderline personality disorder: a proposed model. *British Journal of Psychiatry*, **170**, 82–87.

Schauer M, Neuner F, Elbert T (2005) *Narrative Exposure Therapy: A Short-Term Intervention for Traumatic Stress Disorders after War, Terror, or Torture.* Hogrefe.

Schore AN (2001) The effects of early relational trauma on right brain development, affect regulation, and infant mental health. *Infant Mental Health Journal*, **22**, 201–269.

Shapiro F (1995) *Eye Movement Desensitization and Reprocessing (EMDR): Basic Principles, Protocols, and Procedures.* Guilford Press.

Van der Kolk BA (1989) The compulsion to repeat the trauma: re-enactment, revictimisation and masochism. *Psychiatric Clinics of North America*, **12**, 389–411.

Van der Kolk BA (1996) The body keeps the score: approaches to the psychobiology of post traumatic stress disorder. In *Traumatic Stress: The Effects of Overwhelming Experience on Mind, Body, and Society* (eds BA Van der Kolk, AC McFarlane, L Weisaeth), pp. 214–241. Guilford Press.

Van der Kolk BA (2005) Developmental trauma disorder. *Psychiatric Annals*, **35**, 401–408.

Van Ijzendoorn MH, Bakermans-Kranenberg MJ (1997) Intergenerational transmission of attachment: a move to the contextual level. In *Attachment and Psychopathology* (eds L Atkinson, KJ Zucker), pp. 135–170. Guilford Press.

Wang S (1997) Traumatic stress and attachment. *Acta Physiologica Scandinavica*, **161**, 164–169.

World Health Organization (1992) *The ICD-10 Classification of Mental and Behavioural Disorders: Clinical Descriptions and Diagnostic Guidelines.* WHO.

Yalom I D (1995) *The Theory and Practice of Group Psychotherapy* (4th edn). Basic Books.

Yehuda R (1997) Sensitisation of the hypothalamic–pituitary axis in posttraumatic stress disorder. In *Psychobiology of Posttraumatic Stress Disorder* (eds R Yehuda & AC McFarlane), pp. 57–75. New York Academy of Sciences.

Yehuda R, Halligan SL, Bierer LM (2002) Cortisol levels in adult offspring of Holocaust survivors: relation to PTSD symptom severity in the parent and the child. *Psychoneuroendocrinology*, **27**, 171–180.

Yehuda R, Engel SM, Brand S, *et al* (2005) Transgenerational effects of posttraumatic stress disorder in babies of mothers exposed to the World Trade Center attacks during pregnancy. *Journal of Clinical Endocrinology and Metabolism*, **90**, 4115–4118.

Zeitlin SD, McNally RJ, Cassidy KC (1993) Alexithymia in victims of sexual assault: an effect of repeated traumatisation. *American Journal of Psychiatry*, **150**, 661–663.

CHAPTER 5

Management of antisocial behaviour in childhood

Sajid Humayun and Stephen Scott

Antisocial behaviour is the most common reason for referral to child mental health services (National Institute for Health and Care Excellence, 2013). It is a clinical problem of considerable importance, because there is a marked tendency for it to persist, and the long-term outcome includes antisocial personality disorder and criminality. Longitudinal studies have shown that children with conduct disorder at the age of 7 are ten times more likely to be criminals in adulthood (Fergusson *et al*, 2005). Effective treatments are now available, although not yet widely used in the UK.

We use the term 'antisocial behaviour' to include children who do not necessarily meet the strict definitions of conduct disorder or oppositional defiant disorder, for which DSM-5 (American Psychiatric Association, 2013) and ICD-10 (World Health Organization, 1993) have quite similar diagnostic criteria. For both schemes, the diagnosis of conduct disorder requires a repetitive and persistent pattern of behaviour in which the basic rights of others or major age-appropriate social norms are violated. DSM-5 stresses that the disturbance must cause clinically significant impairment in social, occupational or academic functioning, which is implicit in ICD-10. DSM-5 requires that three of the symptoms/behaviours in Box 5.1 be present during the preceding 12 months and one during the preceding 6 months, whereas ICD-10 merely specifies that three symptoms must be present, but requires one symptom to have been present within the previous month. For oppositional defiant disorder, both DSM-5 and ICD-10 require four symptoms/behaviours from the list in Box 5.2 to have been present for the preceding six months. Although DSM-5 views oppositional defiant disorder as a common precedent to conduct disorder, ICD-10 regards it as a milder form of conduct disorder, and stipulates that no more than two of the symptoms in Box 5.1 should be present.

The one major change from DSM-IV (American Psychiatric Association, 1994) to DSM-5 is the inclusion of a specifier to designate youths 'with limited prosocial emotions' (American Psychiatric Association, 2013). To meet this criterion, individuals must show two or more characteristics of callous-unemotional traits, such as shallow affect, lack of empathy, lack of remorse or guilt, or lack of concern about their performance at school or work during the preceding 12 months.

Box 5.1 Conduct disorder behaviours (amalgamated from ICD-10 and DSM-5)

- Excessive fighting, with frequent initiation of fights
- Deliberate and repeated destruction of others' property
- Often lies to obtain goods or favours or to avoid obligations
- Repeated stealing outside the home without confrontation (e.g. shoplifting)
- Has stolen while confronting a victim (e.g. purse-snatching, mugging)
- Has used a weapon that can cause serious physical harm to others (e.g. a bat, brick, broken bottle, knife or gun)
- Has broken into someone else's house, building or car
- Frequent truancy from school, beginning before 13 years of age
- Often bullies, threatens or intimidates others
- Has run away from home at least twice overnight, or once for more than one night
- Often stays out after dark, despite parental prohibition, beginning before 13 years of age
- Physical cruelty to other people (e.g. ties up, cuts or burns a victim)
- Cruelty to animals
- Deliberate fire-setting, with a risk or intention of causing serious damage
- Forcing another person into sexual activity against their wishes

(World Health Organization, 1993; American Psychiatric Association, 2013)

For the sake of convenience and since antisocial behaviour is more common in boys, we will use the male pronoun. This chapter focuses mainly on children below 12 years of age, as delinquency in adolescence presents a range of separate problems. The chapter is a brief summary of the key issues involved in the management of childhood antisocial behaviour and readers should refer to national guidelines (e.g. National Institute for Health and Care Excellence, 2013) for more detailed information.

Box 5.2 Oppositional defiant behaviours (amalgamated from ICD-10 and DSM-5)

- Temper tantrums that are unusually frequent and severe for the child's developmental level
- Often argues with adults
- Often actively refuses adults' requests or defies rules
- Often deliberately annoys people
- Often blames others for his or her mistakes or behaviour
- Is often touchy or easily annoyed by others
- Is often angry or resentful
- Is often spiteful or vindictive

(World Health Organization, 1993; American Psychiatric Association, 2013)

Aetiology

Figure 4.1 shows the range of risk factors that need to be considered in understanding a child's antisocial behaviour. Predisposing factors include social adversity, parental background and the child's constitution. The most direct causes can be both precipitating and perpetuating: negative cycles of interaction are often self-maintaining, as indicated by the double-headed arrows in the figure. It is well established that parental disciplinary style is important in the development of antisocial behaviour; but the child also contributes to this interaction (Anderson *et al*, 1986). Parents often become disheartened, feeling criticised by neighbours and professionals, and give up trying to find more effective ways of handling their difficult child. The child elicits more and more criticism from adults around him, and it becomes increasingly difficult for him to think of himself as a success. He slips further behind his peers academically and socially, and eventually resorts to a deviant peer group of others with the same problems, who then encourage each other in antisocial acts.

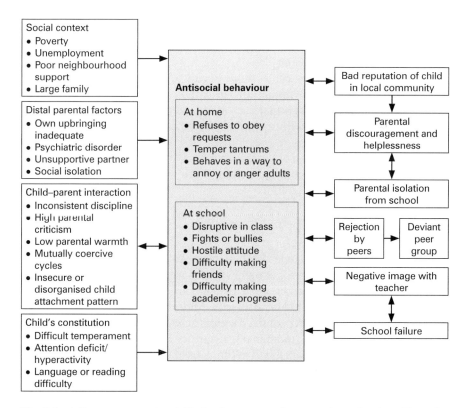

Fig. 5.1 Influences on antisocial behaviour seen at home and at school, and how the consequences may perpetuate it.

Although risk factors are present in multiple domains (for a review see Murray & Farrington, 2010), recent research indicates that there are likely to be three distinct pathways to antisocial behaviour and conduct disorder, each with its own cluster of risk factors (Pardini & Frick, 2013).

First, the timing of onset of antisocial behaviour has been shown to delineate groups of individuals, such that those with early onset (before age 10) appear to constitute a separate group with more severe problems than those whose antisocial behaviour begins in adolescence. Individuals with early-onset antisocial behaviour are more likely to exhibit early hyperactivity and oppositional behaviour (Moffitt, 2006), tend to come from families who use harsh and inconsistent parenting practices (Odgers *et al*, 2008) and are at higher risk of lifetime criminality (Farrington *et al*, 2006: p. 94; Odgers *et al*, 2008) and life failure (Piquero *et al*, 2010).

Second, children with callous-unemotional traits appear to be an aetiologically distinct group with low empathy and high fearlessness. Callous-unemotional traits have higher genetic heritability than conduct disorder (Viding *et al*, 2005) and are associated with a different pattern of neurocognitive deficits, such as reduced amygdala function (Kiehl *et al*, 2001). The presence of callous-unemotional traits in antisocial children has important treatment implications. Studies have shown that these children are more resistant to punishment and are more difficult to treat (Hawes & Dadds, 2005). However, it is not the case that they cannot benefit from treatment (Hawes & Dadds, 2007).

Third, a number of studies have begun to support a causal pathway associated with poor regulation of anger. These are children who misinterpret ambiguous social cues as threatening, which may lead them to respond in an aggressive manner (Orobio de Castro *et al*, 2002). There is often a history of harsh discipline in this group (Pasalich *et al*, 2011). However, the association between harsh discipline and antisocial behaviour seems to be most pronounced among those with a genetic susceptibility (Taylor & Kim-Cohen, 2007).

Assessment

The history should include detailed examples of the child's actions and the parental response, including how everyone felt at the time. Questions should be addressed to the child throughout, and not just to the adults present. Behaviour should be assessed within the context of the child's age and should also be judged on the basis of the level, pattern, persistence and impact of the behaviour (National Institute for Health and Care Excellence, 2013). Box 5.3 lists factors found in the assessment that may need attention.

Developmental history

A difficult temperament from birth ('he wouldn't feed and he kept waking up') may predispose to behaviour problems and permanently impair the

---

Box 5.3 Examples of factors found in the assessment of antisocial behaviour which may need attention

Social factors

- Suitable housing
- Sufficient support in the community
- Presence of specific cultural, ethnic or religious issues

Family factors

- Consistency of discipline and praise-giving
- Joint activity and play
- Parental warmth and criticism
- Whether or not the family is reconstituted
- Whether there is room for improvement in consistency between parents
- Presence of parental psychopathology
- Influence of the grandparents or other relatives
- Whether or not the parent's experience of being a child is relevant to the parenting style
- The relationship of the parent(s) to the teaching staff

School factors

- Academic progress and special educational needs
- Levels of activity, concentration and task completion in the classroom
- Behaviour in the classroom, in the playground and at dinner-time
- Relationships with peers and adults

Child factors

- Temperament
- Nature of attachment to main caregiver
- Presence of medical problems
- Presence of intellectual disabilities or specific learning difficulties
- Comorbid hyperactivity, depression or anxiety

---

affection of the mother for her child. Maternal postnatal depression may compound this and contribute to attachment difficulties. Attachment problems may also result from significant conflict between parents (such as violence or repeated separations and reconciliations) witnessed or experienced by the child in the first few years of his life. Language delay can lead to frustration and is associated with increased conduct problems.

Family history

A genogram is well worth the time spent on it. There is often a family history of behaviour problems or hyperactivity, and a history of harsh and inconsistent parenting is often present in the families of children with early-onset antisocial behaviour. Repeating patterns can sometimes be seen after gleaning minimal information about the grandparents' generation, or the parents' experience of being parented.

Interaction patterns within the nuclear family are more easily grasped from a diagram: is a younger sister perceived to be everything that her older brother is not, or is the eldest son credited by his mother with all the bad qualities of his long-departed father or criminal uncle?

A problem-saturated description

Assessment and treatment are normally regarded as separate processes, but the way the assessment is done can have either a restraining or a liberating effect on treatment options. The first stages of treatment must be part of the initial session, and the way questions are asked may have a major impact on how members of the family see the difficulties they present with, so that the enquiry itself can be seen as part of the treatment (Tomm, 1987). There are many techniques for engaging families (Carpenter & Treacher, 1983), and these are often especially important with the families of antisocial children. Any opportunity should be taken for praising parents and framing in a positive light attempts to manage a difficult situation. It is all too easy, as a psychiatrist, to adopt an expert role, which can make parents feel in a 'one-down' position. They may, for instance, hear the message that they have been doing things wrong for years. It is therefore important to establish a collaborative relationship. Parents are, after all, experts on their own children, and have already conducted many experiments as to what works and what does not.

The danger of inviting the parent(s) to give an account of the problems in front of the child is that a predominantly negative picture is built up, confirming the child's already negative self-image. There are several ways round this. One is to see the parent(s) without the child. Some workers do this as a routine way of starting the assessment; but it may increase parental self-blame, and may therefore be best left until the parent(s) suggest it. Another is to forgo a detailed description of the problem areas, at least initially, and focus instead on relationships within the family and with friends. A third is to adopt a solution-focused approach (de Shazer *et al*, 1987) and emphasise the positive aspects, especially the exceptions to repeated difficulties. Examples might include paying particular attention to times when the child has controlled his temper, or occasions when adults have acted effectively in achieving compliance. The 'miracle' question can be very useful in eliciting unachievable goals: 'If you were to wake up tomorrow morning and find that everything was all right, what would be different?' Much smaller, achievable goals can then be generated. Finally, it is always useful to get the parent(s) to describe the positive attributes of the child with the child present.

Individual interview

It is easy, but foolhardy, to justify not paying individual attention to the child by lack of time, resources or the need to take a family approach. Without an individual interview, it is difficult to understand the child's point of view, and there is some information, such as the revelation of abuse, that is likely to emerge only in the absence of parents.

Some children with conduct disorder refuse to be seen on their own at all. With insecure children, a worthwhile interview of the child can sometimes be done in the presence of the parent(s). Some children have particular difficulty putting their feelings into words; others volunteer untruthful answers. In either case, non-verbal techniques may be particularly useful, such as drawing a picture of the family or playing with figures.

Areas of success in school may be the least threatening topic for initial enquiry. Closest friends, after-school activities and peer contact outside school are also fruitful avenues for exploration. A question about bullying should be included in every assessment, although the older the child, the greater is the reluctance to admit to being bullied (Dawkins & Hill, 1995); older children are even less likely to admit to being a bully.

A child may find it difficult to be open about life within the family, particularly in a first interview. This may be out of loyalty, or for fear that his comments will be fed straight back to his parents. Questions about relationships between two other family members, such as a sibling and a parent, may be easier than questions about his own relationships.

A child's view of himself is particularly important. A parent's or teacher's repeated criticisms of the child may contribute to low self-esteem, which is so commonly seen in conduct disorder. In extreme cases, this may make it impossible for the child to hear praise from parents or teachers, and he may repeatedly describe himself as 'no good'.

At least one suitably worded question should be asked about physical and sexual abuse. It is also important to ask about symptoms of depression and suicidal ideation. In older children, routine questioning should cover the use of drugs, alcohol and cigarettes.

Contributions from other informants

Telephoned or written enquiry to the child's school, after parental consent, is an essential part of assessment. There is a low correlation between reports from home and school, but in children with severe problems there is usually more agreement.

It is useful to have separate opinions on ability and performance, emphasising particular skills, and perhaps including specific attainment target scores. Contact with the educational psychologist can often help the assessment, as well as fostering cooperation between different professionals for the child's benefit.

Peer relationships can be particularly important. Children developing conduct disorder are often noticeable at school entry for their difficulty with learning in groups and impaired ability to make friends. They may respond to other children's social overtures with aggression, simply because they know no other way. The teacher's observations of emotional difficulties can reveal signs of anxiety, social withdrawal or low self-esteem.

In some cases, attendance may be an issue, and it may then be worthwhile communicating with the educational welfare officer. Information from other professionals who are involved, such as social workers, is vital in giving insights into the family from a different perspective – for example, what sort of professional help has worked or not worked so far, previous parental difficulties, and whether there is an entry on the child protection register.

Comorbid problems

Assessment of comorbid conditions and problems is essential. It is extremely common, its presence changes the nature of the problem to be addressed and it is often remediable.

Hyperactivity

Clinical experience suggests that the more symptoms of hyperkinetic disorder the child shows, the more difficult it is for parents, teachers and mental health professionals to make behavioural management techniques work. The techniques may be more effective in combination with medication.

It should be a routine with any child referred for antisocial behaviour to think and ask about problems of inattention, overactivity and impulsivity. Standardised questionnaires such as the Strengths and Difficulties Questionnaire (SDQ), which is brief, are very helpful and just as effective at detecting hyperactivity as longer instruments (Goodman & Scott, 1999). If the diagnostic criteria for hyperkinetic disorder are met, then a trial of medication should be considered (National Institute for Health and Clinical Excellence, 2009).

Reading problems

The association between specific reading difficulties and disruptive behaviour in primary school is well established. This may partly be due to the frustration of not being able to read and partly due to attention problems (Maughan *et al*, 2006), which may be either a cause or a consequence of the reading delay. It is therefore important to include an appraisal of reading, spelling and writing (since these often go together) in the assessment of any child referred with conduct disorder. The teacher's opinion may be sufficient. Adequate remedial teaching will improve reading skills (Snowling, 1996) and is likely to improve academic attainments and self-esteem, as well as reducing frustration in class and disaffection with what school stands for.

Other intellectual disabilities

Other intellectual disabilities, such as language disorders, may contribute to disruptive behaviour and are easily missed. Late diagnosis of pervasive developmental disorders such as autism, and to an even greater extent

Asperger syndrome, is not uncommon. The degree of disruptive behaviour is very variable, but can pose major management difficulties.

Emotional problems

An emotional dimension to conduct disorder is much more common than an accompanying substantive emotional disorder such as depression or anxiety. However, the antisocial behaviour can act as a smokescreen, and prevent the psychiatrist from being sensitive to the child's sadness, worry or anger.

A particular example of emotional problems underlying antisocial behaviour is seen in child sexual abuse. Children may have very strong negative feelings about the abuse, but feel unable to disclose it to anyone. Sexualised behaviour is often a feature, but may be absent. Boys who have been sexually abused are at risk of abusing other boys. Children who have been physically abused may present with aggressive behaviour or bullying.

Treatment

Intervention principles

Rates of drop out from treatment for families of children with conduct problems are high – often up to 60% (Kazdin, 1996a; Nock & Ferriter, 2005). Practical measures such as helping with travel and providing child care are all likely to improve retention. Forming a good alliance with the family is especially important: for example, Prinz & Miller (1994) found that showing parents that the therapist clearly understood their viewpoint led to increased attendance at treatment sessions. Once engaged, the quality of the therapist's alliance with the family affects treatment success: in one meta-analysis it accounted for 15% of the variance in outcome (Shirk & Karver, 2003).

If possible, interventions should specifically address each context. For example, improvements in the home arising from a successful parent training programme will not necessarily lead to less antisocial behaviour at school (Scott, 2002). If the child has pervasive problems that include fights with peers, individual work on anger management and social skills should be added. The National Health Service (NHS) has insufficient resources to treat all antisocial behaviour in childhood, so the mental health professional must decide whether other agencies can be involved. A number of third (voluntary) sector bodies now provide parent training, and schools may be able to set up suitable behavioural programmes.

Identifying the strengths of both the child and the family is crucial. This helps engagement and increases the chances of effective treatment. Encouraging prosocial activities may lead to increased achievements, heightened self-esteem and greater hope for the future. Treatment involves more than the reduction of antisocial behaviour – positive behaviours need to be taught too. Specific intellectual disabilities such as reading retardation, which is particularly common in these children, need to be addressed, as do more general difficulties such as planning homework.

Making use of existing guidelines is important. The American Academy of Child and Adolescent Psychiatry has drawn up sensible practice parameters for the assessment and treatment of conduct disorder (Steiner & Work Group on Quality Issues, 1997), and NICE has published an appraisal of the clinical efficacy and cost-effectiveness of parent training programmes (National Institute for Health and Clinical Excellence, 2006) and clinical guidelines on the treatment of conduct disorder (National Institute for Health and Care Excellence, 2013).

Most of the interventions described below are intended for out-patient or community settings. The key principles of these interventions are listed in Box 5.4. Admission to psychiatric hospital is very rarely necessary: there is no evidence that in-patient admissions lead to gains that are maintained after the child goes home.

Specific interventions

Parent management training

Programmes have been designed to improve parents' behaviour management skills and the quality of the parent–child relationship (see Box 5.5 for examples of good practice). Most target skills, but interventions may also address less direct factors likely to inhibit change, such as parental drug or alcohol misuse, maternal depression and violence between parents. Treatment can be delivered in individual parent–child sessions or in a parenting group. Individual approaches offer the advantages of live observation of the parent–child dyad and therapist coaching and feedback regarding progress. Group treatment is equally effective, and offers opportunities for parents to share their experience with others who are struggling with a disruptive child.

Box 5.4 Intervention principles

- Engage the family
- Select the treatment and who delivers it
- Develop strengths
- Treat comorbid conditions
- Promote social and scholastic learning
- Use guidelines
- Treat in the natural environment

Efficacy

Parent management training is the most extensively studied treatment for children's conduct problems, and there is considerable empirical support for its efficacy (Furlong *et al*, 2013). Several programmes are considered well established according to American Psychological Association criteria, after multiple randomised trials (e.g. Patterson *et al*, 1982; Webster-Stratton *et al*, 2001) and replications by independent research groups (e.g. Scott *et al*, 2001). Randomised trials have shown the efficacy of the Triple P-Positive Parenting Program (e.g. Bor *et al*, 2002; Sanders *et al*, 2000*b*), and there is at least one independent replication supporting the parent–child interaction therapy model (Nixon *et al*, 2003). These studies suggest that behavioural parent training leads to short-term reduction in antisocial behaviour. Follow-up studies suggest enduring effects at up to 6 years after treatment (Hood & Eyberg, 2003; Reid *et al*, 2003). It should be noted that the wider terms 'parenting support' and 'parenting programmes' cover a broad range of approaches, many of which are not evidence based and therefore cannot be advocated.

Established parent training programmes have been less successful with children who have callous-unemotional traits, seemingly because these children are less responsive to discipline (Hawes & Dadds, 2005). However, a number of recent studies have shown support for treatment models that focus on improving the parent–child bond (Somech & Elizur, 2012) and emotion recognition skills in children (Dadds *et al*, 2012).

Child therapies

The most common targets of cognitive–behavioural and social skills therapies for children are aggressive behaviour, social interactions, self-evaluation and emotion dysregulation (Box 5.5). These interventions may be delivered in individual or group therapy. Although groups offer several advantages (e.g. opportunities to practise peer interactions), they may have iatrogenic effects (Dishion *et al*, 1999). These appear to be particularly

---

Box 5.5 Examples of good practice

Parent management training

- The Helping the Non-compliant Child programme (McMahon & Forehand, 2003)
- Parent–child interaction therapy (PCIT; Eyberg, 1988)
- Incredible Years Programme (Webster-Stratton, 1981)
- Positive Parenting Program (Triple P; Sanders *et al*, 2000*a*)

Child therapies

- Problem-solving skills training with *in vivo* practice (PSST–P; Kazdin, 1996*b*)
- Coping Power Program (Lochman & Wells, 2002)

common in larger groups and those with inadequate therapist supervision, where children learn deviant behaviour from their peers and encourage each other to act antisocially.

Efficacy

In two randomised controlled trials, Kazdin *et al* (1987, 1989) found that problem-solving skills training (PSST) resulted in significant decrease in deviant behaviour and increase in prosocial behaviour. Outcomes were superior to a client-centred, relationship-based treatment and were maintained at 1-year follow-up. The addition of both real-life ('*in vivo*') practice and a parent training component enhanced outcomes. Evaluations of the Coping Power Program found reductions in aggression and substance use, and improved social competence (e.g. Lochman & Wells, 2002). Treatment effects were maintained at 1 year, particularly for those whose parents also received parent training (Lochman & Wells, 2004).

School interventions

Typically, teachers are taught techniques to promote positive behaviour for use with all children in their classes, not just those exhibiting the most antisocial behaviour. Successful approaches use proactive strategies and focus on positive behaviour and group interventions, combining instructional strategies with behavioural management. However, other techniques are classroom specific. For example, establishing and teaching rules and procedures involves setting rules such as 'use a quiet voice', 'listen when others are speaking', 'keep your hands and feet to yourself' and 'use respectful words'. Note that these rules are all expressed positively, describing what the child should do, rather than what he should not. Striepling-Goldstein (1997) offers six 'rules for making rules':

1 make few rules (between three and six)
2 negotiate them with the children
3 state them behaviourally and positively
4 make a contract with the children to adhere to them
5 post them on the classroom wall
6 send a copy to parents.

Crucial to all this is a systematic and consistent response to children following or not following the rules. Rewards can be social (teacher praise), material (stickers) or privileges (extra computer time). Mild punishments include reprimands, losing privileges or points, and time out.

Interventions are also used to promote academic engagement and learning. These include self-management and self-reinforcement training programmes that help children, for example, to spend more time on a task.

Efficacy

An older review of 16 studies found moderate to large effects for such school-based programmes (Nelson *et al*, 1991), and subsequent trials uphold this finding (e.g. Levendoski & Cartledge, 2000). A number of programmes build on the idea that antisocial children who are failing at school often have parents who do not get involved in their academic schoolwork and indeed may not value it highly. Approaches include removing barriers to home–school cooperation by training parents to view teachers positively and, equally, training teachers to be constructive in solving children's difficulties and helping parents engage in academic activities with their children. Although there are good descriptions of such programmes (e.g. Christenson & Buerkle, 1999), rigorous evaluations are lacking.

Medications

No pharmacological intervention is currently approved as a primary treatment specifically for conduct disorder. Pharmacological approaches are not recommended by the World Health Organization (2012) and are suggested only as a potential second-line strategy by NICE when all other strategies have failed (National Institute for Health and Care Excellence, 2013). Guidance in the USA (Steiner & Work Group on Quality Issues, 1997) is less clear, but highlights a lack of adequate efficacy studies.

The best-studied pharmacological interventions for children and young people with oppositional defiant disorder or conduct disorder are psycho-stimulants (methylphenidate and dexamfetamine) used for comorbid attention-deficit hyperactivity disorder (ADHD). In these circumstances, there is good evidence that reduction in hyperactivity/impulsivity will also result in reduced conduct problems (Taylor & Sonuga-Barke, 2008). There is insufficient reliable evidence to decide whether stimulants reduce aggression in the absence of ADHD: Klein *et al* (1997) found that improvements in conduct disorder symptoms were independent of ADHD symptom reduction, whereas Taylor *et al* (1987) did not.

Other pharmacological approaches for antisocial behaviour in young people have tended to target reactive aggression and overarousal, primarily in highly aggressive individuals in a hospital setting. Medications used in these conditions include antipsychotics and mood stabilisers (Scotto Rosato *et al*, 2012). In the past few years, the use of the newer antipsychotics in out-patient settings has been increasing. However, there is only modest evidence for their effectiveness for conduct disorder in children of normal IQ without ADHD. Furthermore, these drugs, while not especially sedating, have substantial side-effects. For example, risperidone typically causes considerable weight gain, and the prevalence of long-term movement disorders is unknown. A NICE meta-analysis of antipsychotics for oppositional defiant disorder or conduct disorder (National Institute for Health and Care Excellence, 2013) found only three suitable trials, and these were of moderate quality only. The mean effect size as rated by parents was 0.49 s.d., but researcher/clinician and teacher ratings showed no significant effects; no study used independent observation; and the majority of the children had comorbid ADHD. In contrast, the

69

meta-analysis by Scotto Rosato *et al* (2012) included studies involving children with ADHD, intellectual disabilities and autism. It reported an overall effect size of 0.72 over a mean period of 8 weeks' treatment, during which the children (average age 9 years) gained on average 1.8 kg. This review recommends that if antipsychotics do not work, a mood stabilising medication should be added. Thus, Scotto Rosato *et al* take a very different stance on treatment with medication from that taken by NICE, stating that 'The evidence on the effect of psychosocial interventions on maladaptive aggression is limited'. It should be noted that many of the authors disclosed payments from drug companies.

Despite the lack of reliable evidence, medication is used relatively frequently and increasingly for conduct disorder in the USA (Steiner *et al*, 2003; Turgay, 2004). Primary care physicians are often required to manage such medication, and concerns have been raised because many lack adequate training in developmental psychopathology and do not have time to carry out thorough assessment and monitoring (Vitiello, 2001).

Conclusion

The trend in current research is towards combining different modes of treatment for antisocial behaviour, so that the various components of the disorder all improve concurrently. For instance, a research programme might combine parent training, child cognitive–behavioural training and a school-based intervention. Such costly combinations are beyond the reach of most clinical services in the UK, but services for children with conduct disorder can be improved bit by bit. Thorough assessment which detects comorbid conditions and problems will allow many children to benefit. Many clinics in the UK are offering parent training, and this is clearly a feasible option. Additional components can be added as staff training and resources allow.

References

American Psychiatric Association (1994) *Diagnostic and Statistical Manual of Mental Disorders (4th edn) (DSM-IV)*. APA.

American Psychiatric Association (2013) *Diagnostic and Statistical Manual of Mental Disorders (5th edn) (DSM-5)*. APA.

Anderson KE, Lytton H, Romney DM (1986) Mothers' interactions with normal and conduct-disordered boys: who affects whom? *Developmental Psychology*, **22**, 604–609.

Bor W, Sanders MR, Markie-Dadds C (2002) The effects of the Triple P-Positive Parenting Program on preschool children with co-occurring disruptive behavior and attentional/hyperactive difficulties. *Journal of Abnormal Child Psychology*, **30**, 571–587.

Carpenter J, Treacher A (1983) On the neglected but related arts of convening and engaging families and their wider systems. *Journal of Family Therapy*, **5**, 337–358.

Christenson SL, Buerkle K (1999) Families as educational partners for children's school success: suggestions for school psychologists. In *The Handbook of School Psychology* (3rd edn) (eds CR Reynolds, TB Gutkin), pp. 709–744. John Wiley & Sons.

Dadds MR, Cauchi AJ, Wimalaweera S, *et al* (2012) Outcomes, moderators, and mediators of empathic-emotion recognition training for complex conduct problems in childhood. *Psychiatry Research*, **199**, 201–207.

Dawkins J, Hill P (1995) Bullying: another form of abuse. In *Recent Advances in Paediatrics* (ed T David), pp. 103–122. Churchill Livingstone.

de Shazer S, Berg IK, Lipchik E, *et al* (1987) Brief therapy: focused solution development. *Family Process*, **25**, 207–221.

Dishion TJ, McCord J, Poulin F (1999) When interventions harm: peer groups and problem behavior. *American Psychologist*, **54**, 755–764.

Eyberg S (1988) Parent–child interaction therapy. *Child and Family Behavior Therapy*, **10**, 33–46.

Farrington DP, Coid JW, Harnett LM, *et al* (2006) *Criminal Careers up to Age 50 and Life Success up to Age 48: New Findings from the Cambridge Study in Delinquent Development* (2nd edn). Home Office Research, Development and Statistics Directorate.

Fergusson DM, Horwood LJ, Ridder EM (2005) Show me the child at seven. II: Childhood intelligence and later outcomes in adolescence and young adulthood. *Journal of Child Psychology and Psychiatry*, **46**, 850–858.

Furlong M, McGilloway S, Bywater T, *et al* (2013) Cochrane Review: behavioural and cognitive-behavioural group-based parenting programmes for early-onset conduct problems in children aged 3 to 12 years. *Evidence-Based Child Health: A Cochrane Review Journal*, **8**, 318–692.

Goodman R, Scott S (1999) Comparing the Strengths and Difficulties Questionnaire and the Child Behavior Checklist: is small beautiful? *Journal of Abnormal Child Psychology*, **27**, 17–24.

Hawes DJ, Dadds MR (2005) The treatment of conduct problems in children with callous-unemotional traits. *Journal of Consulting and Clinical Psychology*, **73**, 737–741.

Hawes DJ, Dadds MR (2007) Stability and malleability of callous-unemotional traits during treatment for childhood conduct problems. *Journal of Clinical Child and Adolescent Psychology*, **36**, 347–355.

Hood KK, Eyberg SM (2003) Outcomes of parent–child interaction therapy: mothers' reports of maintenance three to six years after treatment. *Journal of Clinical Child and Adolescent Psychology*, **32**, 419–429.

Kazdin AE (1996a) Dropping out of child psychotherapy: issues for research and implications for practice. *Clinical Child Psychology and Psychiatry*, **1**, 133–156.

Kazdin AE (1996b) Problem solving and parent management in treating aggressive and antisocial behavior. In *Psychosocial Treatments for Child and Adolescent Disorders: Empirically-Based Strategies for Clinical Practice* (eds ES Hibbs, PS Jensen), pp. 377–408. American Psychological Association.

Kazdin AE, Esveldt-Dawson K, French NH, *et al* (1987) Problem-solving skills training and relationship therapy in the treatment of antisocial child behavior. *Journal of Consulting and Clinical Psychology*, **55**, 76–85.

Kazdin AE, Bass D, Siegel T, *et al* (1989) Cognitive–behavioral therapy and relationship therapy in the treatment of children referred for antisocial behavior. *Journal of Consulting and Clinical Psychology*, **57**, 522–535.

Kiehl KA, Smith AM, Hare RD, *et al* (2001) Limbic abnormalities in affective processing by criminal psychopaths as revealed by functional magnetic resonance imaging. *Biological Psychiatry*, **50**, 677–684.

Klein RG, Abikoff H, Klass E, *et al* (1997) Clinical efficacy of methylphenidate in conduct disorder with and without attention deficit hyperactivity disorder. *Archives of General Psychiatry*, **54**, 1073–1108.

Levendoski LS, Cartledge G (2000) Self-monitoring for elementary school children with serious emotional disturbances: classroom applications for increased academic responding. *Behavioral Disorders*, **25**, 211–224.

Lochman JE, Wells KC (2002) Contextual social-cognitive mediators and child outcome: a test of the theoretical model in the coping power program. *Development and Psychopathology*, **14**, 945–967.

Lochman JE, Wells KC (2004) The coping power program for preadolescent aggressive boys and their parents: outcome effects at the 1-year follow-up. *Journal of Consulting and Clinical Psychology*, **72**, 571–578.

Maughan B, Pickles A, Hagell A, *et al* (2006) Reading problems and antisocial behaviour: developmental trends in comorbidity. *Journal of Child Psychology and Psychiatry*, **37**, 405–418.

McMahon RJ, Forehand R (2003) *Helping the Noncompliant Child: A Clinician's Guide to Effective Parent Training*. Guilford Press.

Moffitt TE (2006) Life-course persistent versus adolescence-limited antisocial behavior. In *Developmental Psychopathology: Risk, Disorder, and Adaptation* (2nd edn) (eds D Cicchetti, J Cohen), pp. 570– 598). John Wiley & Sons.

Murray J, Farrington DP (2010) Risk factors for conduct disorder and delinquency: key findings from longitudinal studies. *Canadian Journal of Psychiatry*, **55**, 633–642.

National Institute for Health and Clinical Excellence (2006) *Parent-Training/Education Programmes in the Management of Children with Conduct Disorders* (NICE Technology Appraisal Guidance 102). NICE.

National Institute for Health and Clinical Excellence (2009) *Antisocial Personality Disorder: Treatment, Management and Prevention* (NICE Clinical Guideline 77). NICE.

National Institute for Health and Care Excellence (2013) *Antisocial Behaviour and Conduct Disorders in Children and Young People: Recognition, Intervention and Management* (NICE Clinical Guideline 158). NICE.

Nelson JR, Smith DJ, Young RK, *et al* (1991) A review of self-management outcome research conducted with students who exhibit behavioral disorders. *Behavioral Disorders*, **16**, 168–179.

Nixon RD, Sweeney L, Erickson DB, *et al* (2003) Parent–child interaction therapy: a comparison of standard and abbreviated treatments for oppositional defiant preschoolers. *Journal of Consulting and Clinical Psychology*, **71**, 251–260.

Nock MK, Ferriter C (2005) Parent management of attendance and adherence in child and adolescent therapy: a conceptual and empirical review. *Clinical Child and Family Psychology Review*, **8**, 149–166.

Odgers CL, Moffitt TE, Broadbent JM, *et al* (2008) Female and male antisocial trajectories: from childhood origins to adult outcomes. *Development and Psychopathology*, **20**, 673–716.

Orobio de Castro B, Veerman JW, Koops W, *et al* (2002) Hostile attribution of intent and aggressive behavior: a meta-analysis. *Child Development*, **73**, 916–934.

Pardini D, Frick PJ (2013) Multiple developmental pathways to conduct disorder: current conceptualizations and clinical implications. *Journal of the Canadian Academy of Child and Adolescent Psychiatry*, **22**, 20–25.

Pasalich DS, Dadds MR, Hawes DJ, *et al* (2011) Do callous-unemotional traits moderate the relative importance of parental coercion versus warmth in child conduct problems? An observational study. *Journal of Child Psychology and Psychiatry*, **52**, 1308–1315.

Patterson GR, Chamberlain P, Reid JB (1982) A comparative evaluation of a parent-training program. *Behavior Therapy*, **13**, 638–650.

Piquero AR, Farrington DP, Nagin DS, *et al* (2010) Trajectories of offending and their relation to life failure in late middle age: findings from the Cambridge Study in Delinquent Development. *Journal of Research in Crime and Delinquency*, **47**, 151–173.

Prinz RJ, Miller GE (1994) Family-based treatment for childhood antisocial behavior: experimental influences on dropout and engagement. *Journal of Consulting and Clinical Psychology*, **62**, 645–650.

Reid MJ, Webster-Stratton C, Hammond M (2003) Follow-up of children who received the Incredible Years intervention for oppositional-defiant disorder: maintenance and prediction of 2-year outcome. *Behavior Therapy*, **34**, 471–491.

Sanders MR, Markie-Dadds C, Turner KMT (2000a) Theoretical, scientific, and clinical foundations of the Triple P-Positive Parenting Program: a population approach to the promotion of parenting competence. *Parenting Research and Practice Monograph*, **1**, 1–21.

Sanders MR, Markie-Dadds C, Tully LA, *et al* (2000*b*) The Triple P-Positive Parenting Program: a comparison of enhanced, standard, and self-directed behavioral family intervention for parents of children with early onset conduct problems. *Journal of Consulting and Clinical Psychology*, **68**, 624–640.

Scott S (2002) Parent training programmes. In *Child and Adolescent Psychiatry* (4th edn) (eds M Rutter, E Taylor), pp. 949–967. John Wiley & Sons.

Scott S, Spender Q, Doolan M, *et al* (2001) Multicentre controlled trial of parenting groups for childhood antisocial behaviour in clinical practice. *BMJ*, **323**, 1–7.

Scotto Rosato N, Correll CU, Pappadopulos E, *et al* (2012) Treatment of maladaptive aggression in youth: CERT guidelines II. Treatments and ongoing management. *Pediatrics*, **129**, e1577–1586.

Shirk SR, Karver M (2003) Prediction of treatment outcome from relationship variables in child and adolescent therapy: a meta-analytic review. *Journal of Consulting and Clinical Psychology*, **71**, 452–464.

Snowling MJ (1996) Annotation: contemporary approaches to the teaching of reading. *Journal of Child Psychology and Psychiatry*, **37**, 139–148.

Somech LY, Elizur Y (2012) Promoting self-regulation and cooperation in pre-kindergarten children with conduct problems: a randomized controlled trial. *Journal of the American Academy of Child & Adolescent Psychiatry*, **51**, 412–422.

Steiner H, Work Group on Quality Issues (1997) Practice parameters for the assessment and treatment of children and adolescents with conduct disorder. *Journal of the American Academy of Child & Adolescent Psychiatry*, **36** (issue 10 suppl.), 122S–139S.

Steiner H, Saxena K, Chang K (2003) Psychopharmacologic strategies for the treatment of aggression in juveniles. *CNS Spectrums*, **8**, 298–308.

Striepling-Goldstein SH (1997) The low-aggression classroom: a teacher's view. In *School Violence Intervention: A Practical Handbook* (eds AP Goldstein, JC Conoley), pp. 23–45. Guilford Press.

Taylor A, Kim-Cohen J (2007) Meta-analysis of gene–environment interactions in developmental psychopathology. *Development and Psychopathology*, **19**, 1029–1037.

Taylor E, Sonuga-Barke E (2008) Disorders of attention and activity. In *Rutter's Child and Adolescent Psychiatry* (5th edn) (eds M Rutter, D Bishop, D Pine, *et al*), pp. 519–542. Wiley-Blackwell.

Taylor E, Schachar R, Thorley G, *et al* (1987) Which boys respond to stimulant medication? A controlled trial of methylphenidate in boys with disruptive behaviour. *Psychological Medicine*, **17**, 121–143.

Tomm K (1987) Interventive interviewing: Part II. Reflexive questioning as a means to enable self-healing. *Family Process*, **26**, 167–183.

Turgay A (2004) Aggression and disruptive behavior disorders in children and adolescents. *Expert Review of Neurotherapeutics*, **4**, 623–632.

Viding E, Blair RJR, Moffitt TE, *et al* (2005) Evidence for substantial genetic risk for psychopathy in 7-year-olds. *Journal of Child Psychology and Psychiatry*, **46**, 592–597.

Vitiello B (2001) Psychopharmacology for young children: clinical needs and research opportunities. *Pediatrics*, **108**, 983–989.

Webster-Stratton C (1981) Modification of mothers' behaviors and attitudes through a videotape modeling group discussion program. *Behavior Therapy*, **12**, 634–642.

Webster-Stratton C, Reid MJ, Hammond M (2001) Preventing conduct problems, promoting social competence: a parent and teacher training partnership in Head Start. *Journal of Clinical Child Psychology*, **30**, 283–302.

World Health Organization (1993) *The ICD-10 Classification of Mental and Behavioural Disorders: Diagnostic Criteria for Research*. WHO.

World Health Organization (2012) *Pharmacological interventions for children with Disruptive Behaviour Disorders or Conduct Disorder or Oppositional Defiant Disorder*. WHO (http://www.who.int/mental_health/mhgap/evidence/resource/child_q8.pdf).

CHAPTER 6

Pharmacology for attention-deficit hyperactivity disorder, Tourette syndrome and autism spectrum disorder

David Coghill and Eugenia Sinita

Historically, paediatric pharmacology in general and paediatric psychopharmacology in particular have received much less research interest and funding than their adult counterparts. As a consequence, relatively few drugs are licensed for use in child and adolescent populations.

One of the greatest obstacles to evidence-based clinical practice is the time taken to translate research findings into treatment recommendations that are effective and usable in a general out-patient setting. Unfortunately, there are also several clear examples of changes in clinical practice outstripping the available evidence. In this chapter and the next, we describe some of the recent advances and current controversies in child and adolescent psychopharmacology. With the exception of attention-deficit hyperactivity disorder (ADHD) in this chapter, they are organised by disorder rather than drug class. The section on ADHD is organised by class of drug as this best reflects the ways in which clinical decisions are made about individual patients.

Attention-deficit hyperactivity disorder

There has been more research into the use of medication for the treatment of ADHD than any other area of child and adolescent psychopharmacology, and most clinicians are now comfortable with the idea of using medications as a part of their treatment of ADHD. There have, however, been key advances in knowledge and several new treatment options introduced over the past few years. In addition, more basic science studies have helped clarify the relationship between the pharmacokinetics and misuse potential of stimulant medications (Volkow et al, 1995) and raised interesting questions about the relationship between core ADHD symptoms and cognition (Coghill et al, 2007). Clinical studies have started to address the similarities and differences between different medications as well as their effect on non-core aspects of functioning and quality of life (Coghill, 2010). In view of the quantity of trial data and the fact that most clinicians are used to working with these drugs, we focus here on newer medications and current controversies.

Evidence-based treatment and the MTA study

The end of 1999 saw the publication of the primary findings from the Multimodal Treatment of Attention Deficit Hyperactivity Disorder (MTA) multisite study, which was funded by the US National Institute of Mental Health. These findings, and the ensuing commentaries and criticisms of the study, marked a milestone in child and adolescent psychiatry research. The MTA study's primary findings have been extensively reported (for a full discussion see Swanson et al, 2008a,b) and we will not discuss them in detail. However, several of the secondary papers and results from the longer-term follow-up have clinical relevance and will be discussed below.

The MTA study involved almost 600 children aged 7–9, who were randomly allocated to one of four treatment modes: intensive medication management alone; intensive behavioural treatment alone; a combination of both; or routine community care (the control group). Unlike previous studies, the active treatments in the MTA studies were continued for 14 months.

One of the more interesting initial findings from the MTA study was the superiority of the intensive medication management arm over the community treatment arm (within which most patients also received medication). It seems likely that the medication management algorithm used in the study was responsible for these differences. It utilised highly organised titration and continuing care protocols and aimed for maximal effect with 'no room for improvement', allowing a dose decrease only for moderate to severe side-effects. As a consequence of this protocol, those in the medication arm received higher doses of medication and were usually on thrice-daily doses of immediate-release medication, in contrast to the community group who were usually on twice daily doses. They had also had an initial intensive forced dose titration to optimal dose and had treatment changes informed by detailed feedback from both parents and teachers. All of these approaches can be integrated into day-to-day clinical practice and can aid treatment optimisation. It seems likely that it was the withdrawal of this structured support, rather than decreased efficacy of medication over time, that resulted in the falling back that was reported at both the 3- and 8-year follow-ups for the patients initially randomised to the medication management and the combined treatment (Jensen et al, 2007; Banaschewski et al, 2009; Molina et al, 2009). In our view, this emphasises the need for continued high-quality monitoring of medication effects in ADHD. Unfortunately, this is not yet standard clinical practice in the UK.

Another important finding from the MTA study that has a large impact on clinical guidance in Europe comes from a reanalysis of the primary

75

outcome data by Santosh *et al* (2005). All of those included in the MTA study met criteria for combined type ADHD as defined by DSM-IV (American Psychiatric Association, 1994). The reanalysis focused on comparing outcomes for those who did and did not meet the more restrictive criteria required for a diagnosis of hyperkinetic disorder as defined by ICD-10 (which can be considered as severe, pervasive and impairing ADHD; World Health Organization, 1992). Although for those with the more restrictive hyperkinetic disorder, the medication and combination arms were clearly superior to the behavioural and community arms (as was reported for the whole group in the original papers), for those with combined type ADHD but not meeting the criteria for hyperkinetic disorder the differences between the four arms were much less. As a consequence, the UK's National Institute for Health and Care Excellence (NICE; National Collaborating Centre for Mental Health, 2008) and other European guidelines (Taylor *et al*, 2004) differ from their North American counterparts. The NICE guideline recommends that, although medication should be the first-line treatment for those with hyperkinetic disorder, individuals with less severe ADHD should be first offered non-pharmacological treatments, with medication reserved for those who do not benefit from or cannot take these. It is possible that these recommendations will change in view of a recent meta-analysis of non-pharmacological treatments for ADHD, which suggests that the evidence for their efficacy is less strong than previously assumed (Sonuga-Barke *et al*, 2013).

Stimulant medications

Methylphenidate

The short half-lives of immediate-release stimulant medications and their short duration of action (about 4 hours) give rise to a number of problems. These include: a loss of effect at the most unstructured times of the day, such as lunch-time, break-times and travelling home from school; reduced adherence to dosing regimens, particularly in teenagers; reluctance on the part of schools to administer medications; and stigmatisation and teasing by peers when medication is administered at school.

As a consequence, several long-acting stimulant preparations have been developed, several of which are available for use in the UK and much of mainland Europe (Table 6.1). Understandably, these preparations now account for the bulk of the ADHD drug market. However, in the Dundee ADHD clinic we still prefer the flexibility and shorter duration of action (in case of adverse effects) of immediate-release methylphenidate during the titration period, especially for primary school children. Indeed, some patients elect to remain on medication three times a day rather than switch to extended-release preparations.

The extended-release methylphenidate preparations, all of which are supported by efficacy data from randomised controlled trials (RCTs)

Table 6.1 Long-acting stimulant preparations licensed for the treatment of attention-deficit hyperactivity disorder in the UK and mainland Europe

Medication	Tablets, mg	Dose range, mg/day	IR/ER proportions	Duration of action, h
Methylphenidate				
OROS-methylphenidate, Concerta®	18, 27, 36	18–54	22/78	12
Equasym XL®	10, 20, 30	20–60	30/70	8
Medikinet®	10, 20, 30, 40	20–60	50/50	8
Amfetamine				
Lisdexamfetamine	30, 50, 70	30–70	NA	12–13

ER, extended release; IR, immediate release; NA, not applicable.

(Banaschewski *et al*, 2006), use various techniques to deliver an immediate-release bolus followed by an extended-release dose. This design ensures a relatively fast onset of action followed by a sustained action, giving a combined duration of action of 8–12 hours. The profile of release of most of the extended-release methylphenidate preparations includes an ascending plasma drug level across the day until late afternoon. This profile was informed by an important series of studies that demonstrated that, when administered in such a way as to ensure a flat pharmacokinetic profile across the day (i.e. similar drug levels in the morning and afternoon), afternoon doses of methylphenidate result in an attenuated response compared with the same dose given in the morning (Swanson *et al*, 1999). This has been interpreted as showing the development of acute tolerance, which wears off by the next day, although there may be other explanations, such as a diurnal variation in either symptoms or drug response. Whatever the reason, the increasing plasma drug levels have been shown to help continued clinical response across the day. Other studies have used a laboratory school methodology to demonstrate that the profile of clinical response for these extended-release methylphenidate preparations closely mirrors the pharmacokinetic profile (e.g. Sonuga-Barke *et al*, 2004).

Importantly, the methylphenidate studies do not suggest that one preparation is better than the others. They do, however, help us to understand the differences between the various preparations. It is therefore important that clinicians make themselves familiar with the details of these preparations, as they will otherwise encounter difficulties. A detailed discussion of these issues can be found in Banaschewski *et al* (2006).

As all preparations were designed so that the extended-release portion would continue the initial effects of the immediate-release portion, the most effective way to establish optimal treatment is to carefully titrate against the immediate-release response. To aid switching between preparations we have developed a table that compares the immediate-release components of each of the commonly used doses of the various methylphenidate preparations licensed in the UK and mainland Europe (Table 6.2). We have also developed the Dundee Difficult Times of Day Scale (D-DTODS) (Fig. 6.1), a clinical communication tool that helps identify particularly difficult times of the day and then tailor treatment accordingly.

Table 6.2 The Dundee chart for switching between different methylphenidate preparations

Medication	Immediate release (first 4 h)	Extended release (Equasym XL and Medikinet XL up to 8 h; Concerta XL up to 12 h)	
Equasym XL 10 mg	3 mg	7 mg	± MPH IR
Concerta XL 18 mg	4 mg	14 mg	
Methylphenidate IR 5 mg twice/three times daily	5 mg	5 mg	5 mg
Medikinet XL 10 mg	5 mg	5 mg	± MPH IR
Equasym XL 20 mg	6 mg	14 mg	± MPH IR
Concerta XL 27 mg	6 mg	21 mg	
Concerta XL 36 mg	8 mg	28 mg	
Equasym XL 30 mg	9 mg	21 mg	± MPH IR
Methylphenidate IR 10 mg twice/three times daily	10 mg	10 mg	10 mg
Medikinet XL 20 mg	10 mg	10 mg	± MPH IR
Concerta XL 45 mg	10 mg	35 mg	
Equasym XL 40 mg	12 mg	28 mg	± MPH IR
Concerta XL 54 mg	12 mg	42 mg	
Concerta XL 63 mg	14 mg	49 mg	
Methylphenidate IR 15 mg twice/three times daily	15 mg	15 mg	15 mg
Medikinet XL 30 mg	15 mg	15 mg	± MPH IR
Equasym XL 50 mg	15 mg	35 mg	± MPH IR
Concerta XL 72 mg	16 mg	56 mg	
Equasym XL 60 mg	18 mg	42 mg	
Methylphenidate IR 20 mg twice/three times daily	20 mg	20 mg	20 mg
Medikinet XL 40 mg	20 mg	20 mg	± MPH IR

ER, extended release; IR, immediate release; MPH, methylphenidate.
© University of Dundee.

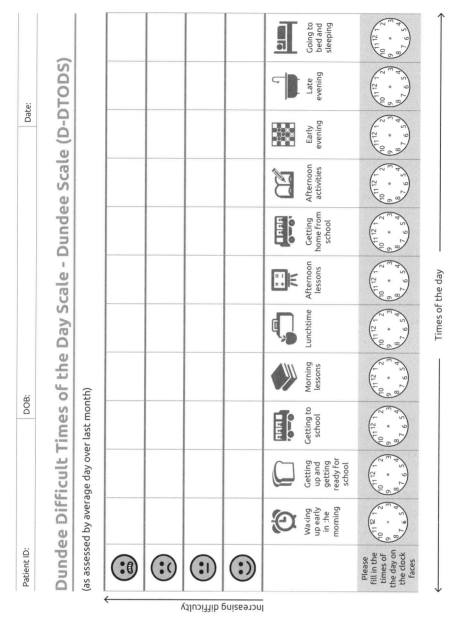

Fig. 6.1 The Dundee Difficult Times of Day Scale. © University of Dundee, 2006–2013.

Amfetamine

Although dexamfetamine has been available for many years in the UK as a treatment for ADHD, it has been used relatively infrequently and, since the introduction of atomoxetine, a non-stimulant treatment for the disorder, its use has declined even more. This is unfortunate as, notwithstanding the decision of NICE not to include any of the dexamfetamine trials in their most recent guidance (National Collaborating Centre for Mental Health, 2008), dexamfetamine is very effective. Recent meta-analyses suggest similar effect sizes for amfetamines and methylphenidate (Faraone & Buitelaar, 2010) and direct comparisons between the two suggest that around 70% respond to either methylphenidate or dexamfetamine, around 40% to both and up to 95% to one or the other (Hodgkins *et al*, 2013). This would suggest that, at the very least, dexamfetamine ought to be considered for those who do not have an adequate response to methylphenidate. One of the reasons that dexamfetamine is used less than would be predicted from the clinical trials data is the concern that it may be misused. In part this arises from a misunderstanding about the differences between dex- and metamfetamine. The latter is indeed a drug of misuse with considerable potential for illegal use. Dexamfetamine, however, like methylphenidate, is not associated with a 'drug high' unless injected or snorted intranasally. For methylphenidate, the introduction of the extended-release preparations reduced the risk of misuse considerably. In the USA, extended-release amfetamine preparations such as Adderall XR® have been available for several years, but this preparation is not licensed in Europe and will not be introduced in the future because of complex regulatory requirements.

The development of lisdexamfetamine, a dexamfetamine prodrug, makes an effective long-acting amfetamine preparation available to European clinicians for the first time. Lisdexamfetamine is taken orally and the prodrug is readily absorbed from the upper intestine. It is then cleaved by enzymes on the surface of the red blood cells into lysine and dexamfetamine, the active drug. An added benefit of lisdexamfetamine over methylphenidate preparations is that it is readily soluble and can be dissolved in water and drunk. Clinical trials have shown lisdexamfetamine to be at least as effective as methylphenidate, with a similar adverse effect profile (e.g. Coghill *et al*, 2013). In Europe, lisdexamfetamine has been licensed for use only in cases where there is an inadequate response to methylphenidate.

Non-stimulant medications

Atomoxetine

Although stimulant medications are effective in the majority of those with ADHD, there remains a significant minority who either do not respond or cannot tolerate the two available stimulant options. Atomoxetine (a specific noradrenaline reuptake inhibitor) was licensed for the treatment of ADHD in the UK in 2004 and subsequently across much of the rest of Europe. Early trials showed it to be both effective and safe in treating ADHD in adults (Spencer *et al*, 1998) and children (Michelson *et al*, 2001) and also that it has a low misuse potential. Atomoxetine is not as immediately effective as the stimulant medications, and although some patients get very clear benefits in the first few weeks, it can take up to 12 weeks for clinically relevant effects to be seen. Dosing is simpler than for the stimulants, with a starting dose of 0.5 mg/kg/day for 1 week, increased to the usual clinical dose of 1.2 mg/kg/day thereafter (sometimes increasing up to 1.8 mg/kg/day if there has been a partial response at the lower dose). The initial clinical trials with atomoxetine were all relatively short and yielded effect sizes between 0.6 and 0.7, significantly lower than those for stimulants (around 1.0). More recently, the results of longer-term studies have been published (Montoya et al, 2009; Svanborg et al, 2009). These suggest that clinical effects continue to develop over at least the first 3 months of treatment and that if one waits this long, the effect sizes also increase to values more comparable to those shown for short-term trials of stimulants.

Although it is almost certainly true that some patients respond best when on a combination of atomoxetine and a stimulant, there are legitimate safety concerns about this combination and we do not support their use together. If clinicians choose to use this combination, they should ensure that there is very close monitoring, particularly of blood pressure, pulse and other cardiac signs and symptoms.

Alpha-2 agonists

Extended-release preparations of the alpha-2 agonists clonidine and guanfacine have been licensed for the treatment of ADHD in the USA, and studies are ongoing with a guanfacine preparation in Europe. Both drugs have been shown to be efficacious as stand-alone treatments, but it is perhaps their potential as adjunctive treatments, alongside the stimulant preparations, that is most clinically relevant. A meta-analysis of 11 clonidine trials published between 1980 and 1999 in children and adolescents with ADHD (often with other comorbid disorders) reported a combined effect size of 0.58 (Connor et al, 1999). More recently, two pivotal RCTs of an extended-release clonidine preparation supported the efficacy of clonidine in children and adolescents with ADHD. Unfortunately, these results have not been published in a peer-reviewed journal. Two large, but still rather short (5–6 weeks), RCTs of extended-release guanfacine in children and adolescents with non-comorbid ADHD both found clinically relevant improvements at doses of 0.05–0.08 mg/kg/day, with additional benefits evident up to a dose of 0.12 mg/kg/day (Biederman et al, 2008; Sallee et al, 2009). A third study evaluated once-daily extended-release guanfacine in children and adolescents who had a suboptimal response to stimulants. Participants were given guanfacine in combination with a psychostimulant in a large 9-week, double-blind placebo-controlled dose-optimisation study. Symptom improvements at end-point were significantly greater for the extended-release guanfacine–stimulant combination compared with the placebo–stimulant combination for both morning and evening guanfacine dosing, and adverse effects were comparable to those reported in other ADHD drug trials.

Prevention and management of adverse effects

A full discussion of the management of adverse effects of ADHD medications is beyond the scope of this chapter. However, this area has recently been comprehensively reviewed by the European ADHD Guidelines Group (EAGG) (Graham *et al*, 2011; Cortese *et al*, 2013). Arguably the most important issue is the identification of cardiac risk before starting treatment and the ongoing management of cardiovascular adverse effects. Contrary to the suggestion of the American Heart Association (American Academy of Pediatrics & American Heart Association, 2008; Vetter *et al*, 2008), it is not necessary to conduct an electrocardiogram (ECG) for every patient before starting ADHD medications (Graham *et al*, 2011; Hamilton *et al*, 2012). It is, however, important to screen for possible cardiac risk factors. The EAGG has suggested routine enquiry into personal history of cardiac disease, history of sudden death in a close relative before the age of 40 years, symptoms of cardiac disease (effort intolerance, frequent palpitations, frequent syncope – particularly exercise induced) and other medications that could cause cardiac problems. Positive findings should prompt the clinician to consider ECG (12 lead and/or 24-hour tape) and/or a discussion with a cardiologist (Cortese *et al*, 2013). Although the average increases in pulse and blood pressure with ADHD medications are generally modest, a proportion of individuals experience clinically significant increases. The EAGG suggests that a heart rate consistently above 120 beats per minute should not be accepted without review and that a blood pressure above the 95th percentile should be considered abnormal and be followed up. Blood pressure charts that incorporate the EAGG guidelines for managing hypertension in the context of ADHD are freely available online (e.g. Dundee Blood Pressure Chart Female and Dundee Blood Pressure Chart Male, accessed through Healthcare Improvement Scotland at www. healthcareimprovementscotland.org).

Tourette syndrome

Although Tourette syndrome is defined by the presence of motor and vocal tics, it is often complicated by associated difficulties such as obsessions and compulsions, aggressive and oppositional behaviour, ADHD symptoms, mood instability, anxiety and depression. As a consequence, the quality of life in young people with Tourette syndrome is influenced by both the tics themselves, which can cause social, emotional, functional and subjective discomfort (up to severe self-mutilation), and the presence of these common comorbid conditions.

Bernard *et al* (2009) found that, in children and adolescents suffering mild to moderate tics, quality of life was not correlated to tic severity (total of motor and phonic scales) but that ADHD and obsessive–compulsive disorder (OCD), when present, did have a major impact. Eddy *et al* (2011) also investigated the clinical correlates of quality of life in Tourette syndrome and again found that the most significant factors affecting quality of life were comorbid anxiety, ADHD, obsessive–compulsive symptoms, depression and dysthymia. As each of these is a potential treatment target in itself, it is important that the clinician considering pharmacotherapy for Tourette syndrome first identifies the target symptoms to be treated and then seeks to match these symptoms to an appropriate medication. Isolated treatment of tics themselves is often not the main focus of treatment. As a consequence, medications with lower levels of evidence may sometimes be preferred to those with a stronger evidence base if they manage some of the individual's comorbid symptoms. Here we will concentrate mainly on the treatment of tics, but also mention the treatment of some other symptoms in the context of Tourette syndrome.

When thinking about treating tics it is important to take into account the natural history and course of Tourette syndrome, which usually has its onset in early childhood, increases in severity at puberty, attenuates somewhat after puberty and stabilises in adulthood. Tics fluctuate in severity throughout this time with a cycle that lasts, on average, about 3 months. This waxing and waning of tics can make it very difficult to assess the effects of pharmacological interventions and highlights the need for careful recording of the baseline and monitoring of symptoms, both before a new medication is started and during treatment.

It is also important to acknowledge the expectations of the child and the parents, the child's adaptive capacities, coping mechanisms, interpersonal relatedness, impulse control and affect regulation, together with the level of family and social support. These all have an effect on outcome that is at least as important as that of medication.

Medications for tics

Although a wide range of medications have been used to treat tics, there have been relatively few published RCTs of their use. Those studies that have been reported are helpfully summarised by Hartmann & Worbe (2012), and it is to that source that readers may refer for the results discussed in this section. Until recently, haloperidol, pimozide and, in the UK, sulpiride were the mainstay of treatment. In RCTs, all three have been shown to be efficacious in reducing tics (Sallee et al, 1997; Ho et al, 2009). Haloperidol, a typical or first-generation antipsychotic, has the strongest effect, leading to improvement in approximately two-thirds of cases, with pimozide and sulpiride improving tics in just over half. However, haloperidol is associated with frequent adverse reactions, including often disabling extrapyramidal effects. Pimozide, another typical, although associated with fewer adverse events than haloperidol, can lead to ECG abnormalities, particularly prolongation of the QT interval. For this reason and following reports of sudden unexplained death, an ECG is recommended before starting treatment and annually to review the QT interval. Sulpiride, an atypical or second-generation antipsychotic, is also associated with a lower, but not absent, rate of extrapyramidal side-effects.

In the past two decades, there has been much interest in the potential use of other atypical antipsychotics to treat Tourette syndrome. The increase in their use outstripped the available evidence and was initially based on case reports and case series. However, RCTs have now begun to appear in the literature.

Sallee et al (2000) demonstrated that ziprasidone was superior to placebo and, at a mean dose of 30 mg/day, was efficacious in reducing tics by an average of 35% in a group of 28 children and adolescents with moderate to severe tic symptoms. Dion et al (2002) found that risperidone, at a median dose of 2.5 mg/day (range 1–6 mg/day), was significantly superior to placebo in reduction of tics, with 60% in the risperidone group showing clinically significant improvements. Zhao & Zhu (2003), using slightly higher doses (up to 3.5 mg/day) in a small study involving 14 children, achieved a total response rate of 85.7%. Risperidone did not result in an increase in OCD symptoms. Indeed, at least one recent study suggests that it may actually improve OCD and can be used to augment the effects of selective serotonin reuptake inhibitors (Eddy et al, 2011). Bruggeman et al (2001) compared risperidone and pimozide in a comparative double-blind parallel-group study. At the end-point, 54% of the patients on risperidone and 38% of those taking pimozide were rated as having only very mild or no symptoms, and both treatment groups had improved significantly with regard to overall functioning. Symptoms of anxiety and low mood had also improved significantly from baseline in both groups, but improvement in obsessive–compulsive behaviour reached significance only in the risperidone group.

Onofrj et al (2000) reported the results of a very small 52-week double-blind cross-over study of olanzapine v. low-dose pimozide in four adult patients. Although the size of the trial prevents definitive conclusions being drawn, it suggested that olanzapine may be as efficacious as pimozide, with all four patients opting for olanzapine at the end of the study. Compared with haloperidol, olanzapine was similarly efficacious in reducing tics and improving global functioning in a double-blind controlled study involving 60 participants (Ji et al, 2005). Several other open-label studies support these findings and suggest that olanzapine may also reduce aggression and improve ADHD symptoms.

Most recently there has been a lot of interest in aripiprazole, even though the evidence, mostly uncontrolled studies, case reports and expert opinions, is not yet particularly strong (Hartmann & Worbe, 2012). Taken together, it suggests that when administered in doses ranging from 5 to 40 mg/day, aripiprazole has an excellent response rate combined with very good tolerability and few side-effects. Several authorities now suggest that aripiprazole should be considered as a first-line medication for moderate tics, in doses of 2.5–5 mg/day, with the possibility of higher doses in more severe cases (Hartmann & Worbe, 2012). Clearly, however, data from RCTs comparing aripiprazole with placebo or other active compounds would be useful to get a better understanding of the efficacy, range of effects and safety of the drug.

Many authors suggest that atypical antipsychotics have a positive effect on general functioning by improving emotional and behavioural symptoms as well as tics, but there is no real evidence to support this observation (Roessner et al, 2011). Although clinical experience suggests that a significant number of patients are unhappy about the adverse effects, particularly weight gain, of the atypicals, for many clinicians these drugs have become a first-line treatment for tics (Roessner et al, 2011). This reflects not only their efficacy in reducing tics, but also their impact on other target symptoms, such as ADHD, OCD and aggression.

Other pharmacological treatments for tics include: alpha-2 agonists such as clonidine and guanfacine; botulinum toxin; calcium antagonists such as nifedipine, flunarizine (not licensed in the UK or the rest of Europe) and verapamil; benzamides, GABAergic (benzodiazepines) and acetylcholinergic medications, including nicotine; cannabinoids; and the selective androgen receptor antagonist flutamide. All have received some support in open use for decreasing tics, but only flutamide has been shown to do so in an RCT (Hartmann & Worbe, 2012).

Medications for comorbid ADHD symptoms in Tourette syndrome

Children and adolescents with Tourette syndrome and also ADHD can be extremely challenging to treat. Clinical judgement is required to balance the relative impairment from ADHD symptoms and from tics before deciding the best approach to treatment. This is particularly important as it has long been debated whether stimulant medications increase tics. Double-blind placebo-controlled studies have demonstrated that stimulants are highly efficacious in the treatment of core ADHD symptoms in these patients and, in the majority, do not increase tic severity or frequency. It is therefore generally accepted that, when the aim is to control ADHD symptoms, stimulants remain a first-line treatment choice.

Atomoxetine, a non-stimulant treatment for ADHD, does not appear to be associated with increasing tic frequency or severity, and in clinical trials there is some evidence of a reduction in tic severity as well as a reduction in ADHD symptoms (Allen et al, 2005). Atomoxetine may therefore be the first-choice medication for some patients with ADHD and comorbid tics. In cases where a stimulant medication leads to either the de novo appearance of tics or an exacerbation of pre-existing tics, atomoxetine would be the first-choice alternative. Treatment with clonidine might also be considered. Although clonidine is thought to be effective in reducing tics, the results of formal trials are inconsistent

(Roessner *et al*, 2011). The drug does, however, appear to be somewhat effective at reducing ADHD symptoms, irrespective of the presence or absence of tics, although these effects are much less clear than for the stimulants and atomoxetine (Connor *et al*, 1999). As noted above, atypical antipsychotics such as risperidone, olanzapine and aripiprazole are also reported to have a certain effect on behavioural symptoms, although further evidence is required. For more detailed advice on using antipsychotics in children and adolescents see the section on schizophrenia in Chapter 7.

Autism spectrum disorder

In DSM-5, the various aspects of autism are brought together in the single diagnosis of autism spectrum disorder (ASD), the core features of which are deficits in social and communicative functioning as well as repetitive behaviours, interests or activities (American Psychiatric Association, 2013). Differential diagnosis remains challenging and it is clear that, both aetiologically and clinically, ASD is a heterogeneous disorder and our understanding of its complex aetiology remains incomplete. The full clinical picture of ASD includes the core symptoms, as well as associated troublesome behaviours and comorbid disorders. It is these associated behaviours and comorbid symptoms, rather than the core ASD symptoms, that usually become the target for pharmacological and non-pharmacological treatments. Seventy per cent of those with ASD have at least one comorbid disorder and 41% have more than one (Simonoff *et al*, 2008). It is unclear whether some of these emotional and behavioural symptoms represent core, associated or comorbid features in ASD, and whether efficacy of treatment related to a specific target symptom can be related to the disorder itself.

There are, as yet, no medications licensed for treating the core symptoms of ASD. It has been suggested that the clinician- and parent-reported symptoms that are potential targets for intervention can be grouped into seven categories: aggression to others, self-injurious behaviour, property destruction, tantrums, yelling/screaming, stereotypy and hyperactivity/impulsivity/agitation. Of these, the only symptom for which there are medications approved by the Food and Drug Administration (FDA) is irritability (risperidone from 2006, and aripiprazole from 2009). Indeed, irritability in ASD was the first case in which the FDA accepted a symptom, rather than a disorder, as an indication for treatment. Identification of patients' problematic behaviour(s), their translation into target symptoms for intervention and the selection of a treatment according to the existing evidence are the three key steps in providing drug treatment for ASD. Even though the evidence for efficacy/effectiveness and safety of pharmacological treatments for these various target symptoms is rather sparse, a working knowledge of what has been studied is helpful in planning clinical work and we will therefore focus on these key symptom groups.

Medications for irritability, aggression and antisocial behaviour

For many individuals with ASD, irritability and aggression are among the most impairing symptoms. They are also the best studied with respect to pharmacological interventions. Various antipsychotics, mood stabilisers, antidepressants (clomipramine) and other agents (clonidine, amantadine, naltrexone, pentoxifylline) have been investigated for reduction of irritability in the context of ASD. As already mentioned, two drugs have been licensed by the FDA for this indication. Risperidone may be prescribed to children over 5 years of age and a body weight of 20 lb (9.1 kg) and aripiprazole to children older than 6 years. The effect size is around 1.2 for risperidone (0.5–3.5 mg/day) and 0.6–0.9 for aripiprazole (5–15 mg/day) (Marcus *et al*, 2009). Extrapyramidal side-effects, weight gain, dizziness and somnolence are the most important adverse effects associated with these medications. It should be noted, however, that their positive effects on irritability and aggression do not appear to be due to somnolence. Of the drugs prescribed off-label, valproic acid in doses resulting in blood valproate levels of 603–762 µmol/l has been shown to reduce irritability scores on the Clinical Global Impression irritability subscale (CGI-I) in a majority (62.5%) of participants (Hollander *et al*, 2010), and also to confer statistically significant improvements in scores on the irritability subscale of the Aberrant Behavior Checklist (ABC). Clomipramine in doses of 100–150 mg/day did not modify irritability on the ABC irritability subscale (Remington *et al*, 2001). Clonidine resulted in improvements on this subscale, although the evidence is not yet sufficient to make any firm conclusions as the study included only 8 participants (Jaselskis *et al*, 1992). Multiple studies have failed to find clinically significant effects on irritability for both naltrexone and amantadine. Preliminary evidence obtained from a study of pentoxifylline (a xanthine derivative that improves blood flow through peripheral blood vessels) administered in combination with risperidone suggests a significant decrease of irritability on the ABC (Akhondzadeh *et al*, 2010).

Medications for hyperactivity, impulsivity and inattention

Despite considerable debate about the status of ADHD symptoms such as hyperactivity, impulsivity and inattention in children with ASD, it is clear that they are present in 40–50% of young patients with pervasive developmental disorders (Jahromi *et al*, 2009). Until now, nosological convention has been to view and analyse them as ADHD symptoms present in ASD and not ADHD comorbid with ASD. However, this has changed with the publication of DSM-5, which for the first time allows ADHD to be formally diagnosed in the context of an ASD diagnosis. In clinical trials hyperactivity, irritability and impulsivity in ASD are treated as target symptoms that can be influenced by medication, and an ADHD diagnosis has usually not been required for inclusion in such trials.

A reasonably sized trial investigating the efficacy of methylphenidate was conducted by the Research Units on Pediatric Psychopharmacology (RUPP) Autism Network, which is sponsored by the US National Institutes of Health (McDougle *et al*, 2005). It included 72 children, 5–14 years of age, with autism and long-standing moderate to severe hyperactivity. This randomised placebo-controlled cross-over study included an initial 1-week tolerability phase, followed by a 4-week cross-over phase, and 8-week open-label continuation phase. During the 1-week tolerability phase each participant received placebo for 1 day, followed by increasing doses of methylphenidate (low, medium and high doses) that were each given for 2 days. The low, medium and high doses were based on the child's weight, and ranged from 7.5 to 50.0 mg/day in divided doses. There was a response rate of 49% in children with ASD complicated by hyperactivity, compared with 70–80% in typically developing children with ADHD. Similar results were reported from two earlier smaller studies (Quintana *et al*, 1995; Handen *et al*, 2000). Both of these studies reported similar adverse effects (mainly irritability and social withdrawal) in the active treatment arms. There is some evidence to suggest that methylphenidate can also improve social communication and self-regulation (Jahromi *et al*, 2009).

There is some preliminary evidence to suggest that atomoxetine may also be effective in treating ADHD symptoms in those with ASD. An initial very small randomised placebo-controlled cross-over trial ($n = 16$) suggested an effect size comparable to that of methylphenidate (0.90 for decrease of scores on the hyperactivity subscale of the ABC, 1.27 for decrease of hyperactivity/impulsivity DSM-IV ADHD symptoms) (Arnold *et al*, 2006). A larger 8-week randomised controlled trial involving 97 children and adolescents with ADHD and ASD supported a positive effect of atomoxetine on ADHD symptom reduction, but not on the CGI-I, compared with placebo (Harfterkamp *et al*, 2012). Although the effects on symptoms were significant they, and the response rate on the CGI-I, were much less than typically seen in uncomplicated ADHD. In an open-label follow-up of this study, the treatment effects were maintained and indeed ADHD symptoms continued to improve up to 28 weeks (Harfterkamp *et al*, 2013). However, children with severe autism were not thought to benefit significantly from atomoxetine administered for 10 weeks (Charnsil, 2011). Although their overall functioning was improved on the CGI scale, there was no improvement on the primary outcome (a reduction in hyperactivity on the ABC), and symptoms of inattentiveness also remained prominent. Safety observations showed that adverse events caused 25% to be withdrawn from the study. The children also experienced more adverse events than children with less severe autism in other studies. These same problems with tolerability limited the dose to 0.98 mg/kg/day, which may also have influenced treatment efficacy.

Clonidine has also been investigated in the context of ADHD in ASD. Although a small open-label study involving 19 children reported some decrease in hyperactivity, the researchers felt that this effect might have been caused by the improvement of sleep (Ming *et al*, 2008).

Medications for stereotypies and repetitive behaviours

On the basis of various neurobiological hypotheses, antipsychotics, antidepressants and mood stabilisers have been studied as potential treatments for the reduction of stereotypies and repetitive behaviours in children and adolescents with ASD. Randomised controlled trials of aripiprazole (Marcus *et al*, 2009; Owen *et al*, 2009) and risperidone (McDougle *et al*, 2005) both reported significant improvement in more than 50% of study participants. Statistically but not clinically significant response has also been reported for fluoxetine and valproic acid (Hollander *et al*, 2005, 2010), haloperidol and clomipramine (Remington *et al*, 2001). A 12-week trial of citalopram found no improvement on the Children's Yale–Brown Obsessive Compulsive Scale (CY-BOCS) of the CGI (King *et al*, 2009).

Summary

Difficulties in differential diagnosis, various evidence levels for different medications, and variable definitions and interpretations of core symptoms by patients, caregivers and clinicians make an individualised treatment the most appropriate, and probably the only possible approach for ASD in children and adolescents. Evidence shows that antipsychotics (risperidone and aripiprazole) are effective in reducing such symptoms as irritability and repetitive behaviours, while the stimulant methylphenidate (and possibly the non-stimulant atomoxetine) is effective for hyperactivity and broader ADHD symptoms.

Conclusion

All of the disorders reviewed in this chapter are chronic and continue into adult life. Increasing evidence supports the use of medication to manage at least some of the symptoms and reduce the impairments associated with them. Nevertheless, other approaches to treatment have much to offer.

References

Akhondzadeh S, Fallah J, Mohammadi MR, *et al* (2010) Double-blind placebo-controlled trial of pentoxifylline added to risperidone: effects on aberrant behavior in children with autism. *Progress in Neuro-Psychopharmacology & Biological Psychiatry*, **34**, 32–36.

Allen AJ, Kurlan RM, Gilbert DL, *et al* (2005) Atomoxetine treatment in children and adolescents with ADHD and comorbid tic disorders. *Neurology*, **65**, 1941–1949.

American Academy of Pediatrics & American Heart Association (2008) American Academy of Pediatrics/American Heart Association clarification of statement on cardiovascular evaluation and monitoring of children and adolescents with heart disease receiving medications for ADHD: May 16, 2008. *Journal of Developmental and Behavioral Pediatrics*, **29**, 335.

American Psychiatric Association (1994) *Diagnostic and Statistical Manual of Mental Disorders (4th edn) (DSM-IV)*. APA.

American Psychiatric Association (2013) *Diagnostic and Statistical Manual of Mental Disorders (5th edn) (DSM-5)*. APA.

Arnold LE, Aman MG, Cook AM, *et al* (2006) Atomoxetine for hyperactivity in autism spectrum disorders: placebo-controlled crossover pilot trial. *Journal of the American Academy of Child & Adolescent Psychiatry*, **45**, 1196–1205.

Banaschewski T, Coghill D, Santosh P, *et al* (2006) Long-acting medications for the hyperkinetic disorders: a systematic review and European treatment guideline. *European Child & Adolescent Psychiatry*, **15**, 476–495.

Banaschewski T, Buitelaar J, Coghill DR, *et al* (2009) The MTA at 8. *Journal of the American Academy of Child & Adolescent Psychiatry*, **48**, 1120–1121.

Bernard BA, Stebbins GT, Siegel S, *et al* (2009) Determinants of quality of life in children with Gilles de la Tourette syndrome. *Movement Disorders*, **24**, 1070–1073.

Biederman J, Melmed RD, Patel A, *et al* (2008) A randomized, double-blind, placebo-controlled study of guanfacine extended release in children and adolescents with attention-deficit/hyperactivity disorder. *Pediatrics*, **121**, e73–e84.

Bruggeman R, van der Linden C, Buitelaar JK, *et al* (2001) Risperidone versus pimozide in Tourette's disorder: a comparative double-blind parallel-group study. *Journal of Clinical Psychiatry*, **62**, 50–56.

Charnsil C (2011) Efficacy of atomoxetine in children with severe autistic disorders and symptoms of ADHD: an open-label study. *Journal of Attention Disorders*, **15**, 684–689.

Coghill D (2010) The impact of medications on quality of life in attention-deficit hyperactivity disorder: a systematic review. *CNS Drugs*, **24**, 843–866.

Coghill DR, Rhodes SM, Matthews K (2007) The neuropsychological effects of chronic methylphenidate on drug-naive boys with attention-deficit/hyperactivity disorder. *Biological Psychiatry*, **62**, 954–962.

Coghill D, Banaschewski T, Lecendreux M, *et al* (2013) European, randomized, phase 3 study of lisdexamfetamine dimesylate in children and adolescents with attention-deficit/hyperactivity disorder. *European Neuropsychopharmacology*, **23**, 1208–1218.

Connor DF, Fletcher KE, Swanson JM (1999) A meta-analysis of clonidine for symptoms of attention-deficit hyperactivity disorder. *Journal of the American Academy of Child & Adolescent Psychiatry*, **38**, 1551–1559.

Cortese S, Holtmann M, Banaschewski T, *et al* (2013) Current best practice in the management of AEs during treatment with ADHD medications in children and adolescents. *Journal of Child Psychology and Psychiatry*, **54**, 227–246.

Dion Y, Annable L, Sandor P, *et al* (2002) Risperidone in the treatment of Tourette syndrome: a double-blind, placebo-controlled trial. *Journal of Clinical Psychopharmacology*, **22**, 31–39.

Eddy CM, Cavanna AE, Gulisano M, *et al* (2011) Clinical correlates of quality of life in Tourette syndrome. *Movement Disorders*, **26**, 735–738.

Faraone SV, Buitelaar J (2010) Comparing the efficacy of stimulants for ADHD in children and adolescents using meta-analysis. *European Child & Adolescent Psychiatry*, **19**, 353–364.

Graham J, Banaschewski T, Buitelaar J, *et al* (2011) European guidelines on managing adverse effects of medication for ADHD. *European Child & Adolescent Psychiatry*, **20**, 17–37.

Hamilton RM, Rosenthal E, Hulpke-Wette M, *et al* (2012) Cardiovascular considerations of attention deficit hyperactivity disorder medications: a report of the European Network on Hyperactivity Disorders work group, European Attention Deficit Hyperactivity Disorder Guidelines Group on attention deficit hyperactivity disorder drug safety meeting. *Cardiology in the Young*, **22**, 63–70.

Handen BL, Johnson CR, Lubetsky M (2000) Efficacy of methylphenidate among children with autism and symptoms of attention-deficit hyperactivity disorder. *Journal of Autism and Developmental Disorders*, **30**, 245–255.

Harfterkamp M, van de Loo-Neus G, Minderaa RB, *et al* (2012) A randomized double-blind study of atomoxetine versus placebo for attention-deficit/hyperactivity disorder symptoms in children with autism spectrum disorder. *Journal of the American Academy of Child & Adolescent Psychiatry*, **51**, 733–741.

Harfterkamp M, Buitelaar JK, Minderaa RB, *et al* (2013) Long-term treatment with atomoxetine for attention-deficit/hyperactivity disorder symptoms in children and adolescents with autism spectrum disorder: an open-label extension study. *Journal of Child and Adolescent Psychopharmacology*, **23**, 194–199.

Hartmann A, Worbe Y (2102) Pharmacological treatment of Gilles de la Tourette syndrome. *Neuroscience and Biobehavioral Reviews*, **37**, 1157–1161.

Ho CS, Chen HJ, Chiu NC, *et al* (2009) Short-term sulpiride treatment of children and adolescents with Tourette syndrome or chronic tic disorder. *Journal of the Formosan Medical Association*, **108**, 788–793.

Hodgkins P, Shaw M, Coghill D, *et al* (2013) Amfetamine and methylphenidate medications for attention-deficit/hyperactivity disorder: complementary treatment options. *European Child & Adolescent Psychiatry*, **21**, 477–492.

Hollander E, Phillips A, Chaplin W, *et al* (2005) A placebo controlled crossover trial of liquid fluoxetine on repetitive behaviors in childhood and adolescent autism. *Neuropsychopharmacology*, **30**, 582–589.

Hollander E, Chaplin W, Soorya L, *et al* (2010) Divalproex sodium vs placebo for the treatment of irritability in children and adolescents with autism spectrum disorders. *Neuropsychopharmacology*, **35**, 990–998.

Jahromi LB, Kasari CL, McCracken JT, *et al* (2009) Positive effects of methylphenidate on social communication and self-regulation in children with pervasive developmental disorders and hyperactivity. *Journal of Autism and Developmental Disorders*, **39**, 395–404.

Jaselskis CA, Cook EH Jr, Fletcher KE, *et al* (1992) Clonidine treatment of hyperactive and impulsive children with autistic disorder. *Journal of Clinical Psychopharmacology*, **12**, 322–327.

Jensen PS, Arnold LE, Swanson JM, *et al* (2007) 3-year follow-up of the NIMH MTA study. *Journal of the American Academy of Child & Adolescent Psychiatry*, **46**, 989–1002.

Ji W-D, Li Y, Li N, *et al* (2005) Olanzapine for treatment of Tourette Syndrome: a double-blind randomized controlled trial. *Chinese Journal of Clinical Rehabilitation*, **9**, 66–68.

King BH, Hollander E, Sikich L, *et al* (2009) Lack of efficacy of citalopram in children with autism spectrum disorders and high levels of repetitive behavior: citalopram ineffective in children with autism. *Archives of General Psychiatry*, **66**, 583–590.

Marcus RN, Owen R, Kamen L, *et al* (2009) A placebo-controlled, fixed-dose study of aripiprazole in children and adolescents with irritability associated with autistic disorder. *Journal of the American Academy of Child & Adolescent Psychiatry*, **48**, 1110–1119.

McDougle CJ, Scahill L, Aman MG, *et al* (2005) Risperidone for the core symptom domains of autism: results from the study by the autism network of the research units on pediatric psychopharmacology. *American Journal of Psychiatry*, **162**, 1142–1148.

Michelson D, Faries D, Wernicke J, *et al* (2001) Atomoxetine in the treatment of children and adolescents with attention-deficit/hyperactivity disorder: a randomized, placebo-controlled, dose-response study. *Pediatrics*, **108**, E83.

Ming X, Gordon E, Kang N, *et al* (2008) Use of clonidine in children with autism spectrum disorders. *Brain and Development*, **30**, 454–460.

Molina BS, Hinshaw SP, Swanson JM, *et al* (2009) The MTA at 8 years: prospective follow-up of children treated for combined-type ADHD in a multisite study. *Journal of the American Academy of Child & Adolescent Psychiatry*, **48**, 484–500.

Montoya A, Hervas A, Cardo E, *et al* (2009) Evaluation of atomoxetine for first-line treatment of newly diagnosed, treatment-naive children and adolescents with attention deficit/hyperactivity disorder. *Current Medical Research and Opinion*, **25**, 2745–2754.

National Collaborating Centre for Mental Health (2008) *Attention Deficit Hyperactivity Disorder: The NICE Guideline on Diagnosis and Management of ADHD in Children, Young People and Adults* (National Clinical Practice Guideline Number 72). British Psychological Society & Royal College of Psychiatrists.

Onofrj M, Paci C, D'Andreamatteo G, et al (2000) Olanzapine in severe Gilles de la Tourette syndrome: a 52-week double-blind cross-over study vs. low-dose pimozide. *Journal of Neurology*, **247**, 443–446.

Owen R, Sikich L, Marcus RN, et al (2009) Aripiprazole in the treatment of irritability in children and adolescents with autistic disorder. *Pediatrics*, **124**, 1533–1540.

Quintana H, Birmaher B, Stedge D, et al (1995) Use of methylphenidate in the treatment of children with autistic disorder. *Journal of Autism and Developmental Disorders*, **25**, 283–294.

Remington G, Sloman L, Konstantareas M, et al (2001) Clomipramine versus haloperidol in the treatment of autistic disorder: a double-blind, placebo-controlled, crossover study. *Journal of Clinical Psychopharmacology*, **21**, 440–444.

Roessner V, Plessen KJ, Rothenberger A, et al (2011) European clinical guidelines for Tourette syndrome and other tic disorders. Part II: pharmacological treatment. *European Child & Adolescent Psychiatry*, **20**, 173–196.

Sallee FR, Nesbitt L, Jackson C, et al (1997) Relative efficacy of haloperidol and pimozide in children and adolescents with Tourette's disorder. *American Journal of Psychiatry*, **154**, 1057–1062.

Sallee FR, Kurlan R, Goetz CG, et al (2000) Ziprasidone treatment of children and adolescents with Tourette's syndrome: a pilot study. *Journal of the American Academy of Child & Adolescent Psychiatry*, **39**, 292–299.

Sallee FR, McGough J, Wigal T, et al (2009) Guanfacine extended release in children and adolescents with attention-deficit/hyperactivity disorder: a placebo-controlled trial. *Journal of the American Academy of Child & Adolescent Psychiatry*, **48**, 155–165.

Santosh PJ, Taylor E, Swanson J, et al (2005) Refining the diagnoses of inattention and overactivity syndromes: a reanalysis of the multimodal treatment study of attention deficit hyperactivity disorder (ADHD) based on ICD-10 criteria for hyperkinetic disorder. *Clinical Neuroscience Research*, **5**, 307–314.

Simonoff E, Pickles A, Charman T, et al (2008) Psychiatric disorders in children with autism spectrum disorders: prevalence, comorbidity, and associated factors in a population-derived sample. *Journal of the American Academy of Child & Adolescent Psychiatry*, **47**, 921–929.

Sonuga-Barke EJ, Swanson JM, Coghill D, et al (2004) Efficacy of two once-daily methylphenidate formulations compared across dose levels at different times of the day: preliminary indications from a secondary analysis of the COMACS study data. *BMC Psychiatry*, **4**, 28.

Sonuga-Barke EJ, Brandeis D, Cortese S, et al (2013) Nonpharmacological interventions for ADHD: systematic review and meta-analyses of randomized controlled trials of dietary and psychological treatments. *American Journal of Psychiatry*, **170**, 275–289.

Spencer T, Biederman J, Wilens T, et al (1998) Effectiveness and tolerability of tomoxetine in adults with attention deficit hyperactivity disorder. *American Journal of Psychiatry*, **155**, 693–695.

Svanborg P, Thernlund G, Gustafsson PA, et al (2009) Efficacy and safety of atomoxetine as add-on to psychoeducation in the treatment of attention deficit/hyperactivity disorder: a randomized, double-blind, placebo-controlled study in stimulant-naive Swedish children and adolescents. *European Child & Adolescent Psychiatry*, **18**, 240–249.

Swanson J, Gupta S, Guinta D, et al (1999) Acute tolerance to methylphenidate in the treatment of attention deficit hyperactivity disorder in children. *Clinical Pharmacology & Therapeutics*, **66**, 295–305.

Swanson J, Arnold LE, Kraemer H, et al (2008a) Evidence, interpretation, and qualification from multiple reports of long-term outcomes in the Multimodal Treatment Study of

Children with ADHD (MTA). Part I: executive summary. *Journal of Attention Disorders,* **12**, 4–14.

Swanson J, Arnold LE, Kraemer H, *et al* (2008*b*) Evidence, interpretation, and qualification from multiple reports of long-term outcomes in the Multimodal Treatment Study of Children with ADHD (MTA). Part II: supporting details. *Journal of Attention Disorders,* **12**, 15–43.

Taylor E, Dopfner M, Sergeant J, *et al* (2004) European clinical guidelines for hyperkinetic disorder: first upgrade. *European Child & Adolescent Psychiatry,* **13** (suppl 1), I7–30.

Vetter VL, Elia J, Erickson C, *et al* (2008) Cardiovascular monitoring of children and adolescents with heart disease receiving stimulant drugs: a scientific statement from the American Heart Association Council on Cardiovascular Disease in the Young Congenital Cardiac Defects Committee and the Council on Cardiovascular Nursing. *Circulation,* **117**, 2407–2423.

Volkow ND, Ding YS, Fowler JS, *et al* (1995) Is methylphenidate like cocaine? Studies on their pharmacokinetics and distribution in the human brain. *Archives of General Psychiatry,* **52**, 456–463.

World Health Organization (1992) *The ICD-10 Classification of Mental and Behavioural Disorders: Clinical Descriptions and Diagnostic Guidelines.* WHO.

Zhao H, Zhu Y (2003) Risperidone in the treatment of Tourette Syndrome. *Chinese Mental Health Journal,* **17**, 30–40.

CHAPTER 7

Pharmacology for anxiety and obsessive–compulsive disorders, affective disorders and schizophrenia

Eugenia Sinita and David Coghill

This chapter has been written as a companion to Chapter 6. Here we focus on current pharmacological approaches to the treatment of anxiety disorders, obsessive–compulsive disorder, affective disorders and schizophrenia in children and adolescents.

Anxiety disorders

Despite being the most common psychiatric illness in childhood and adolescence, affecting somewhere between 5 and 18% of young people, early-onset anxiety disorders remain poorly understood. They can, however, cause serious disruption to children's lives and are often persistent over time, leading to increased risks of continued anxiety disorders in adulthood as well as major depression, substance misuse and educational underachievement. The use of medication to manage child and adolescent anxiety disorders remains contentious, with many clinicians arguing that these disorders are always most appropriately treated with psychosocial interventions. However, as success rates for cognitive and behavioural interventions fall in the range of 70–80%, significant numbers of children require further treatments.

Benzodiazepines and tricyclic antidepressants

The first drugs to be studied in the treatment of child and adolescent anxiety were benzodiazepines and tricyclic antidepressants. Benzodiazepines should be considered only when other pharmacological approaches have failed, and they should be prescribed for weeks rather than months. Dose adjustments should be made gradually, both when starting and when tapering off treatment (Velosa & Riddle, 2000). There have been several randomised controlled trials (RCTs) of tricyclic antidepressants in the treatment of paediatric anxiety. Unfortunately, the positive results from initial studies have not been sustained (Velosa & Riddle, 2000) and tricyclics should not be considered as first-line treatments for anxiety disorders in this age group. Several open-label studies have shown buspirone, a non-benzodiazepine anxiolytic reported effective in adults, to be comparable in efficacy to the benzodiazepines, with fewer adverse events, in childhood anxiety disorders. However, no controlled data are available for either safety or efficacy.

Selective serotonin reuptake inhibitors

The selective serotonin reuptake inhibitors (SSRIs) are now the first-choice pharmacological treatment for child and adolescent anxiety disorders. As in depression (see below), their use increased before firm data on their efficacy were available. However, there are now RCT data for fluvoxamine, fluoxetine, sertraline, paroxetine and venlafaxine.

The first RCT data were published by the Research Unit on Pediatric Psychopharmacology Anxiety Study Group (2001). The group conducted a well-designed, large-scale RCT that compared fluvoxamine (up to a maximum dose of 300 mg/day) with placebo in 128 children and adolescents with social phobia, separation anxiety disorder or generalised anxiety disorder, all of whom had failed to respond to 3 weeks of psychological therapy. From the beginning of the third week, children in the fluvoxamine group showed greater reductions on both the Pediatric Anxiety Rating Scale (PARS) and the Clinical Global Impression Improvement (CGI-I) scale than those receiving placebo. Clinical improvement reached its maximum in week 6, with little change afterwards. Effect size was calculated to be 1.1 for fluvoxamine. Few participants dropped out from either group as a result of adverse events, suggesting that fluvoxamine is an efficacious and safe treatment for anxiety in this population.

A smaller RCT compared fluoxetine at a dose of 20 mg/day with placebo (Birmaher et al, 2003). Fluoxetine was effective in reducing anxiety symptoms and improving functioning on all measures, with an effect size of 0.53 and number needed to treat (NNT, how many need to be treated for one to truly respond) of 4. A further small RCT comparing sertraline at a dose of up to 50 mg/day and placebo in 22 children and adolescents with generalised anxiety disorder also reported significant global improvements and a decrease in anxiety symptoms beginning after 4 weeks of treatment (Rynn et al, 2001). The rate of adverse effects in the active treatment arm was no higher than for placebo.

There has been one RCT comparing paroxetine with placebo in children and adolescents with social anxiety. Interestingly, comorbid conditions, such as specific phobia, generalised anxiety and separation anxiety disorders, were also allowed, so results may generalise somewhat. This trial included a total of 322 young people randomised to paroxetine or placebo for 16 weeks (Wagner et al, 2004). Rates of withdrawal due to adverse events were low in both groups, and efficacy of the active compound was observed in the first 4 weeks of treatment, with an effect size of 0.88. *Post hoc* analysis found a remission rate of 47.2% for those receiving paroxetine *v.* 13.3% for placebo, with an NNT of 3.

The efficacy of venlafaxine was evaluated in two RCTs (March *et al*, 2007; Rynn *et al*, 2007), with treatment lasting 8 and 16 weeks respectively and good-sized samples (293 and 320 participants). Venlafaxine was superior to placebo in both studies, with effect sizes of 0.45 and 0.57, and NNT of 6 and 5. Several adverse effects, such as asthenia, anorexia, pain, somnolence, as well as statistically significant changes in height, weight, blood pressure, pulse and cholesterol levels, were greater in those taking the extended-release venlafaxine (Rynn *et al*, 2007).

Long-term safety of SSRIs

All of these studies were short-term trials, lasting a maximum of 16 weeks and often much less. Despite the absence of clear evidence, concerns have been expressed about the long-term safety of SSRIs for children and adolescents. Animal studies raise the possibility of long-term negative effects on brain and development. The administration of SSRIs to juvenile rodents has in some studies been shown to induce long-term changes in serotonergic transmission in the cortex and hippocampus. However, these concerns must be balanced against the finding that chronic stress, such as that associated with ongoing anxiety, also results in unwanted long-term changes to neurochemistry and neuronal development.

Only one clinical study has investigated long-term treatment. The Child/Adolescent Anxiety Multimodal Study (Walkup *et al*, 2008; Compton *et al*, 2010) investigated both short-term efficacy (12 weeks) and long-term persistence of effect (36 weeks) in four treatment groups: cognitive–behavioural therapy (CBT); sertraline; combined therapy (CBT + sertraline); and placebo. This was a large study that included 488 children and adolescents. The inclusion criteria allowed for comorbid conditions such as attention-deficit hyperactivity disorder (ADHD), major depression and dysthymia, which helps with the generalisation of the results to clinic populations. It was found that 80.7% of patients receiving combined therapy had a significant improvement on the CGI-I, compared with 59.7% of those receiving CBT alone and 54.9% receiving sertraline. Effect sizes based on the PARS were 0.86 for combined therapy, 0.45 for sertraline and 0.31 for CBT; NNT were 2 for combined therapy, 3 for sertraline and 3 for CBT. Again, there were no differences in adverse event rates between the sertraline and placebo groups. Clearly, further studies investigating the long-term safety and efficacy of SSRIs in paediatric anxiety disorders are required, as well as research to clarify the effects of both stress and SSRIs on human brain and development.

Psychological or pharmacological treatment?

As already mentioned, although initial psychological treatments are effective for up to 80% of young patients with anxiety disorders, a significant proportion will benefit from pharmacological treatments. Indeed, effect sizes and response rates for medications seem to be greater for children and adolescents with anxiety disorders than for adults. Unfortunately, it is not yet possible predict which young people will respond to either psychological or pharmacological treatments (Nilsen *et al*, 2013). The complex neurobiological basis of anxiety spectrum disorders makes clinical decision-making even more difficult, as agents capable of suppressing one type of anxiety may not work for other types. When using medication, the SSRIs should be seen as the first-line treatment for anxiety disorders in children and adolescents. Clinicians should allow at least 3 weeks at an adequate dose (Table 7.1) before deciding whether there has been a response. In cases of non-response it would be appropriate to switch to an alternative SSRI before changing to a drug from a different class. Even where a pharmacological approach is chosen it should usually be combined with a psychotherapeutic approach, as this has been demonstrated to increase response rates and clinical improvement.

Anxiety disorders in ADHD

Many children with ADHD present with comorbid anxiety disorders. There has been uncertainty as to whether these children respond as well to methylphenidate as do children with ADHD alone. Initial studies suggested that anxiety may blunt the response to methylphenidate, but several good-quality studies undertaken more recently question these

Table 7.1 Doses and indications for medications used to treat depression, anxiety and obsessive–compulsive disorder (OCD) in children and adolescents

Name	Indication	Age, years	Average daily dose, mg	BNFC recognised indication
Buspirone	Anxiety	Not stated	Not stated	No
Clomipramine	OCD	Not stated	Not stated	No
Fluoxetine	Major depression	8–18	10–20	Yes
Fluvoxamine	OCD	8–18	25–100	Yes
	Anxiety	Not stated	Not stated	No
	Depression	Not stated	Not stated	No
Paroxetine	Anxiety, depression	Not stated	Not stated	Unfavourable
Sertraline	OCD	6–12	25–200	Yes
		12–18	50–200	
	Major depression	12–18	50–200	Unfavourable
Venlafaxine	Anxiety, depression	Not stated	Not stated	Unfavourable

BNFC, *British National Formulary for Children* (BMJ Group *et al*, 2013).

97

findings. Initial reports from the Multimodal Treatment of Attention Deficit Hyperactivity Disorder (MTA; discussed in Chapter 6, pp. 75–76) reported that children with ADHD and anxiety disorders showed enhanced responses to a behavioural intervention, both when given alone and when given in combination with medication. They did not, however, display a reduced response to medication when it was given alone. Secondary, more detailed analyses of these data confirmed both the importance of psychosocial treatment for children with anxiety disorders and ADHD and that anxiety has no adverse effect on the response to stimulant medication (March *et al*, 2000). Another study found that, compared with those treated with placebo, children and adolescents with ADHD and anxiety treated with atomoxetine showed reductions in both ADHD and anxiety symptoms, suggesting that atomoxetine may be a good choice for this group (Geller *et al*, 2007). Children with combined ADHD, anxiety and either oppositional defiant disorder or conduct disorder seem to benefit particularly from combined psycho-social interventions and medication.

Obsessive–compulsive disorder

Compared with generalised anxiety there is a much stronger evidence base to support the use of drug treatments for early-onset OCD. Current theories of OCD stress the role of dysregulation in central serotonin sub-systems, with target areas of dysfunction including the basal ganglia and orbitofrontal cortex. Although the true situation is likely to be rather more complex and involve other brain regions and neurotransmitters, it is not surprising that serotonin-enhancing agents such as the SSRIs and clomipramine are efficacious treatments for this disorder. The overall effect size for pharmacotherapy in children and adolescents is medium at 0.48, and the NNT is 6, with some variation between different medications (Watson & Rees, 2008). These figures are similar to those reported for adults.

The tricyclic antidepressant clomipramine has been shown in several RCTs to be the most efficacious drug in treating child and adolescent OCD, and multivariate regression has demonstrated its superiority to each of the SSRIs. This anti-obsessional effect is independent of antidepressant effect and is not seen with other tricyclics (Grados *et al*, 1999). Notwithstanding its superiority in efficacy, concern over the safety of clomipramine led to increased interest in the use of the SSRIs in early-onset OCD. A number of RCTs have found positive effects *v.* placebo for fluoxetine, fluvoxamine, paroxetine and sertraline. Clomipramine is still recommended for OCD in the presence of comorbid psychiatric conditions or following poor response to an initial trial of an SSRI or SSRI combined with CBT (National Collaborating Centre for Mental Health, 2005*a*). Average daily doses of fluvoxamine and sertraline are shown in Table 7.1.

Duration of treatment and response rates

There are now ten published RCT comparisons for early-onset OCD. These trials are of variable quality, but they include several large methodologically sound studies and it seems reasonable to conclude that the SSRIs are both safe and efficacious in the short- and medium-term treatment of paediatric OCD, either as a single disorder or where accompanied by tic disorder/ Tourette syndrome or ADHD (March *et al*, 1998; Geller *et al*, 2001; Riddle *et al*, 2001; Watson & Rees, 2008). The time taken to respond to treatment varies between the studies and, even though Riddle *et al* (2001) reported significant responses after only 1 week of treatment, most authors suggest titration over 6–8 weeks to maximum doses in partial or non-responders.

Obsessive–compulsive disorder is recognised as a chronic condition that persists into early adulthood in about 50% of early-onset cases. Several studies report that long-term treatment with SSRIs is not only well tolerated and effective at maintaining improvement, but also results in continued improvement for up to 1 year (Cook *et al*, 2001; Thomsen *et al*, 2001). Treatment continued after this time appears to remain effective but does not result in further improvements. Optimal duration of treatment for children with OCD is unknown. Obsessional symptoms may relapse on discontinuation of treatment, but it is suggested that treatment should be withdrawn after 1–1.5 years and restarted if significant symptoms reoccur.

Although these results are encouraging it has been suggested that, as a group, children and adolescents with OCD may not respond as well to some SSRIs as do adults. In one small study, around 25% showed no improvement after a trial of an SSRI, and for those who did respond, most reported a 20–50% improvement in symptoms; only 20–25% of those treated with medication alone were symptom-free at the end of a course of treatment (Thomsen, 2000). It has been suggested that early-onset OCD is a subtype of OCD that is more difficult to treat effectively. As a significant proportion of those with paediatric OCD are thought to develop obsessive–compulsive personality disorder, rather than true obsessive–compulsive disorder, as adults, it is possible that these individuals would be more resistant to treatment from an early age. Whatever the explanation, it is important that medication is not viewed in isolation: it should usually be given in combination with CBT. Interestingly, medication and CBT appear to have additive effects, with the effect size for combined treatment being similar to the arithmetic sum of that of the component treatments given separately (Pediatric OCD Treatment Study (POTS) Team, 2004).

Non-response

If the patient does not respond to medication, it is important to assess treatment adherence and to ensure that other factors, such as family discord, other psychosocial stressors and comorbid disorders, have been adequately addressed. Earlier age at onset, longer duration of OCD and specific symptom subtypes seem to predict a lower response. As individuals respond differently to particular SSRIs, it is recommended that a second SSRI should be introduced if there is no response to the initial one and that this be augmented by CBT. In adults with OCD, augmentation strategies using antipsychotics have been efficacious in cases of partial response. These strategies have not been studied in children and adolescents.

Affective disorders

Depressive episodes

The National Institute for Health and Care Excellence (NICE) reports that psychotherapeutic interventions, particularly CBT and interpersonal therapy, have been shown to be effective in the treatment of many children and adolescents with depressive symptoms and mild to moderate depressive episodes (National Collaborating Centre for Mental Health, 2005b). Although the NICE guidance takes a very conservative approach to the use of antidepressant medications in treating child and adolescent depression, the limited availability of therapists trained in CBT and interpersonal therapy, and the fact that a psychotherapeutic approach is sometimes unsuitable or ineffective, particularly in more severe cases, means that pharmacological treatments often need to be considered.

As a consequence of an influential Cochrane review (Hazell & Mirzaie, et al, 2013) that showed tricyclic antidepressants to be of unlikely benefit and to have significant adverse events, the early 2000s saw a rapid increase in the use of SSRIs in children and adolescents. This increased use significantly outstripped the evidence base. Fortunately, several RCTs have now compared SSRIs with placebo, CBT and CBT plus SSRI, and one good-quality trial investigated treatment strategies for those who fail to respond to first-line therapies. There are consistently positive RCTs for fluoxetine (Emslie et al, 1997, 1998; March et al, 2004) in children and adolescents, mixed results for sertraline, citalopram and escitalopram (all reviewed in Usala et al, 2008), and negative results for paroxetine, venlafaxine, nefazodone (not licensed in the UK) and mirtazapine (all unpublished 'data on file'). The excellent meta-analysis by Usala et al (2008) reports a pooled odds ratio of 1.57 for the SSRIs, but only fluoxetine appeared to offer a moderately significant benefit profile, with an odds ratio of 2.39. Bridge et al (2007) calculated an overall NNT of 14 for children and 8 for adolescents. For the children under 12 years of age, it was again only fluoxetine that showed benefit over placebo. Bridge et al (2007) looked at the risk of reported suicidal ideation and suicide attempts among children and adolescents receiving these antidepressants for major depressive disorder, OCD and non-OCD anxiety disorders. Although the risk of suicidal ideation/suicide attempt across all trials and all therapeutic indications was greater for antidepressants than for placebo, with a number needed to harm (NNH, how many need to be treated for one to suffer harm) of 143, the pooled risk differences within each indication were not statistically significant for depression, OCD or non-OCD anxiety disorders and there were no completed suicides in any of the trials.

The publicly funded Treatment for Adolescents with Depression Study (TADS) in the USA (March *et al*, 2004) and the ADAPT study in the UK (Goodyer *et al*, 2007) investigated combination treatment with CBT and an SSRI (in TADS this was fluoxetine, in ADAPT it was most often fluoxetine) compared with the SSRI alone (in both studies), CBT alone (TADS only) and placebo (TADS only). In the 12-week TADS, both combination treatment and fluoxetine alone were more effective than placebo, with the combination being the most effective treatment. In TADS, CBT alone was less effective than fluoxetine and no more effective than placebo. In the 28-week ADAPT study both the SSRI and SSRI + CBT groups improved, but there was no significant difference between the two groups. The TADS team also investigated suicidality during treatment. Suicidality decreased substantially with any treatment, and improvement in suicidality was greatest for the combined treatment and least for fluoxetine alone. Importantly, however, fluoxetine did not increase suicidal ideation. The interpretation was that suicide-related adverse events are uncommon, but may occur more often in fluoxetine-treated patients, and that CBT may protect against suicide-related adverse events in fluoxetine-treated patients.

It is estimated that only around 60% of young people with depression will respond adequately to initial treatment with an SSRI. The Treatment of Resistant Depression in Adolescents (TORDIA) trial, funded by the National Institute of Mental Heath (NIMH) in the USA, was designed to investigate alternative treatments for the other 40%. The aim was to recruit adolescents whose depression had not responded to an 'adequate trial' of an SSRI and assess them twice, 2 weeks apart, to eliminate those who were in fact responders and then randomise true non-responders to one of four treatments in a 2 × 2 balanced design. The four treatments were: switch to another SSRI; switch to venlafaxine; switch to another SSRI + CBT; switch to venlafaxine + CBT. Response was assessed at 6, 12, 24, 48 and 72 weeks (Brent *et al*, 2008; Emslie *et al*, 2010).

Over the first 12 weeks, just under 50% of participants had responded to the switch in treatment. The combination of CBT and a switch to another antidepressant resulted in a higher rate of clinical response than did a medication switch alone. For those who had a simple switch of medication, a switch to another SSRI was just as effective as a switch to venlafaxine and resulted in fewer adverse effects (Brent *et al*, 2008). At week 12, responders continued in their assigned treatment arm and non-responders received open treatment (medication and/or CBT) for 12 more weeks. The outcome assessed at 24 weeks was remission, as opposed to response. Remission was defined as at least 3 consecutive weeks without clinically significant depressive symptoms. Of the 334 adolescents enrolled in the study, 38.9%

achieved remission by 24 weeks. Initial treatment assignment did not affect rates of remission, but likelihood of remission was much higher (61.6% *v.* 18.3%) and time to remission was much shorter among those who had already demonstrated clinical response by week 12 (Emslie *et al*, 2010). All participants were treated naturalistically from week 24 onwards. The remission rate had risen to 50% by week 48 and to 61% by week 72. However, 72% of participants still had at least one residual symptom of depression, such as irritability or low self-esteem, at week 72, and 11% met diagnostic criteria for major depression. The overall conclusions are that clinicians should pay significant attention to patients who do not respond in the first 6 weeks of treatment and consider either a combination treatment or switching to another SSRI in such cases. For doses of antidepressants in children and adolescents see Table 7.1.

Manic episodes and bipolar affective disorder

In the UK, a diagnosis of bipolar disorder is still rarely made in children and younger adolescents, although the situation in the USA has become very different. The DSM-IV diagnoses bipolar II disorder and bipolar disorder not otherwise specified (BP-NOS) have frequently been used to diagnose adolescents presenting with exacerbations of disruptive behaviour, moodiness, low frustration tolerance and explosive anger followed by guilt, and difficulty sleeping at night, very often in the context of ADHD (American Psychiatric Association, 1994). Mood stabilisers and antipsychotics are frequently used to manage these children who in the UK would be more likely to be given other diagnostic labels. In DSM-5 it is likely that many of these children will be diagnosed as suffering from disruptive mood dysregulation disorder, a new disorder introduced, at least in part, to reduce the inappropriate use of the bipolar disorder (American Psychiatric Association, 2013). What is not clear is how they will be treated.

The NICE guideline (National Collaborating Centre for Mental Health, 2006) recommends that diagnoses of bipolar II disorder and BP-NOS are reserved for adults, but acknowledge that bipolar I disorder is a valid, if still uncommon, diagnosis in adolescents and rare but possible in children. Liu *et al* (2011) conducted a systematic review and meta-analysis of pharmacological approaches to the treatment of bipolar disorder in children and adolescents. They identified 29 open-label trials and 17 RCTs. The overall odds ratio of 2.23 was significantly greater than 1. This was mainly accounted for by the highly significant effect of the second-generation antipsychotics, and there was positive evidence from RCTs for aripiprazole, olanzapine, quetiapine, risperidone and ziprasidone. The meta-analysis effects were not significant for divalproex (sodium valproate) and only mildly positive for topiramate and oxcarbazepine (a derivative of carbamazepine).

Although there is some evidence that lithium is also effective in treating bipolar I disorder in children and adolescents, it is low in quality and findings are mixed. The US Food and Drug Administration (FDA) has indicated that: risperidone, quetiapine and aripiprazole can be used in bipolar disorder for children aged 10 and over; lithium for children over 12; and olanzapine for children over 13 years of age. None of these drugs are yet licensed for use in the UK and the rest of Europe, but this may change. The *British National Formulary for Children* (BNFC; BMJ Group *et al*, 2013: section 4.2.3) suggests that 'Atypical antipsychotic drugs (normally olanzapine, quetiapine, or risperidone) [...] are useful in acute episodes of mania and hypomania; if the response to antipsychotic drugs is inadequate, lithium or valproate may be added. An antipsychotic drug may be used concomitantly with lithium or valproate in the initial treatment of severe acute mania'. This is similar to the recommendations of NICE (National Collaborating Centre for Mental Health, 2006) that atypical antipsychotics are the treatment of choice for severe mania, whereas lithium or sodium valproate may be considered for less severe cases. The NICE guideline recommends starting treatment with lower initial doses than would be used in adults and that the clinician regularly checks weight and prolactin levels. It also recommends that lithium or valproate can be added if there is inadequate response to an antipsychotic. For doses of antipsychotics in children and adolescents see Table 7.2.

Longer-term management

The BNFC suggests that 'atypical antipsychotics are the treatment of choice for the long-term management of bipolar disorder in children and adolescents; if the patient has frequent relapses or continuing functional impairment, consider concomitant therapy with lithium or valproate. An atypical antipsychotic that causes less weight gain and does not increase prolactin levels is preferred' (BMJ Group *et al*, 2013: section 4.2.1). The NICE guideline recommends atypical antipsychotics as first-line prophylaxis and lithium (girls and boys) or valproate (boys) as second-line prophylaxis (National Collaborating Centre for Mental Health, 2006). Clearly, in addition to pharmacological treatment it is important for the clinician to support parents and carers in helping the patient maintain a regular lifestyle and to give schools advice on managing the patient's bipolar disorder. For more detailed advice on using antipsychotics in children and adolescents see the next section ('Schizophrenia').

Schizophrenia

Early-onset schizophrenia, used in this context to refer to the development of psychotic symptoms before the age of 18 years, is associated with severe functional impairments and poor outcomes. It leads to loss of promise and fulfilment as well as frequent hospital admissions and usually heralds the beginning of a long career as a psychiatric patient. The identification and treatment of children and young people at an early stage of transition

Table 7.2 Doses and indications for antipsychotics in children and adolescents

Name	Indication	Age, years	Average daily dose, mg	BNFC recognised indication
Haloperidol	Schizophrenia; psychosis	12–18	5–10	Yes
	Tic disorders	5–12	0.125–10	No
Pimozide	Schizophrenia	12–18	2–20	Yes
	Tic disorders	Not stated	Not stated	No
Sulpiride	Schizophrenia	14–18	800–2400	Yes
	Tourette syndrome	12–18	50–400	Yes
Clozapine	Schizophrenia	12–18	200–450	Yes
Aripiprazole	Schizophrenia	13–18	10–30	Yes
	Mania	13–18	10–30	Yes
	Repetitive behaviour in autism	Not stated	Not stated	No
	Tourette syndrome	Not stated	2.5–5	No[a]
Olanzapine	Schizophrenia	12–18	5–20	Yes
	Mania	12–18	5–20	Yes
	Tourette syndrome	Not stated	Not stated	No
Quetiapine	Schizophrenia	12–18	400–600	Yes
	Mania	12–18	400–600	Yes
Risperidone	Schizophrenia; psychosis	12–18	4–6	Yes
	Autism	5–18 (15–20 kg in weight)	0.25–1	No[b]
		18 (>20 kg in weight)	0.25–2.5	
	Aggression in conduct disorders	5–18	0.5–1	Yes
	Mania in bipolar disorder	12–18	5	Yes
	Tourette syndrome	Not stated	3	No[c]
Ziprasidone	Tourette syndrome	Not stated	30	No[d]

BNFC, *British National Formulary for Children* (BMJ Group *et al*, 2013).
a. Hartmann & Worbe (2013).
b. US Food and Drug Administration indication (Levin, 2012).
c. Zhao & Zhu (2003).
d. Sallee *et al* (2000).

to frank psychosis or at the beginning of a first psychotic episode can not only facilitate normal development, but also affect the course of the illness. Unfortunately, as schizophrenia in young people is often insidious in onset, diagnosis and treatment are often delayed. Nevertheless, antipsychotic treatment should not usually be started if the clinical manifestations are not sufficient to make a clear diagnosis of either a psychotic state or schizophrenia, or if the aim is to prevent the possible development of psychosis (National Institute for Health and Clinical Excellence, 2013).

Pharmacological treatments should always be given within the context of a multidisciplinary team able to offer a broad range of supportive therapies. Although there are countless trials providing clear and unambiguous evidence that antipsychotics reduce symptoms of schizophrenia in adults, very few studies have included children or young people, although some are starting to appear. As a consequence, treatment of both the acute psychotic episode and the longer-term maintenance phase is currently based mainly on experience and the extrapolated results from adult studies. Fortunately, there seems to be considerable continuity in drug response between early- and adult-onset schizophrenia. However, it is important that further studies are conducted to confirm both the effectiveness and safety of antipsychotics in early-onset schizophrenia. As this is often a life-long condition requiring long-term treatment, studies of both short and long duration are needed.

The evidence base

The research that has been conducted in both adults and children suggests that almost all antipsychotic medications are of similar efficacy and result in similar rates and patterns of symptom reduction. The main effects centre on reduction of positive symptoms, while effects on negative symptoms are relatively minor. As a consequence, it is the adverse effects profile that has the biggest influence in clinical decision-making. Unfortunately, there is little evidence to predict the differential development of adverse effects in the paediatric population prior to initiating treatment.

Several controlled trials have reported on the efficacy of traditional (typical or first-generation) antipsychotics in early-onset schizophrenia. Haloperidol was found to be clinically and statistically superior to placebo by Spencer *et al* (1992) and to be more efficacious than placebo and equally as efficacious as loxitane (not licensed in the UK) by Pool *et al* (1976). These traditional antipsychotics are, of course, limited in their use by their serious long-term side-effects, especially extrapyramidal symptoms and tardive dyskinesia. There are also now some very short-term studies investigating the next generation, so-called atypical, antipsychotics in early-onset schizophrenia. Positive effects in short-term trials *v.* placebo have been demonstrated for olanzapine (Kryzhanovskaya *et al*, 2009), aripiprazole (Findling *et al*, 2008), risperidone (Haas *et al*, 2009) and quetiapine (Findling *et al*, 2012), with NNTs similar to those in adults (between 5 and 10).

In adult psychiatry in the West, typical antipsychotics have pretty much been displaced by the atypicals, which are reputed to be at least as effective at treating positive symptoms, more effective at treating negative symptoms and less likely to lead to extrapyramidal symptoms. Nevertheless, the Treatment of Early-Onset Schizophrenia Spectrum Disorders (TEOSS) study, a relatively large comparative study of 119 children in the USA who were randomly assigned to an 8-week treatment with either a typical (molindone, which is not licensed in the UK) or an atypical (olanzapine or risperidone) antipsychotic reported high withdrawal rates among the patients receiving the atypical (Sikich *et al*, 2008). The study's authors question the now almost exclusive use of atypicals in view of the high likelihood of metabolic side-effects and the impact these may have on an individual who is still developing. Taken together, studies suggest that response rates, which range from 34 to 50%, are not significantly different for any of the available antipsychotics, and that side-effects are common for both the typicals and the atypicals. For the typicals, the most common are neurological (e.g. extrapyramidal symptoms, akathisia), and for the atypicals they are metabolic (e.g. weight gain, and relative increase in total cholesterol, insulin, alanine aminotransferase (ALT) and aspartate aminotransferase (AST)). A systematic review found an average response rate of 55.7% across 8 studies of atypicals, compared with a rate of 72.3% across 13 studies of typicals (although the effect size for typicals was larger than that for atypicals) (Armenteros & Davies, 2006).

For treatment-resistant schizophrenia, clozapine is the best studied of the atypicals in adults. Although there are relatively few studies investigating the use of clozapine in children and adolescents, there is some indication that it may be more efficacious than haloperidol (Kumra *et al*, 1996) and olanzapine (Shaw *et al*, 2006; Kumra *et al*, 1996) at treating both positive and negative symptoms. However, in the haloperidol *v.* clozapine trial by Kumra *et al*, 5 of the 21 young people on clozapine developed significant neutropenia and 2 had seizures. So despite the evidence of efficacy, the use of clozapine in children and adolescents is severely limited by its association with serious adverse events, including neutropenia, and the need for regular blood testing. Large long-term systematic studies of the efficacy, effectiveness and safety of the atypicals are needed before clear evidence-based statements can be made about their use.

Treatment

The recent NICE guideline (National Institute for Health and Clinical Excellence, 2013) avoids naming any of the antipsychotics, which is understandable in light of the evidence, but not particularly helpful for clinicians making choices. However, as there is no evidence, other than for clozapine, to suggest that any one antipsychotic is better than another in treating psychosis, the choice is generally made on the basis of potencies and side-effect profiles (Table 7.2).

The NICE guideline suggests that the following baseline investigations should be carried out before starting any antipsychotic: weight and height (both plotted on a growth chart), waist and hip circumference, pulse and blood pressure, blood glucose, glycosylated haemoglobin (HbA1c), blood lipid profile and prolactin levels, assessment of any movement disorders, assessment of nutritional status, diet and level of physical activity, and electrocardiogram (ECG). When initiating treatment with an antipsychotic, it is important to ensure that the patient has an adequate trial (6 weeks) at an adequate dose. If there is no response after this time, a different antipsychotic should be tried.

Clozapine should be reserved for patients who have failed to respond to at least two adequate trials of other antipsychotic agents, at least one of which was an atypical, or who have experienced significant drug-induced side-effects (e.g. tardive dyskinesia). Efficacy assessment, together with a safety assessment similar to baseline investigations, should be repeated systematically during the treatment according to the following scheme: weight (plotted on a growth chart) weekly for the first 6 weeks, at 12 weeks and then every 6 months; height (plotted on a growth chart) every 6 months; waist and hip circumference (plotted on a percentile chart) every 6 months; pulse and blood pressure (plotted on a percentile chart) at 12 weeks and then every 6 months; fasting blood glucose, HbA1c, blood lipid and prolactin levels at 12 weeks and then every 6 months.

The choice of which antipsychotic medication to use and in which order is complex, and dependent not only on the relative efficacy of treatments and their adverse effects, but also on a range of complex social, educational, psychological and medical factors. As suggested above, the current level of evidence is not sufficient to allow for clear recommendations about which drug to use when. Practitioners should make themselves familiar with the different adverse effect profiles of the various antipsychotics and consider these when discussing treatment options with patients and their families (Table 7.3).

Conclusion

Although there remain many unanswered questions, the evidence base for the pharmacological treatment of child and adolescent psychiatric disorders is growing. Psychological and psychosocial therapies remain the first-line treatments for some disorders (such as anxiety and autism spectrum disorders) and they are an important component of a comprehensive treatment package for others. It is important, however, that clinicians develop an understanding of the potential role that medication can play, especially when psychological treatments have been unsuccessful in adequately reducing symptoms. It is also important to recognise the limitations of the current evidence and to alert patients and their families to these uncertainties when suggesting the use of medication.

More good-quality treatment trials are needed. This will require collaboration between academics and clinicians across a wide range of settings and also support from funding bodies and managers within healthcare, who must ensure that these studies are recognised as an essential component of healthcare provision.

Table 7.3 Adverse effect profiles of haloperidol and second-generation (atypical) antipsychotics in children and adolescents

Adverse effect	Onset	Haloperidol	Aripiprazole	Clozapine	Olanzapine	Quetiapine	Risperidone	Ziprasidone
Anticholinergic	Early	–	–	+++	++	–/+	–	–
Acute Parkinsonism	Early	+++	+	–	+	–	++	+
Akathisia	Early/intermediate	+++	++	+	+	+	+	+
Tardive dyskinesia	Late	++	–/+	–	–/+	–/+	–/+	–/+
Withdrawal dyskinesia	During switch	++	++	–	–/+	–/+	+	+
Diabetes	Late	–/+	–/+	+++	+++	++	+	–/+
Increased lipids	Early/intermediate	–/+	–/+	++	++	+	+	–/+
Weight gain	Intermediate	+	+	+++	+++	++	++	+
Increased prolactin/ sexual dysfunction	Early	++	–	–	++	–	+++	+
Decreased prolactin	Early	–	++	–	–	–	–	–
Sedation	Early	–/+	–/+	+++	++	++	+	–/+
Increased QTc	Throughout	–/+	–/+	+	–/+	+	+	++
Postural hypotension	Early	–	+/–	+++	++	++	+	–
Neutropenia	Early/intermediate	–/+	–/+	++	–/+	–/+	–/+	–/+

–, not present; –/+, minimal; +, mild; ++, moderate; +++, severe.

References

American Psychiatric Association (1994) *Diagnostic and Statistical Manual of Mental Disorders (4th edn) (DSM–IV)*. APA.

American Psychiatric Association (2013) *Diagnostic and Statistical Manual of Mental Disorders (5th edn) (DSM-5)*. APA.

Armenteros JL, Davies M (2006) Antipsychotics in early onset schizophrenia: systematic review and meta-analysis. *European Child & Adolescent Psychiatry*, **15**, 141–148.

Birmaher B, Axelson DA, Monk K, *et al* (2003) Fluoxetine for the treatment of childhood anxiety disorders. *Journal of the American Academy of Child & Adolescent Psychiatry*, **42**, 415–423.

BMJ Group, Royal Pharmaceutical Society, Royal College of Paediatrics and Child Health, *et al* (2013) *BNF for Children: 2013–2014*. Pharmaceutical Press.

Brent D, Emslie G, Clarke G, *et al* (2008) Switching to another SSRI or to venlafaxine with or without cognitive behavioral therapy for adolescents with SSRI-resistant depression: the TORDIA randomized controlled trial. *JAMA*, **299**, 901–913.

Bridge JA, Iyengar S, Salary CB, *et al* (2007) Clinical response and risk for reported suicidal ideation and suicide attempts in pediatric antidepressant treatment: a meta-analysis of randomized controlled trials. *JAMA*, **297**, 1683–1696.

Compton SN, Walkup JT, Albano AM, *et al* (2010) Child/Adolescent Anxiety Multimodal Study (CAMS): rationale, design, and methods. *Child and Adolescent Psychiatry and Mental Health*, **4**, 1.

Cook EH, Wagner KD, March JS, *et al* (2001) Long-term sertraline treatment of children and adolescents with obsessive–compulsive disorder. *Journal of the American Academy of Child & Adolescent Psychiatry*, **40**, 1175–1181.

Emslie GJ, Rush AJ, Weinberg WA, *et al* (1997) A double-blind, randomized, placebo-controlled trial of fluoxetine in children and adolescents with depression. *Archives of General Psychiatry*, **54**, 1031–1037.

Emslie GJ, Rush AJ, Weinberg WA, *et al* (1998) Fluoxetine in child and adolescent depression: acute and maintenance treatment. *Depression and Anxiety*, **7**, 32–39.

Emslie GJ, Mayes T, Porta G, *et al* (2010) Treatment of Resistant Depression in Adolescents (TORDIA): week 24 outcomes. *American Journal of Psychiatry*, **167**, 782–791.

Findling RL, Robb A, Nyilas M, *et al* (2008) A multiple-center, randomized, double-blind, placebo-controlled study of oral aripiprazole for treatment of adolescents with schizophrenia. *American Journal of Psychiatry*, **165**, 1432–1441.

Findling RL, McKenna K, Earley WR, *et al* (2012) Efficacy and safety of quetiapine in adolescents with schizophrenia investigated in a 6-week, double-blind, placebo-controlled trial. *Journal of Child and Adolescent Psychopharmacology*, **22**, 327–342.

Geller DA, Hoog SL, Heiligenstein JH, *et al* (2001) Fluoxetine treatment for obsessive–compulsive disorder in children and adolescents: a placebo-controlled clinical trial. *Journal of the American Academy of Child & Adolescent Psychiatry*, **40**, 773–779.

Geller D, Donnelly C, Lopez F, *et al* (2007) Atomoxetine treatment for pediatric patients with attention-deficit/hyperactivity disorder with comorbid anxiety disorder. *Journal of the American Academy of Child & Adolescent Psychiatry*, **46**, 1119–1127.

Goodyer I, Dubicka B, Wilkinson P, *et al* (2007) Selective serotonin reuptake inhibitors (SSRIs) and routine specialist care with and without cognitive behaviour therapy in adolescents with major depression: randomised controlled trial. *BMJ*, **335**, 142.

Grados M, Scahill L, Riddle MA (1999) Pharmacotherapy in children and adolescents with obsessive–compulsive disorder. *Child and Adolescent Psychiatric Clinics of North America*, **8**, 617–634.

Haas M, Unis AS, Armenteros J, *et al* (2009) A 6-week, randomized, double-blind, placebo-controlled study of the efficacy and safety of risperidone in adolescents with schizophrenia. *Journal of Child and Adolescent Psychopharmacology*, **19**, 611–621.

Hartmann A, Worbe Y (2013) Pharmacological treatment of Gilles de la Tourette syndrome. *Neuroscience and Biobehavioral Reviews*, **37**, 1157–1161.

Hazell P, Mirzaie M (2013) Tricyclic drugs for depression in children and adolescents. *Cochrane Database of Systematic Reviews*, issue 6, CD002317.

Kryzhanovskaya L, Schulz SC, McDougle C, *et al* (2009) Olanzapine versus placebo in adolescents with schizophrenia: a 6-week, randomized, double-blind, placebo-controlled trial. *Journal of the American Academy of Child & Adolescent Psychiatry*, **48**, 60–70.

Kumra S, Frazier JA, Jacobsen LK, *et al* (1996) Childhood-onset schizophrenia: A double-blind clozapine-haloperidol comparison. *Archives of General Psychiatry*, **53**, 1090–1097.

Levin RL (2012) *20272-S-65 Cross-Discipline Team Leader Review Memo.* Food and Drug Administration (http://www.fda.gov/downloads/drugs/developmentapprovalprocess/developmentresources/ucm322381.pdf). Accessed 2 Dec 2013.

Liu HY, Potter MP, Woodworth KY, *et al* (2011) Pharmacologic treatments for pediatric bipolar disorder: a review and meta-analysis. *Journal of the American Academy of Child & Adolescent Psychiatry*, **50**, 749–762.

March JS, Biederman J, Wolkow R, *et al* (1998) Sertraline in children and adolescents with obsessive–compulsive disorder: a multicenter randomized controlled trial. *JAMA*, **280**, 1752–1756.

March JS, Swanson, JM, Arnold LE, *et al* (2000) Anxiety as a predictor and outcome variable in the multimodal treatment study of children with ADHD (MTA). *Journal of Abnormal Child Psychology*, **28**, 527–541.

March J, Silva S, Petrycki S, *et al* (2004) Fluoxetine, cognitive–behavioral therapy, and their combination for adolescents with depression: Treatment for Adolescents with Depression Study (TADS) randomized controlled trial. *JAMA*, **292**, 807–820.

March JS, Entusah AR, Rynn M, *et al* (2007) A randomized controlled trial of venlafaxine ER versus placebo in pediatric social anxiety disorder. *Biological Psychiatry*, **62**, 1149–1154.

National Collaborating Centre for Mental Health (2005a) *Obsessive-Compulsive Disorder: Core Interventions in the Treatment of Obsessive-Compulsive Disorder and Body Dysmorphic Disorder* (Clinical Guideline 31). National Institute for Health and Clinical Excellence.

National Collaborating Centre for Mental Health (2005b) *Depression in Children and Young People: Identification and Management in Primary, Community and Secondary Care* (Clinical Guideline 28). National Institute for Health and Clinical Excellence.

National Collaborating Centre for Mental Health (2006) *Bipolar Disorder: The Management of Bipolar Disorder in Adults, Children and Adolescents, in Primary and Secondary Care* (National Clinical Practice Guideline Number 38). British Psychological Society and Gaskell.

National Institute for Health and Clinical Excellence (2013) *Psychosis and Schizophrenia in Children and Young People: Recognition and Management* (NICE Clinical Guideline 155). NICE.

Nilsen TS, Eisemann M, Kvernmo S (2013) Predictors and moderators of outcome in child and adolescent anxiety and depression: a systematic review of psychological treatment studies. *European Child & Adolescent Psychiatry*, **22**, 69–87.

Pediatric OCD Treatment Study (POTS) Team (2004) Cognitive–behavior therapy, sertraline, and their combination for children and adolescents with obsessive–compulsive disorder: the Pediatric OCD Treatment Study (POTS) randomized controlled trial. *JAMA*, **292**, 1969–1976.

Pool D, Bloom W, Mielke DH, *et al* (1976) A controlled evaluation of loxitane in seventy-five adolescent schizophrenic patients. *Current Therapeutic Research: Clinical and Experimental*, **19**, 99–104.

Research Unit on Pediatric Psychopharmacology Anxiety Study Group (2001) Fluvoxamine for the treatment of anxiety disorders in children and adolescents. *New England Journal of Medicine*, **344**, 1279–1285.

Riddle MA, Reeve EA, Yaryura-Tobias JA, *et al* (2001) Fluvoxamine for children and adolescents with obsessive–compulsive disorder: a randomized, controlled, multicenter trial. *Journal of the American Academy of Child & Adolescent Psychiatry*, **40**, 222–229.

Rynn MA, Siqueland L, Rickels K (2001) Placebo-controlled trial of sertraline in the treatment of children with generalized anxiety disorder. *American Journal of Psychiatry*, **158**, 2008–2014.

Rynn MA, Riddle MA, Yeung PP, et al (2007) Efficacy and safety of extended-release venlafaxine in the treatment of generalized anxiety disorder in children and adolescents: two placebo-controlled trials. *American Journal of Psychiatry*, **164**, 290–300.

Sallee FR, Kurlan R, Goetz CG, et al (2000) Ziprasidone treatment of children and adolescents with Tourette's syndrome: a pilot study. *Journal of the American Academy of Child & Adolescent Psychiatry*, **39**, 292–299.

Shaw P, Sporn A, Gogtay N, et al (2006) Childhood-onset schizophrenia: a double-blind, randomized clozapine–olanzapine comparison. *Archives of General Psychiatry*, **63**, 721–730.

Sikich L, Frazier JA, McClellan J, et al (2008) Double-blind comparison of first- and second-generation antipsychotics in early-onset schizophrenia and schizo-affective disorder: findings from the treatment of early-onset schizophrenia spectrum disorders (TEOSS) study. *American Journal of Psychiatry*, **165**, 1420–1431.

Spencer EK, Kafantaris V, Padron-Gayol MV, et al (1992) Haloperidol in schizophrenic children: early findings from a study in progress. *Psychopharmacology Bulletin*, **28**, 183–186.

Thomsen PH (2000) Obsessive–compulsive disorder: pharmacological treatment. *European Child & Adolescent Psychiatry*, **9** (suppl 1), S76–S84.

Thomsen PH, Ebbesen C, Persson C (2001) Long-term experience with citalopram in the treatment of adolescent OCD. *Journal of the American Academy of Child & Adolescent Psychiatry*, **40**, 895–902.

Usala T, Clavenna A, Zuddas A, et al (2008) Randomised controlled trials of selective serotonin reuptake inhibitors in treating depression in children and adolescents: a systematic review and meta-analysis. *European Neuropsychopharmacology*, **18**, 62–73.

Velosa JF, Riddle MA (2000) Pharmacologic treatment of anxiety disorders in children and adolescents. *Child and Adolescent Psychiatric Clinics of North America*, **9**, 119–133.

Wagner KD, Berard R, Stein MB, et al (2004) A multicenter, randomized, double-blind, placebo-controlled trial of paroxetine in children and adolescents with social anxiety disorder. *Archives of General Psychiatry*, **61**, 1153–1162.

Walkup JT, Albano AM, Piacentini, J, et al (2008) Cognitive behavioral therapy, sertraline, or a combination in childhood anxiety. *New England Journal of Medicine*, **359**, 2753–2766.

Watson HJ, Rees CS (2008) Meta-analysis of randomized, controlled treatment trials for pediatric obsessive–compulsive disorder. *Journal of Child Psychology and Psychiatry*, **49**, 489–498.

Zhao H, Zhu Y (2003) Risperidone in the treatment of Tourette Syndrome. *Chinese Mental Health Journal*, **17**, 30–40.

CHAPTER 8

Pharmacological management of core and comorbid symptoms in autism spectrum disorder

Rachel Elvins and Jonathan Green

Autism spectrum disorders (ASD) are frequently grouped as pervasive developmental disorders to include childhood autism, atypical autism and Asperger syndrome. They are recognised as complex neurodevelopmental disorders, often becoming clinically apparent in the second or third year of life. The diagnosis is based on disturbance in the domains of reciprocal social interactions, communication, restricted interests and stereotyped patterns of behaviour. Up to two-thirds of affected individuals will present with a degree of global intellectual disability, although some may have a very uneven profile of abilities. Accurate diagnosis, usually made by a combination of direct observation of behaviour and informant history, is complicated by considerable heterogeneity in the manifestation of these core deficits, by variation in ability level and by developmental changes. However, it is clear that ASD usually persist across the lifespan, resulting in varied and complex needs in adult life. The course of development into old age is, as yet, largely unknown.

The prevalence of ASD in children is about 1.2% (Baird *et al*, 2009). There are no accurate prevalence figures available for adults, but in 2011 it was estimated there were 5.3 million adults with diagnosed ASD across Europe, the USA and Japan (Nightingale, 2012). A male excess of between 3:1 and 4:1 is generally observed. Maladaptive behaviours and comorbid psychiatric symptoms are common. Autism is thus a relatively common, chronic, potentially substantially disabling disorder, with significant costs to both the affected individual and family members. Recent guidance from the National Institute for Health and Care Excellence (NICE) has addressed assessment and management in both young people and adults (National Institute for Health and Clinical Excellence, 2011, 2012; National Institute for Health and Care Excellence & Social Care Institute for Excellence, 2013) and the Autism Act 2009, which extends to England and Wales, has been a landmark in statutory legislation. These developments, along with acknowledgement of the life-time needs imposed by the disorder in the context of normal-range intellectual ability as well as disability, will lead to a great increase in referrals to adult psychiatry services, with a need for service adaptations.

Medication management in autism

Educational and psychosocial interventions are the mainstay of treatment, with the aim of improving language acquisition and maximising communication and social skills. However, medication management, particularly of maladaptive behaviours, is common and possibly increasing. Such behaviours, and the symptoms of comorbid psychiatric disorders, may interfere with socialisation and educational progress, and severely impair the quality of life of affected individuals and their families. A UK study revealed that up to 75% of adults with autism and intellectual disabilities were prescribed at least one psychotropic medication (Tsakanikos *et al*, 2006). Factors associated with increasing medication use include greater age, poorer functioning and higher levels of challenging behaviour (Aman *et al*, 2005). The aim of this chapter is to discuss and summarise clinical pharmacotherapy for ASD based on target domains of behaviour (Table 8.1). Such symptoms, which are difficult to manage, are often the reason that families seek medical treatments. We first evaluate treatments targeted at the underlying core social deficit of autism and then address certain target clusters of comorbid or co-occurring symptoms such as stereotypical and compulsive/ritualistic behaviours, and serious aggressive and self-injurious behaviour.

It should be noted that many drugs are not licensed for children because there are few trials in that age group. Nevertheless, they are used quite widely by specialists (child psychiatrists and paediatricians with expertise in mental health) with the view that parents should be made aware of this off-label use and give consent for it.

Pharmacotherapy for the core symptoms

Social deficits

The detailed underlying pathophysiology of social impairments in ASD is still unclear. Their treatment has been subject to many 'false dawns' in the literature, with therapeutic approaches based on questionable theory heavily promoted. Rigorous trials have on occasion reduced interest in approaches despite such active promotion; for instance, secretin, a gastrointestinal peptide, and fenfluramine, an indirect 5-HT partial agonist, have been widely studied, with nearly 500 children with ASD being recruited to randomised controlled trials (RCTs) for secretin alone. Both drugs were initially claimed to have prosocial effects in autism, but larger placebo-controlled trials failed to replicate these improvements (Volkmar *et al*, 1983; Sandler *et al*, 1999). Robust trials can have an important function in disproving treatment claims.

113

Table 8.1 Selected medication for behavioural domains in autism[a]

Symptom cluster	Medications	Common/important adverse effects	Reference (first-named author)
Stereotypical and compulsive/repetitive behaviours	SSRI (fluoxetine, fluvoxamine)	Irritability, activation, insomnia, gastrointestinal upset, potential increase in suicidal ideation	McDougle, 1996;[b] Hollander, 2005; Posey, 2006a
	Second generation antipsychotic (risperidone, aripiprazole)	Appetite increase, weight gain, sedation, glucose dysregulation, extrapyramidal symptoms, QTc prolongation, NMS	Scahill, 2002; McDougle, 2005; Ching, 2012
Irritability, aggression and self-injury	Second generation antipsychotic (risperidone and aripiprazole)	As above	McDougle, 1998;[b] Shea, 2004; Ching, 2012
	Opiate antagonist (naltrexone)	Headaches and dizziness	Symons, 2004
	Typical antipsychotic (haloperidol)	Extrapyramidal symptoms, akathisia, weight gain, QTc prolongation, NMS	Remington, 2001
Hyperkinesis and inattention	Immediate-release methylphenidate	Appetite suppression, weight loss, insomnia, rebound hyperkinesis, tachycardia, hypertension	RUPPAN, 2005a
	Alpha-2 agonist (clonidine)	Fatigue, hypotension	Jaselskis, 1992
	Atomoxetine	Gastrointestinal upset, fatigue, appetite suppression, liver dysfunction, suicidal ideation, hypertension, tachycardia	Arnold, 2006; Zeiner, 2011
	Antipsychotic (aripiprazole, risperidone)	As above	Aman, 2009; Ching, 2012
Depressive symptoms	SSRI	As above	Posey, 2006a
Manic symptoms	Anticonvulsant mood stabiliser (valproate/divalproex)	Weight gain, sedation, gastrointestinal upset, platelet suppression, liver dysfunction, pancreatitis, teratogenicity	Hollander, 2001
	Second generation antipsychotics	As above	Joshi, 2012
Anxiety symptoms	SSRI	As above	Posey, 2006a
	Buspirone	Dyskinesia	Buitelaar, 1998
Sleep dysfunction	Melatonin	Somnolence	Owens, 2005
	Antihistamine	Irritability, somnolence	Owens, 2005

NMS, neuroleptic malignant syndrome; RUPPAN, Research Units on Pediatric Psychopharmacology Autism Network; SSRI, selective serotonin reuptake inhibitor.
a. See the *British National Formulary for Children* (BMJ Group *et al*, 2013) for licensed prescription. Off-label use should be initiated and monitored by specialists (child psychiatrists and paediatricians with expertise in mental health) with the parents' consent.
b. Study in adults only.

Diet

There is widespread interest in exclusion diets, particularly among families of children with autism, but the theory behind their value has been generally unconvincing and there is a dearth of good-quality RCTs. Vitamins and minerals have been widely trialled, with broadly disappointing results. A Cochrane review of RCTs studying the use of vitamin B6 and magnesium (Nye & Brice, 2005) concluded that the available evidence does not support their use in ASD and that larger, better designed studies are needed.

Immune function

Infectious and immune mechanisms have been popular proposed aetiological agents in autism (with little justification to date from basic science). A limited number of related treatment studies have been carried out. One trial of vancomycin (Sandler *et al*, 2000) showed that improvements in communication returned to baseline when the drug was stopped. Pentoxifylline (a methylxanthine that has immunological and serotonergic effects) has been shown to improve irritability and social withdrawal in combination with risperidone, an antipsychotic drug (Akhondzadeh *et al*, 2010). Other drugs that have a direct effect on immune function have not yet undergone RCTs in autism.

This there is at present no place for immunotherapy in the management of autism. There is also no reliable evidence that anti-fungal treatments are effective in the treatment of ASD. Vaccinations, particularly the combined measles, mumps and rubella (MMR) vaccine, have been the subject of controversy; however, an accumulation of several large-scale studies has clearly disproved a causal link between MMR and the development of autism (Godlee *et al*, 2011).

Antidepressants and antipsychotics

Clinical studies (mostly open label) of selective serotonin reuptake inhibitors (SSRIs) and second-generation antipsychotics such as risperidone suggest that some individuals with autism show improvement in aspects of social relatedness following treatment (McDougle *et al*, 2006). Risperidone does have a proven effect on arousal states and behaviour (see below), and any effect on prosocial behaviour is likely to be secondary to this, thus an indirect outcome. Aripiprazole, a partial D_2 dopamine agonist, has also resulted in improvements in measures of social withdrawal and inappropriate speech (Owen *et al*, 2009). The caveats that need to accompany these positive results relate to the inconsistent quality of the evidence (because of sample size and heterogeneity) and the balancing facts of the substantial unwanted effects associated with antipsychotics, including increased risk of adverse events, weight gain, prolactin concentration and leptin levels.

Glutamate-active medication

Glutamatergic function has been the focus of recent extensive research in neuropsychiatric disorders. Glutamate is the primary excitatory amino

115

acid in the brain and is thought to be important in regulating neuronal plasticity and higher cognitive functions (Carlsson, 1998). Both ASD and schizophrenia are postulated to be hypoglutamatergic disorders and parallels have been drawn between the negative symptoms of schizophrenia and the social impairment in autism (Nikolov *et al*, 2006). Further interest has been excited by a large pooled genetic analysis (Autism Genome Project Consortium, 2007) which used linkage and copy number variation analysis respectively to implicate candidate gene loci on chromosome 11p12-p13 and neurexins. Neurexins and neuroligins (independently linked with autism in other analyses) are implicated in glutamatergic synaptogenesis, highlighting glutamate-related genes as promising candidates in ASD. One glutamate-active drug of interest is D-cycloserine (a partial agonist at the *n*-methyl-D-aspartic acid (NMDA) receptor complex). When added to conventional antipsychotics it can reduce negative symptoms in schizophrenia, and this benefit has been associated with enhanced temporal lobe function (Yurgelun-Todd *et al*, 2005). Recent trials of D-cycloserine have shown that it does not improve social relatedness in young children. Large-scale neurobiological and pharmaceutical trials involving this drug are under development, particularly by C. J. McDougle and D. J. Posey's team from Indiana University School of Medicine in the USA.

Other drugs currently undergoing trials include amantadine and memantine, which act as non-competitive antagonists at the NMDA receptor. Open-label and retrospective studies of memantine have had mixed results in the domain of social relatedness (Owley *et al*, 2006; Chez *et al*, 2007) and side-effects have included irritability and excessive sedation. One small controlled trial of amantadine in children (King *et al*, 2001) showed a trend towards greater treatment response based on Clinical Global Improvement (CGI) scale ratings. Other studies have been less optimistic, for example lamotrigine (an anticonvulsant which attenuates cortical glutamate release) was found to be no better than placebo on any outcome measure employed in a small RCT involving children (Belsito *et al*, 2001). However, work is still at a preliminary stage and at present the available evidence would not support the clinical use of glutamate-active medications in autism.

Stereotypical and ritualistic/compulsive behaviours

These behaviours are defined as part of the core of autism. They include verbal and motor rituals, obsessive questioning, rigid adherence to routine, preoccupation with details and obsessive desire for maintenance of sameness. Such symptoms are commonly the most functionally impairing aspect of the syndrome and interfere significantly with an individual's progression in educational and socialisation programmes. They have similarities with obsessive–compulsive disorder (OCD) phenomena and thus medications such as tricyclic antidepressants and SSRIs with known efficacy in OCD are obvious candidate drugs.

Antidepressants

Clomipramine is a non-selective tricyclic antidepressant that affects uptake of serotonin, noradrenaline and dopamine. Two cross-over RCTs using children and young adults provide some evidence that clomipramine is superior to placebo on measures such as anger and obsessive symptoms. However, there were no gains in areas such as hyperactivity and global symptom severity (Remington et al, 2001). Concerns about adverse effects of clomipramine make this drug less widely used than SSRIs.

Using the SSRI fluvoxamine, a short-term RCT in adults with autism showed improvements in both compulsive and prosocial behaviour (McDougle et al, 1996). Trials with children have had more mixed results. A short-term RCT involving children with ASD showed that fluvoxamine had no advantage over placebo (McDougle et al, 2000). Adverse effects were noted in 78%. More encouragingly, another 12-week cross-over RCT involving 18 children with ASD judged that 10 were treatment responders on the CGI. However, a placebo response rate is not recorded, and adverse events occurred in 7 (39%), although this was not considered significant (Sugie et al, 2005).

Two very small cross-over RCTs of fluoxetine in adults (Buchsbaum et al, 2001) and children (Hollander et al, 2005) reported improvements in repetitive behaviours. There were no differences in side-effects between drug and placebo in the children. Unpublished data of a large-scale RCT of fluoxetine in children showed that repetitive behaviours were reduced in those taking either placebo or fluoxetine but there were no statistically significant differences in response between the two groups (Autism Speaks, 2009). Large-scale trials of fluoxetine aiming to identify responders and non-responders to SSRIs are in development (Nightingale, 2012).

Evidence regarding other antidepressant use is scant and of lower quality. Open-label trials of sertraline, citalopram and escitalopram in children and adults have showed benefits in reducing aggression and repetitive behaviours. Studies of paroxetine have not shown ongoing benefit in adults and there are no studies using paroxetine in children as yet. A larger RCT of citalopram in children with ASD and repetitive behaviours showed no significant differences in response between the citalopram- and placebo-treated groups, although both groups showed improvements. Citalopram was more likely to be associated with adverse events such as increased energy levels and insomnia (King et al, 2009). Open-label studies of venlafaxine have suggested efficacy for repetitive behaviours in some children and adults (Hollander et al, 2000). It is possible that SSRIs are more effective and give rise to fewer side-effects in adolescents and adults than in children (Erickson et al, 2007).

Antipsychotics

Large multi-site trials involving children (e.g. McDougle et al, 2005) showed that risperidone was significantly more effective than placebo for reducing stereotypical and ritualistic behaviours. However, in smaller

RCTs with preschool children with ASD, risperidone was not meaningfully superior to placebo (Luby *et al*, 2006). Adverse effects of second-generation antipsychotics include increased appetite and weight gain, dyslipidaemia and insulin resistance, somnolence, extrapyramidal symptoms and prolactin elevation. One study looking at long-term risperidone treatment used a pooled database of prolactin levels in 700 children over the course of 12 months (Dunbar *et al*, 2004). Mean levels were found to increase and peak in the first 1–2 months and then return to near normal by 3–5 months. There was no associated delay in growth or sexual maturation. Prolongation of the QTc interval with risperidone has been reported, but studies in both adults and children did not find prolongation beyond the threshold accepted as being associated with *torsade de pointes* or other significant electrocardiogram (ECG) changes.

Summary

Despite the considerable and ongoing efforts described above to improve core features of autism with pharmacotherapy, there has been no signal success to date. Additionally, the adverse effects of many agents have to be taken in the balance. Consequently, recent clinical guidelines from the National Institute for Health and Care Excellence & Social Care Institute for Excellence (2013) do not to recommend any medication as effective specifically for core symptoms. The situation however is rather different in relation to comorbidity, to which we now turn.

Comorbid psychiatric symptoms

Autism spectrum disorders have a high prevalence of both psychiatric and physical comorbidities. These tend to emerge in middle childhood and wax and wane according to circumstance. At a theoretical level it is not always clear that such symptoms constitute a true psychiatric comorbidity; commonly, symptoms will co-occur with autism because of the interaction between the developmental disorder and concurrent stressors. These may include increased social demands, inadequately adapted schooling, a sense of rejection or poor self-image, bullying or family conflict. It is important to understand these symptoms, as they are often as functionally impairing and yet more tractable than the core disorder, and are often a key target for intervention.

Accurate diagnosis of comorbid psychiatric disorders can be difficult. Modifications of diagnostic criteria may be necessary to account for differing clinical presentations in individuals with developmental disability. 'Diagnostic overshadowing' may prevent accurate detection of symptoms; even if detected, they may be spuriously attributed to the core disorder. Deciding whom and when to treat may be largely based on functional impairment. Conditions such as depression and anxiety may be eminently treatable and tackling them may vastly improve the quality of life of patients and families.

There is some evidence for treating symptoms of hyperkinetic disorder in autism but sparse high-quality data concerning other psychiatric comorbidities. Most of the available data come from trials designed to assess core and behavioural symptoms associated with autism, but which also found improvements in other domains such as depressive or anxious symptoms. There is no evidence that pharmacological treatment of OCD, tic disorders and sleep problems should differ from that used for each disorder alone. The use of haloperidol, clonidine and risperidone for tics, clomipramine or SSRIs for obsessions and compulsions, and melatonin for sleep is well described in the literature and in NICE guidance.

Maladaptive aggression and self-injury

Self-injurious behaviour and aggression can severely disrupt the management of autism. Many pharmacological treatments have undergone trials. Evidence for alpha-2 agonists such as clonidine and beta-blockers is limited to small RCTs and case reports.

Second-generation antipsychotics are the most frequently used psychotropic medication for aggression and serious self-injury in people with autism. Moderately sized RCTs of risperidone in both adults and children have described beneficial effects. Open-label studies with a double-blind discontinuation component have suggested both longer-term benefits and tolerance (e.g. Research Units on Pediatric Psychopharmacology Autism Network, 2005b). In 2006, the US Food and Drug Administration approved risperidone for the symptomatic treatment of irritability (including aggression and self-injury) in children and adolescents. In the UK, a Cochrane review (Jesner et al, 2007) concluded that risperidone can be beneficial, but that the lack of a single standardised outcome measure did not allow direct comparison of studies. Aripiprazole has demonstrated improvements in irritability, aggression and self-injury, and a recent Cochrane review (Ching & Pringsheim, 2012) concluded that it is effective in the short-term treatment of irritability, hyperactivity and repetitive movements in children. However, the long-term safety of aripiprazole needs further investigation and, given its considerable extra cost, it is not established to be cost-effective over risperidone.

Evidence of efficacy of other antipsychotics is very preliminary. One small RCT of olanzapine found it to be effective in about 50% of children (Hollander et al, 2006). However, olanzapine is strongly associated with weight gain and other physical morbidity. Open-label trials of quetiapine indicate that the response rate and tolerability are poor (e.g. Martin et al, 1999). Clozapine and ziprasidone are rarely used because of the risk of blood dyscrasias and QTc prolongation respectively. Several large, well-designed RCTs (e.g. Remington et al, 2001) have studied haloperidol and found it efficacious in both children and adults with autism and behaviour problems. Adverse events including dyskinesia and sedation are common, however, and it is therefore more often reserved for treatment-refractory symptoms.

The NICE guidelines recommend consideration of antipsychotic medication for treatment of challenging behaviour if psychosocial management has been insufficient or the problem is so severe as to preclude such management (National Institute for Health and Clinical Excellence, 2008; National Institute for Health and Care Excellence & Social Care Institute for Excellence, 2013).

Opiate antagonists

Initial findings of open-label studies of naltrexone seemed promising but subsequent placebo-controlled studies showed no positive effects on the core social deficits. The most consistent finding is a modest reduction in hyperactivity. A quantitative review of the literature suggests that naltrexone might be beneficial for reducing self-injurious behaviours in individuals with intellectual disabilities ('mental retardation'), including those with ASD (Symons et al, 2004).

Mood stabilisers

Evidence regarding the effects of anti-epileptic medication is mixed. A small RCT of valproate (Hellings et al, 2005) for aggression in 30 adolescents could not demonstrate a significant difference between the drug and placebo. Trials of divalproex indicate that it confers benefits on measures of irritability (Hollander et al, 2010).

Published data for carbamazepine are limited to case reports. Hepatotoxicity, weight gain, sedation and teratogenicity are important side-effects for this group of drugs. There are no controlled trials of lithium for ASD.

Hyperkinesis and inattention

Symptoms of hyperkinetic disorder (inattention, impulsivity, distractibility and hyperactivity) are very common in ASD, particularly in children and adolescents (Lee & Ousley, 2006). Traditionally in UK diagnostic schemes such as ICD-10 (World Health Organization, 1992), a diagnosis of hyperkinetic disorder is not made if it occurs exclusively during the course of an ASD (the diagnostic hierarchy concept). However, these symptoms may severely impair an individual's functioning and warrant treatment in their own right. It is likely that ICD-11, which is due in 2015, will relax this strictly hierarchical approach to diagnostic formulation.

Psychostimulants

Randomised controlled trials of methylphenidate have demonstrated improvement in childhood autism (Research Units on Pediatric Psychopharmacology Autism Network, 2005a). This applies to immediate-release preparations, but it is unclear whether the results can be applied to other stimulants. Trials suggest that the response rate in people with autism is lower than that in people without autism, and that side-effects such as irritability and poor appetite are more common. One trial suggested that patients with Asperger syndrome may respond more positively than those with other ASD, but not better than neurotypical individuals (Stigler *et al*, 2004). However, a subsequent large open-label study in children with attention-deficit hyperactivity disorder found no statistically significant difference in degree of response or adverse events between those with ASD and those without (Santosh *et al*, 2006). Psychostimulants may have a positive effect on some aspects of social communication, such as joint attention initiations, in children with ASD and hyperactivity.

Atomoxetine

Atomoxetine is a selective noradrenaline inhibitor. Open-label studies (Posey *et al*, 2006*b*) and a small pilot RCT (Arnold *et al*, 2006) have suggested efficacy for hyperactivity, impulsivity and oppositional behaviour in ASD. Atomoxetine is often well tolerated, but common side-effects include nausea, increased heart rate and fatigue.

Alpha-2 adrenergic agonists

Two very small RCTs involving a total of 17 patients (Fankhauser *et al*, 1992) have suggested modest benefits of clonidine, and one small cross-over study suggests similar effects for lofexidine (Niederhofer *et al*, 2002). A small cross-over RCT in children indicates that guanfacine may also be helpful for hyperactivity (Handen *et al*, 2008). Common side-effects include sedation and hypotension.

Amantadine

One RCT of amantadine for children (King *et al*, 2001) showed some improvements in hyperactivity and impulsivity on observer measures but not on parent-scored measures. Amantadine may therefore be useful in modulating behaviour in some young patients, but it is not clear whether this is because of its glutamatergic activity or enhancement of dopaminergic neurotransmission.

Antipsychotics

Aripiprazole has demonstrated short-term improvements in measures of hyperactivity in RCTs in children (Ching & Pringsheim, 2012). Open-label trials of risperidone also indicate that it may be helpful in this domain, particularly when combined with behavioural therapy (Aman *et al*, 2009) or other drugs, for example mood stabilisers such as topiramate (Rezaei *et al*, 2010).

Mood disorders

Patients with autism have been reported to be at increased risk of depression (which has a prevalence of about 2% in all ASD), particularly those who are more cognitively able (Ghaziuddin *et al*, 2002). However, one follow-up study suggests that the incidence of mood disorder may be no different from that in the general population (Hutton *et al*, 2008). Nevertheless, depressive symptoms remain an important treatable cause of deterioration in functioning.

Mood disorder tends to emerge from middle childhood and it is often associated clinically with the child's increased self-awareness of difference and the increasing social demands of peers. As in other childhood mood disorders, psychosocial management is the first-line approach, and adaptation of the social and educational environment is often a first-line target (National Collaborating Centre for Mental Health, 2005).

For persistent and/or severe depressive disorder, open-label trials of SSRIs, including fluoxetine, fluvoxamine, sertraline, citalopram and escitalopram, in children and adults have been associated with improvements in a depressive phenotype that includes such symptoms as social withdrawal, irritability, sadness or crying, decreased energy and weight loss. Systematic reviews have confirmed that SSRIs should be considered for the treatment of depressive symptoms in ASD (Posey *et al*, 2006*a*).

Anticonvulsants such as divalproex have been posited to be useful for mood lability (Myers, 2007). Several case reports describe patients with autism and atypical bipolar disorder who responded well to open-label treatment with lithium (e.g. Kerbeshian *et al*, 1987). Open-label trials of second-generation antipsychotics suggest no difference in response to treatment for bipolar disorder in those with ASD and those without (Joshi *et al*, 2012).

Anxiety disorders

Individuals with ASD show an increased risk of anxiety disorders (Kim *et al*, 2000). The anxiety is often particularly intense and sometimes atypical; in some, it can interact with core symptomatology to mimic thought disorder. One double-blind trial shows evidence of efficacy using fluvoxamine (McDougle *et al*, 1996), and case reports indicate improvement in anxiety symptoms with other SSRIs (Posey *et al*, 2006*a*).

An open-label study as well as case reports suggest that buspirone (a 5-HT agonist) may be effective for anxiety (Buitelaar *et al*, 1998). Beta-blockers may be appropriate where panic is a component symptom (Famularo *et al*, 1988).

Clinical implications

The core social impairments in ASD remain relatively intractable. In childhood and adolescence, psychosocial and education management strategies should be the first line in management. The current small evidence base for a pharmacological approach to long-term disabilities means that at present medication management does not have a significant place in practice.

Severe maladaptive aggression and self-injury can be the most disturbing and impairing of comorbid symptoms in autism, particularly in individuals with intellectual disabilities. Antipsychotics, particularly risperidone and aripiprazole, have a consistent evidence base, and are increasingly prescribed. Principles of careful targeting, frequent review and minimum necessary dosing should be applied in use of antipsychotics.

In children with any form of developmental disability, hyperactivity and inattention are more complex to treat than in neurotypical children: response is more idiosyncratic and unwanted effects are more common. Thus far, immediate-release methylphenidate has the most consistent evidence base for symptoms of motor hyperactivity and inattention in children and adolescents, although there is increasing interest in antipsychotics. The NICE guidelines on ADHD state that drug treatments should be offered as first-line treatment to school-age children and young people only if they have severe symptoms or impairment, and always in combination with psychosocial interventions (National Institute for Health and Clinical Excellence, 2008: para. 1.5.3.1). Methylphenidate, dexamfetamine and atomoxetine are all regarded as options for management.

Anxiety management strategies and desensitisation for behavioural avoidance can usefully be combined with SSRIs, as can psychotherapeutic interventions for mood disorder.

Medication management should be carefully monitored; doses should be titrated up from a low base to the 'minimum effective dose' using frequent detailed symptom monitoring. Specific medications should not be continued if there is no evidence of their benefit, but withdrawal should be slow and judicious to avoid withdrawal effects.

Conclusion

Research in many of the areas discussed is still in its early phases, and it is important that clinicians remember the ongoing limitations of the evidence and intrinsic difficulties of measurement when discussing things with often well-informed and frustrated families. There is the inherent difficulty of studying pharmacological response in developmental disorders themselves. Measuring change in ASD is complex and must take into account day-to-day fluctuations, powerful placebo effects and idiosyncratic responses. These issues are more widely recognised now and researchers are attempting to address them. However, the field awaits a critical mass of larger, more robust clinical trials with more specific measurements and sophisticated analyses of clinical effectiveness. Clinicians will need to carefully interpret the clinical evidence and make active adjustments in applying it to the specific situation of their patients. Despite the limitations, however, both the quantity and quality of medication trials targeting symptom domains in ASD have increased in recent years. There remains a lack of important information on long-term safety and efficacy of drugs, and the standard of

---

Box 8.1 Important considerations when prescribing for autism spectrum disorder

To make informed decisions about a potential role for medication, the prescriber must:

- clarify characteristics of the challenging behaviours, including frequency, intensity, duration and degree of interference with functioning
- be clear about the target symptoms to be treated (differentiate core from comorbid symptoms)
- identify exacerbating and ameliorating factors, including response to psycho-therapeutic interventions
- assess existing and available health, educational and social supports, and the strengths of the family (e.g. the family's ability to support the individual)
- assess comorbid physical problems by thorough history and examination, and consider their impact on presentation and treatment of the challenging behaviours
- consider potential adverse events and drug interactions
- avoid polypharmacy
- use a 'start low and go slow' treatment strategy.

---

evidence so far does not allow for definitive treatment protocols for various symptom clusters. However, the aggregation of data suggests that SSRIs, risperidone and immediate-release methylphenidate can be of great value within the domains discussed. There are as yet no proven treatments for the underlying social deficit in autism.

We have emphasised that medication management is only one strand of intervention for people with ASD, and the mainstay of treatment remains educational and psychosocial. Pharmacological management needs to be undertaken by thorough assessment, accurate diagnosis and regular monitoring of target symptom clusters, comorbid diagnoses and response to treatment (Box 8.1).

Researchers are beginning to consider the value of a more formal combination of behavioural and medical interventions in complex treatment trials designed to alter the developmental trajectory of those with autism. Advances in neurophysiology and genetics, such as stem cell therapy, may also make it possible to delineate subgroups that may be particularly responsive to particular treatments. Such developments may pave the way for a more integrated consensus on an overall approach to treatment of ASD across the lifespan.

References

Akhondzadeh S, Falleh J, Mohammadi MR, *et al* (2010) Double-blind placebo-controlled trial of pentoxifylline added to risperidone: effects on aberrant behaviour in children with autism. *Programme of Neuropsychopharmacological and Biological Psychiatry*, **34**, 32–36.

Aman MG, Lam KSL, Van Bourgondien ME (2005) Medication patterns in patients with autism: temporal, regional, and demographic influences. *Journal of Child and Adolescent Psychopharmacology*, **15**, 116–126.

Aman MG, McDougle CJ, Scahill L, *et al* (2009) Medication and parent training in children with pervasive developmental disorders and serious behavior problems: results from a randomized clinical trial. *Journal of the American Academy of Child & Adolescent Psychiatry*, **48**, 1143–1154.

Arnold LE, Aman MG, Cook AM, *et al* (2006) Atomoxetine for hyperactivity in autism spectrum disorders: placebo-controlled crossover pilot trial. *Journal of the American Academy of Child and Adolescent Psychiatry*, **45**, 1196–1205.

Autism Genome Project Consortium (2007) Mapping autism risk loci using genetic linkage and chromosomal rearrangements. *Nature Genetics*, **39**, 319–328.

Autism Speaks (2009) *Autism Speaks announces results reported for the study of fluoxetine in autism (SOFIA)*. Autism Speaks (http://www.autismspeaks.org/press/as_announces_sofia_results.php). Accessed 22 Jan 2014.

Baird, G, Simonoff, E, Pickles, A, *et al* (2009) Prevalence of disorders of the autism spectrum in a population cohort of children in South Thames: the Special Needs and Autism Project (SNAP). *Lancet*, **368**, 210–215.

Belsito KM, Law PA, Kirk KS, *et al* (2001) Lamotrigine therapy for autistic disorder: a randomized, double-blind, placebo-controlled trial. *Journal of Autism and Developmental Disorders*, **31**, 175–181.

BMJ Group, Royal Pharmaceutical Society, Royal College of Paediatrics and Child Health, *et al* (2013) *BNF for Children: 2013–2014*. Pharmaceutical Press.

Buchsbaum MS, Hollander E, Haznedar MM, *et al* (2001) Effect of fluoxetine on regional cerebral metabolism in autistic spectrum disorders: a pilot study. *International Journal of Neuropsychopharmacology*, **4**, 119–125.

Buitelaar JK, van der Gaag RJ, van der Hoeven J (1998) Buspirone in the management of anxiety and irritability in children with pervasive developmental disorders: results of an open-label study. *Journal of Clinical Psychiatry*, **59**, 56–59.

Carlsson ML (1998) Hypothesis: is infantile autism a hypoglutamatergic disorder? Relevance of glutamate–serotonin interactions for pharmacotherapy. *Journal of Neural Transmission*, **105**, 525–535.

Chez MG, Burton Q, Dowling T, *et al* (2007) Memantine as adjunctive therapy in children diagnosed with autistic spectrum disorders: an observation of initial clinical response and maintenance tolerability. *Journal of Child Neurology*, **22**, 574–579.

Ching H, Pringsheim T (2012) Aripiprazole for autistic spectrum disorders (ASD). *Cochrane Database of Systematic Reviews*, **16** (5), CD009043.

Dunbar F, Kusumakar V, Daneman D, *et al* (2004) Growth and sexual maturation during long-term treatment with risperidone. *American Journal of Psychiatry*, **161**, 918–920.

Erickson CA, Posey DJ, Stigler KA, *et al* (2007) Pharmacologic treatment of autism and related disorders. *Pediatric Annals*, **36**, 575–585.

Famularo R, Kinscherff R, Fenton T (1988) Propranolol treatment for childhood posttraumatic stress disorder, acute type: a pilot study. *American Journal of Diseases of Children*, **142**, 1244–1247.

Fankhauser MP, Karumanchi VC, German ML, *et al* (1992) A double-blind, placebo-controlled study of the efficacy of transdermal clonidine in autism. *Journal of Clinical Psychiatry*, **53**, 77–82.

Ghaziuddin M, Ghaziuddin N, Greden J (2002) Depression in persons with autism: implications for research and clinical care. *Journal of Autism and Developmental Disorders*, **32**, 299–306.

Godlee F, Smith J, Marcovitch H (2011) Wakefield's article linking MMR vaccine and autism was fraudulent. *BMJ*, **342**, c7452.

Handen BL, Sahl R, Hardan AY (2008) Guanfacine in children with autism and/or intellectual disabilities. *Journal of Developmental and Behavioral Pediatrics*, **29**, 303–308.

Hellings JA, Weckbaugh M, Nickel EJ, *et al* (2005) A double-blind, placebo-controlled study of valproate for aggression in youth with pervasive developmental disorders. *Journal of Child and Adolescent Psychopharmacology*, **15**, 682–692.

Hollander E, Kaplan A, Cartwright C, *et al* (2000) Venlafaxine in children, adolescents, and young adults with autism spectrum disorders: an open retrospective clinical report. *Journal of Child Neurology*, **15**, 132–135.

Hollander E, Dolgoff Caspar R, Cartwright C, *et al* (2001) An open trial of divalproex sodium in autism spectrum disorders. *Journal of Clinical Psychiatry*, **62**, 530–534.

Hollander E, Phillips A, Chaplin W, *et al* (2005) A placebo controlled crossover trial of liquid fluoxetine on repetitive behaviors in childhood and adolescent autism. *Neuropsychopharmacology*, **30**, 582–589.

Hollander E, Wasserman S, Swanson EN, *et al* (2006) A double-blind placebo-controlled pilot study of olanzapine in childhood/adolescent pervasive developmental disorder. *Journal of Child and Adolescent Psychopharmacology*, **16**, 541–548.

Hollander E, Chaplin W, Soorya L, *et al* (2010) Divalproex sodium vs. placebo for the treatment of irritability in children and adolescents with autism spectrum disorders. *Neuropsychopharmacology*, **35**, 990–998.

Hutton J, Goode S, Murphy M, *et al* (2008) New-onset psychiatric disorders in individuals with autism. *Autism*, **12**, 373–390.

Jaselskis CA, Cook EH, Fletcher KE, *et al* (1992) Clonidine treatment of hyperactive and impulsive children with autistic disorder. *Journal of Clinical Psychopharmacology*, **12**, 322–327.

Jesner OS, Aref-Adib M, Coren E (2007) Risperidone for autism spectrum disorder. *Cochrane Database of Systematic Reviews*, **1**, CD005040.

Joshi G, Beiderman J, Wozniack J, *et al* (2012) Response to second generation antipsychotics in youth with comorbid bipolar disorder and autism spectrum disorder. *CNS Neuroscience and Therapeutics*, **18**, 28–33.

Kerbeshian J, Burd L, Fisher W (1987) Lithium carbonate in the treatment of two patients with infantile autism and atypical bipolar symptomatology. *Journal of Clinical Psychopharmacology*, **7**, 401–405.

Kim JA, Szatmari P, Bryson SE, *et al* (2000) The prevalence of anxiety and mood problems among children with autism and Asperger syndrome. *Autism*, **4**, 117–132.

King BH, Wright DM, Handen BL, *et al* (2001) Double-blind, placebo-controlled study of amantadine hydrochloride in the treatment of children with autistic disorder. *Journal of the American Academy of Child & Adolescent Psychiatry*, **40**, 658–665.

King BH, Hollander E, Sikich L, *et al* (2009) Lack of efficacy of citalopram in children with autism spectrum disorders and high levels of repetitive behavior: citalopram ineffective in children with autism. *Archives of General Psychiatry*, **66**, 583–590.

Lee DO, Ousley OY (2006) Attention-deficit hyperactivity disorder symptoms in a clinic sample of children and adolescents with pervasive developmental disorders. *Journal of Child and Adolescent Psychopharmacology*, **16**, 737–746.

Luby J, Mrakotsky C, Stalets MM, *et al* (2006) Risperidone in preschool children with autistic spectrum disorders: an investigation of safety and efficacy. *Journal of Child and Adolescent Psychopharmacology*, **16**, 575–587.

Martin A, Koenig K, Scahill L, *et al* (1999) Open-label quetiapine in the treatment of children and adolescents with autistic disorder. *Journal of Child and Adolescent Psychopharmacology*, **9**, 99–107.

McDougle CJ, Naylor ST, Cohen DJ, *et al* (1996) A double-blind, placebo-controlled study of fluvoxamine in adults with autistic disorder. *Archives of General Psychiatry*, **53**, 1001–1008.

McDougle CJ, Holmes JP, Carlson DC, *et al* (1998) A double blind placebo controlled study of risperidone in adults with autistic disorder and other pervasive developmental disorders. *Archives of General Psychiatry*, **55**, 633–641.

McDougle CJ, Kresch LE, Posey DJ (2000) Repetitive thoughts and behavior in pervasive developmental disorders: treatment with serotonin reuptake inhibitors. *Journal of Autism and Developmental Disorders*, **30**, 427–435.

McDougle CJ, Scahill L, Aman MG, *et al* (2005) Risperidone for the core symptom domains of autism: results from the study by the Autism Network of the Research Units on Pediatric Psychopharmacology. *American Journal of Psychiatry*, **162**, 1142–1148.

McDougle CJ, Stigler KA, Erickson CA, *et al* (2006) Pharmacology of autism. *Clinical Neuroscience Research*, **6**, 179–188.

Myers SM (2007) The status of pharmacotherapy for autism spectrum disorders. *Expert Opinion in Pharmacotherapy*, **8**, 1579–1603.

National Collaborating Centre for Mental Health (2005) *Depression in Children and Young People: Identification and Management in Primary, Community and Secondary Care* (Clinical Guideline 28). National Institute for Health and Clinical Excellence.

National Institute for Health and Care Excellence & Social Care Institute for Excellence (2013) *Autism: The Management and Support of Children and Young People on the Autism Spectrum* (NICE Clinical Guideline 110). NICE.

National Institute for Health and Clinical Excellence (2008) *Attention Deficit Hyperactivity Disorder: Diagnosis and Management of ADHD in Children, Young People and Adults* (NICE Clinical Guideline 72). NICE.

National Institute for Health and Clinical Excellence (2011) *Autism Diagnosis in Children and Young People: Recognition, Referral and Diagnosis of Children and Young People on the Autism Spectrum* (NICE Clinical Guideline 128). NICE.

National Institute for Health and Clinical Excellence (2012) *Autism: Recognition, Referral, Diagnosis and Management of Adults on the Autism Spectrum* (NICE Clinical Guideline 142). NICE.

Niederhofer H, Staffer W, Mair A (2002) Lofexidine in hyperactive and impulsive children with autistic disorder. *Journal of the American Academy of Child & Adolescent Psychiatry*, **41**, 1396–1397.

Nightingale S (2012) Autism spectrum disorders. *Nature Reviews: Drug Discovery*, **11**, 745–746.

Nikolov R, Jonker J, Scahill L (2006) Autistic disorder: current psychopharmacological treatments and areas of interest for future developments [Portuguese, English]. *Revista Brasileira de Psiquiatria*, **28** (suppl. 1), S39–S46.

Nye C, Brice A (2005) Combined vitamin B6–magnesium treatment in autism spectrum disorder. *Cochrane Database of Systematic Reviews*, **4**, CD003497.

Owen R, Sikich L, Marcus RN, *et al* (2009) Aripiprazole in the treatment of irritability in children and adolescents with autistic disorder. *Pediatrics*, **124**, 1533–1540.

Owens JA, Babcock D, Blumer J, *et al* (2005) The use of pharmacotherapy in the treatment of pediatric insomnia in primary care: rational approaches. A consensus meeting summary. *Journal of Clinical Sleep Medicine*, **1**, 49–59.

Owley T, Salt J, Guter S, *et al* (2006) A prospective open label trial of memantine in the treatment of cognitive, behavioral and memory dysfunction in pervasive developmental disorders. *Journal of Child and Adolescent Psychopharmacology*, **16**, 517–524.

Posey DJ, Erickson CA, Stigler KA, *et al* (2006a) The use of selective serotonin reuptake inhibitors in autism and related disorders. *Journal of Child and Adolescent Psychopharmacology*, **16**, 181–186.

Posey DJ, Wiegand RE, Wilkerson J, *et al* (2006b) Open-label atomoxetine for attention-deficit/hyperactivity disorder symptoms associated with high-functioning pervasive developmental disorders. *Journal of Child and Adolescent Psychopharmacology*, **16**, 599–610.

Remington G, Sloman L, Konstantareas M, *et al* (2001) Clomipramine versus haloperidol in the treatment of autistic disorder: a double-blind, placebo-controlled, crossover study. *Journal of Clinical Psychopharmacology*, **21**, 440–444.

Research Units on Pediatric Psychopharmacology Autism Network (2005a) Randomised, controlled, crossover trial of methylphenidate in pervasive developmental disorders with hyperactivity. *Archives of General Psychiatry*, **62**, 1266–1274.

Research Units on Pediatric Psychopharmacology Autism Network (2005b) Risperidone treatment of autistic disorder: longer term benefits and blinded discontinuation after 6 months. *American Journal of Psychiatry*, **162**, 1361–1369.

Rezaei V, Mohammadi MR, Ghanizadeh A, *et al* (2010) Double-blind, placebo-controlled trial of risperidone plus topiramate in children with autistic disorder. *Programme of Neuropsychopharmacological and Biological Psychiatry*, **34**, 1269–1272.

Sandler AD, Sutton KA, Deweese J, *et al* (1999) A double blind placebo controlled study of synthetic human secretin in the treatment of autism and pervasive developmental disorder. *New England Journal of Medicine*, **341**, 1801–1806.

Sandler RH, Finegold SM, Bolte ER, *et al* (2000) Short-term benefit from oral vancomycin treatment of regressive-onset autism. *Journal of Child Neurology*, **15**, 429–435.

Santosh PJ, Baird G, Pityaratstian N, *et al* (2006) Impact of comorbid autism spectrum disorders on stimulant response in children with attention deficit hyperactivity disorder: a retrospective and prospective effectiveness study. *Child: Care, Health and Development*, **32**, 575–583.

Scahill L, McCracken JT, McGough J, *et al* (2002) Risperidone in children with autism and serious behavioral problems. *New England Journal of Medicine*, **347**, 314–321.

Shea S, Turgay A, Carroll A, *et al* (2004) Risperidone in the treatment of disruptive behavioral symptoms in children with autistic and other pervasive developmental disorders. *Pediatrics*, **114**, e634–641.

Stigler KA, Desmond LA, Posey DJ, *et al* (2004) A naturalistic retrospective analysis of psychostimulants in pervasive developmental disorders. *Journal of Child and Adolescent Psychopharmacology*, **14**, 49–56.

Sugie Y, Sugie H, Fukuda T, *et al* (2005) Clinical efficacy of fluvoxamine and functional polymorphism in a serotonin transporter gene on childhood autism. *Journal of Autism and Developmental Disorders*, **35**, 377–385.

Symons FJ, Thompson A, Rodriguez MC (2004) Self-injurious behavior and the efficacy of naltrexone treatment: a quantitative synthesis. *Mental Retardation and Developmental Disability Research Review*, **10**, 193–200.

Tsakanikos E, Costello H, Holt G, *et al* (2006) Psychopathology in adults with autism and intellectual disability. *Journal of Autism and Developmental Disorders*, **36**, 1123–1129.

Volkmar FR, Paul R, Cohen DJ, *et al* (1983) Irritability in autistic children treated with fenfluramine. *New England Journal of Medicine*, **309**, 187.

World Health Organization (1992) *The ICD-10 Classification of Mental and Behavioural Disorders: Clinical Descriptions and Diagnostic Guidelines*. WHO.

Yurgelun-Todd DA, Coyle JT, Gruber SA, *et al* (2005) Functional magnetic resonance imaging studies of schizophrenic patients during word production: effects of D-cycloserine. *Psychiatry Research*, **138**, 23–31.

Zeiner P, Gjevik E, Weidle B (2011) Response to atomoxetine in boys with high-functioning autism spectrum disorders and attention deficit/hyperactivity disorder. *Acta Paediatrica*, **100**, 1258–1261.

CHAPTER 9

Pharmacological treatment of depression and bipolar disorder

Bernadka Dubicka, Paul Wilkinson, Raphael G. Kelvin and Ian M. Goodyer

Major depressive disorder and bipolar disorder can occur in quite young children. However, since both conditions are more common in adolescence than in childhood, and there is a greater evidence base for medication use in this age group, we focus here primarily on adolescents. Mood disorders in children and adolescents are diagnosed using adult criteria, although this is controversial, particularly in paediatric bipolar disorder. The advent of DSM-5 (American Psychiatric Association, 2013) has brought about few changes in the classification of mood disorders: grief is no longer an exclusion criterion for depression, and increased energy/activity is now regarded as a core symptom of mania and hypomania. A new category, disruptive mood dysregulation disorder (DMDD), has been introduced with the aim of reducing inappropriate diagnosis of bipolar disorder in children and adolescents who have non-cyclical, frequent severe temper outbursts along with a persistent irritable mood. Currently, there is little research regarding the diagnosis and treatment of DMDD, but early studies suggest that it is unlikely to be a precursor of bipolar disorder, so it will not be considered further in this chapter.

Prescribing in depression

Background

The prescribing of newer-generation antidepressants to children and adolescents with depression has been controversial in the UK since the publication of the Committee on Safety of Medicines (CSM) report on selective serotonin reuptake inhibitors (SSRIs) (Committee on Safety of Medicines, 2003). This report highlighted the important matter of the non-publication of negative trial results and questioned both the effectiveness and safety of these medications, particularly an increased risk of suicidality. Before discussing the practicalities of prescribing, we will first review the evidence for the CSM findings. The tricyclic antidepressants will not be discussed here, as the risks associated with these drugs outweigh the relatively small benefits of using them.

Evidence base for pharmacological treatment

The CSM report concluded that, of the new-generation antidepressants (a group which includes the SSRIs and antidepressants such as venlafaxine, a serotonin–noradrenaline reuptake inhibitor or SNRI), only fluoxetine showed a positive risk–benefit ratio in treating depression in young people when compared with a drug placebo (Committee on Safety of Medicines, 2003).

A meta-analysis of 15 randomised controlled trials (RCTs) of new-generation antidepressants compared outcomes of paediatric major depressive disorder, obsessive–compulsive disorder (OCD) and non-OCD anxiety disorders (Bridge *et al*, 2007). It found a pooled difference for response of 11% between drug and placebo in depression that significantly favoured the antidepressants (number needed to treat, NNT = 10). However, this effect was more modest for major depressive disorder than for OCD or anxiety, and only fluoxetine showed a significant benefit. Fluoxetine also showed a larger effect overall (difference 20%, NNT = 5), consistent with the findings of the CSM. The authors concluded that, overall, new-generation antidepressants are efficacious when compared with placebo, but other authors have been more circumspect. For example, in a meta-analysis of 19 depression trials, Hetrick *et al* (2012) highlighted significant methodological problems, and questioned whether the overall modest improvements found are clinically meaningful. There was no evidence of any differential effects between children and adolescents. The authors did not comment on the comparative efficacy of the antidepressants, although fluoxetine and escitalopram had consistent evidence of efficacy across more than one outcome.

What are we to make of these findings? First, although the overall effects appear modest, many of the trials excluded suicidal young people and none included the most severe, complex cases that would commonly be treated with antidepressants by child and adolescent mental health services (CAMHS) in the UK. Therefore, we do not know how the most vulnerable depressed children and adolescents would respond. There is some indication that greater effects are seen in more severe adult depression as a result of a reduced placebo response (Kirsch *et al*, 2008), and increased severity of depression has also been associated with reduced placebo effects in children and adolescents (Bridge *et al*, 2009). Therefore it is possible that antidepressant/placebo differences may be greater for severe paediatric depression.

Second, it can be argued that the overall response seen with antidepressants also needs to take into account the sizeable placebo effect (up to 50% in children and adolescents), since placebos are not normally prescribed in clinical practice .

Finally, although the effect size of antidepressants compared with placebo appears to be modest, do psychological treatments fare any better when compared with placebo? Many psychological treatment trials have used non-active comparators such as waiting lists and have, unsurprisingly, found large effects. Thus far, only one psychological treatment trial involving adolescents has used a pill placebo and this compared cognitive–behavioural therapy (CBT) with both fluoxetine and pill placebo (March *et al*, 2004). At 12 weeks, the overall effect size for depressive symptoms relative to placebo was 0.68 for fluoxetine (a moderate to large effect) and −0.03 for CBT alone (equivalent to placebo); fluoxetine was significantly superior to CBT (effect size: 0.66). Adverse effects are rarely measured in psychological treatment trials, but it cannot be assumed that all such interventions are harmless.

Suicidal thoughts, behaviour and non-suicidal self-harm

In considering this area it should be noted that different trials used different operational criteria, which makes comparison difficult. Meta-analyses conducted since the 2003 CSM report generally indicate a small, increased risk of suicidal ideation/attempts and non-suicidal self-harm with the new-generation antidepressants compared with placebo, but no deaths by suicide have been reported (e.g. Dubicka *et al*, 2006; Bridge *et al*, 2007). A more recent analysis of 17 trials reported an increased risk of suicide-related behaviours and ideation from 25 in 1000 to 40 in 1000 (Hetrick *et al*, 2012), but this increase was not significant for either children or adolescents, and there were no completed suicides. Conversely, a review of observational studies reported an increased risk of completed suicide among adolescents prescribed SSRIs, whereas a decreased risk was found among adults (Barbui *et al*, 2009). Although these findings are concerning, a number of points need to be considered.

First, in most trials suicidal thoughts and behaviour and self-harm were examined retrospectively in clinical notes and there was no agreed definition of these events or standardised way of data collection: weaknesses that undermine the certainty of their findings. The Treatment for Adolescents with Depression Study (TADS) is the only placebo-controlled trial that has examined this risk prospectively. This four-arm study (fluoxetine; CBT; fluoxetine plus CBT; pill placebo) found a reduction in suicidal ideation in all four groups at 12 weeks, with no significant differences between groups for ideation or attempts. However, there did appear to be an overall increased risk of suicidal events in adolescents receiving fluoxetine alone compared with other groups at both 12 and 36 weeks (Emslie *et al*, 2006; March *et al*, 2007).

Second, evidence from other sources does not consistently support an increased risk of suicide attempts and completed suicide. For example, the risk of suicide attempts is highest in the month before treatment is started (Simon *et al*, 2006); longer-term treatment is associated with a reduction in suicide attempts (Valuck *et al*, 2004) and fewer attempts occur if depression has been treated with antidepressants (Gibbons *et al*, 2007). Concerning completed suicide, antidepressants are rarely found in post-mortem examinations of child and adolescent suicides (Cortes *et al*, 2011), and ecological studies do not support an increased risk of suicide with the general rise in antidepressant prescribing (Baldessarini *et al*, 2007). A UK study reported that affective disorder remains the most common psychiatric diagnosis in child and adolescent suicides, and antidepressants had been prescribed to only 8% of those who had taken their lives (Windfuhr *et al*, 2008). Similarly, a review of population-based observational data of adolescent suicides found that only 1.6% (9/574) of those who completed suicide had been exposed to antidepressants; the authors concluded that, given the prevalence of depression associated with youth suicide, most adolescents dying by suicide have not had the potential benefit of antidepressants at the time of their deaths (Dudley *et al*, 2010).

Third, the antidepressant trials excluded the most severely suicidal children and adolescents, so the balance of risks and benefits remains speculative in this group.

Last, it is mental illness that remains untreated owing to a reluctance to seek help that has been most strongly implicated in child and adolescent suicides, rather than the adverse effects of receiving treatment (Moskos *et al*, 2007).

Overall, therefore, the evidence suggests that antidepressants are an important therapeutic option for moderate to severe adolescent depression, but the risk–benefit ratio in mild to moderate depression is likely to be less favourable. Clinicians need to closely monitor the risk of suicidality. Even though the importance of the increased risk of suicide-related behaviours with antidepressants is unclear (Hetrick *et al*, 2012), the risk of completed suicide in untreated depression is likely to be far greater.

Guidelines for pharmacological treatment

The National Institute for Health and Care Excellence (NICE) guidelines on the management of depression in children and adolescents advocate the use of fluoxetine as the first-line pharmacological treatment, with citalopram or sertraline as the second-line choices (National Collaborating Centre for Mental Health, 2005). This is broadly consistent with the guidelines produced by the Texas Consensus Conference Panel on Medication Treatment of Childhood Major Depressive Disorder in the USA (Hughes *et al*, 2007), although the Texas guidelines advise the use of any of these three SSRIs as a first-line medication. However, NICE advises starting SSRIs only in combination with a specific psychological treatment, and only if there has been no response to psychological treatment over 4–6 weeks. The Texas guidelines advise a non-specific treatment intervention initially, which concurs with our findings from the UK Adolescent Depression Antidepressant and Psychotherapy Trial (ADAPT) (Goodyer *et al*, 2007), in which 20% of adolescents with moderate to severe depression responded to our brief 'specialised clinical care' (SCC: see below).

Since the publication of these guidelines, cardiac warnings have been issued regarding the use of citalopram (and escitalopram) in adults.

Moreover, a recent meta-analysis failed to demonstrate a positive effect of citalopram on any outcome in depressed adolescents (Hetrick *et al*, 2012), in contrast to escitalopram, which demonstrated consistently positive outcomes on a number of measures. Sertraline was only effective for severity of depressive symptoms. Currently, escitalopram is the only antidepressant, other than fluoxetine, which is approved by the FDA for adolescent depression, although in light of warnings from the Medicines and Healthcare Products Regulatory Agency (2011) regarding their use in adults, caution should also be exerted in children and adolescents.

Key points of pharmacological treatment guidelines and drug licensing are summarised in Table 9.1.

Specialised clinical care

The elements of specialised clinical care (SCC) used in CAMHS are outlined in Box 9.1. We suggest that SCC be adopted as the initial intervention for depression, before medication or more specialised psychological treatments are added. The duration of initial SCC should depend on the response to treatment and the severity of the presentation. In more severe depression, with continuing significant impairment, suicidality and/or psychosis, we suggest that antidepressant treatment be started after 2–4 weeks of non-response; for patients at high risk, antidepressants might be prescribed even sooner. Individuals who do not wish or are unable to take medication

Table 9.1 Pharmacological treatment for depression in children and adolescents: UK and US guidelines and licensing

Drug	Guideline advice in terms of pharmacological treatment		Minimum age for licensed prescribing, years	
	NICE	Texas[a]	UK	USA
Citalopram	Second-line	First-line	≥18	≥18
Escitalopram	Not discussed	Second-line	≥18	≥12
Fluoxetine	First-line	First-line	≥8[b]	≥8
Paroxetine	Contraindicated by CSM	Second-line[c]	≥18	≥18
Sertraline	Second-line	First-line	≥18	≥18
Venlafaxine	Contraindicated by CSM	Third-line	≥18	≥18

CSM, Committee on Safety of Medicines (2003); NICE, National Institute for Health and Care Excellence's Clinical Guideline 28 (National Collaborating Centre for Mental Health, 2005); Texas, Texas Children's Medication Algorithm Project (Hughes *et al*, 2007).
a. For major depression of sufficient severity to warrant medication.
b. For moderate to severe depression.
c. Adolescents only.

Box 9.1 Specialised clinical care in CAMHS

- Engagement
- Empathic, reflective framework
- Formulation
- Instilling hope and managing expectations
- Psychoeducation
- Mental state monitoring
- Risk assessment and management, especially of suicidality
- Treating comorbid illnesses
- Family work
- Addressing parents' mental health issues
- Context management
- Liaison with schools and services
- Problem-solving
- Addressing alcohol and substance use
- Advising on diet, sleep, exercise and activities
- Relapse prevention work

---

and those with less severe depression who fail to respond to initial SCC should be offered specialised psychological treatment. As recommended in similar frameworks suggested in other guidelines (American Academy of Child and Adolescent Psychiatry, 2007a; Hughes *et al*, 2007), SSRIs should not be given without SCC.

The ADAPT study found that adding CBT to SCC and an SSRI did not confer any additional advantage in terms of improved clinical outcomes or a protective effect against suicidality over and above SCC and an SSRI. This questions the need for more specialised specific psychological treatment as an initial adjunct to medication. In addition, meta-analyses of trials of psychological treatment plus antidepressants have reported limited evidence of the benefit of combined treatment over antidepressants alone, or of a consistent protective effect against suicidality (Dubicka *et al*, 2010; Cox *et al*, 2012).

Principles of prescribing

Starting doses should be low (e.g. fluoxetine 10 mg) and the dose should be gradually titrated according to response and side-effects. Although there is a widely held belief regarding delayed onset of action of antidepressants, this does not concur with trial data for adults, which suggest that 35% of eventual improvement occurs in the first week (Posternak & Zimmerman, 2005). Current evidence suggests that continuing antidepressants for 6 months after an adequate response at 12 weeks significantly reduces the risk of relapse when compared with placebo (Emslie *et al*, 2008). The NICE guidelines (National Collaborating Centre for Mental Health, 2005) recommend continuing treatment for at least 6 months after recovery, defined as full functioning for 8 weeks and no symptoms.

Discontinuation should be gradual to avoid discontinuation symptoms: NICE suggests tapering over 6–12 weeks. Paroxetine and venlafaxine are more likely than fluoxetine to lead to such symptoms, but they are usually self-limiting and of short duration. Before stopping medication, consideration needs to be given to any current stresses that might increase the risk of relapse and make discontinuation inadvisable. In addition, those with a history of chronic depression or recurrence should be considered for longer maintenance treatment of more than a year (American Academy of Child and Adolescent Psychiatry, 2007a). Relapse is most likely to occur within the first 6 months following discontinuation, so close monitoring is recommended during this time.

Adverse effects

The SSRIs are associated with side-effects such as sedation, insomnia and gastrointestinal disturbances, although these are uncommon (<5%). Even more rarely, SSRIs can induce bleeding, serotonin syndrome, mania and agitation (Emslie *et al*, 2006; American Academy of Child and Adolescent Psychiatry, 2007a). Prenatal exposure to SSRIs may be associated with cardiovascular malformations in the first trimester and persistent pulmonary hypertension in later pregnancy. There is some recent evidence that SSRIs can also induce neuroendocrine adverse effects such as weight gain, type 2 diabetes mellitus and dyslipidaemia in children and adolescents, particularly females and children under 12 (Jerrell, 2010), although the implications of this are yet to be fully realised. Finally, citalopram and escitalopram are associated with dose-dependent QT interval prolongation. Although recommendations have not been made for children and adolescents, caution should be exerted when prescribing in this age group.

Predictors of response

About one-third of adolescents fail to show an adequate response to antidepressants for reasons listed in Box 9.2 (see Wilkinson *et al*, 2009). A more favourable response to SSRIs has been found in children and adolescents with anxiety and depression who are homozygous for the more functional long allele of the promoter of the serotonin transporter gene (Kronenberg *et al*, 2007); however, this finding has yet to be confirmed.

The rate of improvement in the early weeks of treatment is a good indicator of eventual remission (Rongrong *et al*, 2009). Before considering alternative treatment strategies, reassessment is required to review possible reasons for non-response. These can include misdiagnosis, comorbidity, inadequate treatment, non-adherence, side-effects and life events (American Academy of Child and Adolescent Psychiatry, 2007a; Maalouf *et al*, 2011). After reassessment, increasing the dose (up to 40 mg with fluoxetine,

135

Box 9.2 Predictors of poorer outcome with treatment in depression

- Older age
- Severity of depression
- Obsessive–compulsive disorder
- Suicidality
- Greater impairment
- Disappointing life events
- Melancholia
- Hopelessness
- Chronicity of depression
- Poor social function
- Two or more comorbid disorders
- Family conflict
- Low expectations
- Anxiety
- Substance abuse
- Maternal depression
- History of abuse

---

depending on the side-effect profile) may be a reasonable first strategy before considering switching.

The NICE guidelines (National Collaborating Centre for Mental Health, 2005) recommend using either sertraline or citalopram if there is no response to fluoxetine, and this advice is consistent with the results of the more recent Treatment of SSRI-Resistant Depression In Adolescents (TORDIA) study (Brent *et al*, 2008). This study found that in adolescents who failed to respond to an SSRI, switching to another SSRI at 12 weeks was as effective as switching to the SNRI venlafaxine, with fewer adverse effects. Nearly half of these treatment-resistant adolescents showed a positive response to a second-line SSRI. Direct switching of SSRIs without a washout period seems to be well tolerated (Anderson *et al*, 2008). The Texas guidelines (Hughes *et al*, 2007) include escitalopram and paroxetine as second-line SSRIs. In the UK paroxetine is currently contraindicated by the CSM for patients under 18 years of age because of its adverse risk–benefit profile (Committee on Safety of Medicines, 2003).

For third-line treatment, the Texas guidelines suggest using an antidepressant from a different class (Hughes *et al*, 2007). However, there have been no positive RCTs of other classes of antidepressant in children and adolescents. Venlafaxine is contraindicated by the CSM in the UK for use in people under 18, owing to its adverse risk–benefit profile (Committee on Safety of Medicines, 2003). The Texas guidelines also suggest augmentation strategies in the event of partial response to an SSRI, but the evidence base for this in children and adolescents is sparse.

Additional treatment strategies

Although NICE advises prescribing SSRIs together with a specialised psychological treatment such as CBT or interpersonal psychotherapy (National Collaborating Centre for Mental Health, 2005), the ADAPT study Goodyer *et al*, 2007) and other treatment guidelines (American Academy of Child and Adolescent Psychiatry, 2007a; Hughes *et al*, 2007; Anderson *et al*, 2008) suggest that this is not always necessary. The TADS group reported an advantage of combining fluoxetine with CBT over fluoxetine alone (without SCC), although this advantage was lost in more severe cases (March *et al*, 2004; Curry *et al*, 2006). The TORDIA study also reported an advantage of combined treatment (Brent *et al*, 2008), but this effect was not consistent on all measures, and has not been consistently replicated in other studies (Dubicka *et al*, 2010). Although TADS indicated that CBT was protective against suicidality when combined with fluoxetine, neither the ADAPT nor TORDIA studies found this effect, and meta-analyses have found a limited effect of combined treatment and limited evidence for a protective effect against suicidality (Dubicka *et al*, 2010; Cox *et al*, 2012). We therefore suggest that an adjunctive specialised psychological treatment should be targeted at children and adolescents who are receiving SCC and do not respond to antidepressants and require either treatment augmentation or a change of treatment.

In psychotic depression the addition of a second-generation antipsychotic may need to be considered. The choice of drug should be determined on an individual basis after a discussion of side-effect profiles with the young person and their family. The dose should be continued for 2–3 months following remission of psychotic symptoms and then slowly discontinued (Hughes *et al*, 2007).

There is some evidence that second-generation antipsychotics may be effective as an augmentation strategy in treatment-resistant depression in adults (Anderson *et al*, 2008) and also from a *post hoc* analysis of the TORDIA study in adolescents (Emslie *et al*, 2010). However, there remains little evidence to guide clinicians in the management of treatment resistance in children and adolescents. Various strategies have been tried with adults but any extrapolation from the adult literature to children and adolescents needs to be carried out with caution.

Prescribing in bipolar disorder

Background

Prepubertal mania is recognised more commonly in the USA than in the UK and more individuals are being diagnosed with an 'atypical' presentation of bipolar disorder. Rates of diagnosis of bipolar disorder have increased dramatically in recent years in the USA, but it is not clear whether this is due to increased recognition, increased prevalence or overly inclusive diagnoses.

This review will focus on the DSM-5 (American Psychiatric Association, 2013) and ICD-10 (World Health Organization, 1992) definitions of bipolar disorder (Box 9.3). The NICE guidelines on bipolar disorder specify: that adult criteria should be used with children and adolescents, but that mania must be present (not just depression and a family history of bipolar disorder); that euphoria should be present most of the time for at least a

---

Box 9.3 Comparative summary of key diagnostic criteria for bipolar affective disorder

DSM-5[a]	ICD-10[b]
Manic episode	*Manic episode*
Mood elation, expansiveness or irritability, *plus increased energy/activity*[c]	Mood elation or irritability or suspiciousness
	Minimum 7 days' duration
Minimum 7 days' duration (less if admitted to hospital)	Several other symptoms should be present in addition to mood change and increased energy (number of symptoms not specified)
Three additional listed symptoms (four if irritability present), e.g. grandiosity, decreased need for sleep, pressured speech, flight of ideas	
	Significant impairment
Marked impairment or hospital admission or psychosis	Psychosis may be present
Mixed episode excluded	
Hypomania	*Hypomania*
Lesser degree of mania (no psychosis)	Lesser degree of mania (no psychosis)
Bipolar I	*Bipolar affective disorder*
Presence of manic episode (can be diagnosed in absence of depression)	At least two episodes where mood (hypomania/mania and depression) and activity levels are significantly disturbed
Bipolar II	
Periods of major depression and hypomania lasting at least 4 days over 2 weeks	
Specifiers	
e.g. rapid cycling, mixed features	
For cases not meeting criteria	
Additional categories available including cyclothymia and 'other'	

a. After American Psychiatric Association (2013)
b. After World Health Organization (1992).
c. This has been added as a core symptom in the DSM-5 revision.

week; and that irritability should not be used as a core criterion, except in older adolescents, since this symptom is non-specific in younger children (National Collaborating Centre for Mental Health, 2006). However, controversy still remains regarding the interpretation of core symptoms, namely elation or grandiosity, as it depends on the subjective view of the clinician. The NICE guidelines also state that bipolar II disorder should not be diagnosed in children and younger adolescents, in view of the uncertainties regarding the diagnostic criteria.

The treatment implications of subthreshold bipolar disorder are still unclear. However, in a study of children and adolescents with bipolar spectrum disorder (the Course and Outcome of Bipolar Youth (COBY) study), young people with clearly defined DSM-IV-TR bipolar disorder not otherwise specified showed lower rates of recovery compared with those with bipolar I or II disorder, and also had similar levels of impairment and suicidality (Birmaher et al, 2009). Nearly half of these young people developed either bipolar I (23%) or bipolar II disorder (22%) within 5 years, particularly if there was a family history of bipolar disorder (Axelson et al, 2011). The use of these broader diagnostic criteria in children remains a topic of much debate and is an area that requires further research.

Evidence base for pharmacological treatment

There have been few studies of pharmacological treatment of bipolar disorder in children and adolescents (Pfeifer et al, 2010; Liu et al, 2011). Those that have been published are problematic as they include few RCTs, most of which have been small and in which treatment response rates have varied widely, partly a result of inconsistent definitions of bipolar disorder and differing response criteria.

Lithium has been the most widely studied pharmacological treatment for mania in children and adolescents and in adults. Trials support its use in adults (Fountoulakis et al, 2012) and early trials in children and adolescents were generally positive, although their conclusions are limited owing to methodological problems (American Academy of Child and Adolescent Psychiatry, 2007b).

Anticonvulsants appear to be more effective for mania in adults than in youths (Correll et al, 2010). Valproate semisodium (divalproex) is less effective than quetiapine and risperidone in children and adolescents with mania (DelBello et al, 2006; Pavuluri et al, 2010), and it does not appear to be more effective than placebo (Wagner et al, 2009).

There have been no placebo-controlled trials of lamotrigine in young people, but open-label data suggest that it may be effective in bipolar depression as well as in controlling manic symptoms (Biederman et al, 2010). There is very little evidence to support the use of carbamazepine in children and adolescents, and placebo-controlled RCTs of oxcarbazepine and topiramate have been negative (DelBello et al, 2005; Wagner et al, 2006). Overall, therefore, there is little evidence currently supporting the

139

use of anticonvulsants for bipolar disorder in children and adolescents, concurring with meta-analytical findings which report that second-generation antipsychotics appear to be more effective for mania than either lithium or anticonvulsants (Correll *et al*, 2010).

First-generation antipsychotics are not currently recommended as first-line treatments for mania in youths because of the increased risk of movement disorders. However, there is increasing evidence from randomised placebo-controlled trials that second-generation antipsychotics are effective in children and adolescents with bipolar disorder, and may be more effective in youths than in adults (Correll *et al*, 2010). In a trial of olanzapine for adolescent mania, the drug was more effective than placebo but weight gain and metabolic adverse effects were a significant problem (Tohen *et al*, 2007). Risperidone has been shown to be more effective than placebo in children and adolescents with mania, with lower doses (<3 mg) demonstrating a better risk–benefit profile than higher doses (Haas *et al*, 2009). Risperidone also appears to be more effective than lithium or divalproex (Pavuluri *et al*, 2010; Geller *et al*, 2012), although in the absence of attention-deficit hyperactivity disorder (ADHD), it has not been found to be more effective than lithium (Vitiello *et al*, 2012). A large placebo-controlled trial of aripiprazole reported that the drug was more effective than placebo in children and adolescents with manic episodes (Findling *et al*, 2009). Although there is evidence that quetiapine is useful in preventing relapse of both poles of bipolar disorder in adults (Fountoulakis *et al*, 2012), a small placebo-controlled study of quetiapine for bipolar depression in adolescents has been negative (DelBello *et al*, 2009), and currently there is only limited evidence for its use in adolescents with mania (DelBello *et al*, 2002).

Guidelines for pharmacological treatment

Owing to the limited evidence base for treatment of bipolar disorder in children and adolescents, guidelines are extrapolated from the adult literature (Fountoulakis *et al*, 2012). As this is a rapidly changing area, clinicians need to keep abreast of the emerging literature. Medication remains the first-line treatment for bipolar disorder that meets diagnostic criteria, although caution should be used, particularly in younger children, as the effectiveness and safety of medication in children and adolescents is still being established.

Pharmacological treatment guidelines and licensing indications for the UK and USA are summarised in Table 9.2. The use of second-generation antipsychotics rather than mood stabilisers as a first-line treatment for acute mania has become increasingly common in clinical practice (Fountoulakis *et al*, 2012) and is supported by the current NICE guidelines (National Collaborating Centre for Mental Health, 2006). These guidelines also suggest concurrent use of a benzodiazepine such as lorazepam to manage agitation if required. If antidepressant medication is being taken,

Table 9.2 Pharmacological treatment for mania/hypomania and bipolar disorder in children and adolescents: UK and US guidelines and licensing[a]

| Drug | Guideline advice[b] | | Age for licensed prescribing in bipolar disorder/mania/hypomania, years | |
	NICE	AACAP	UK	USA
Aripiprazole	Moderate to severe mania, aged 13 years and above, for up to 12 weeks[c]	First-line	≥13 (EMA approval for moderate to severe mania, up to 12 weeks)	≥10 (mania/mixed)
Carbamazepine	Third-line	Second-line (although first-line in another US guideline[d])	≥18 (in non-responders to lithium for prophylaxis of 'manic–depressive psychosis')	≥18 (mania/mixed)
Lamotrigine	Third-line, especially in bipolar II disorder and recurrent depression	Maintenance	≥18 (prevention of depressive episodes in bipolar I disorder if past history of depression)	≥18 (maintenance treatment and acute mood episode)
Lithium carbonate	Second-line for augmentation (first-line only if previously successful); maintenance treatment	First-line, maintenance	12 and over (450 mg lithium carbonate, extended release only; mania and prophylaxis)	≥12 (mania/mixed)
Olanzapine	First-line and maintenance	First-line, maintenance	≥18 (monotherapy in mania, prophylaxis)	≥13 (mania/mixed and maintenance)
Quetiapine	First-line, and chronic and recurrent depression	First-line	≥18 (acute manic and depressive episodes in bipolar disorder; prophylaxis if previous response)	≥10 (mania: standard-release formulation; extended-release formulation for ≥18)

(continued)

Table 9.2 *(continued)*

Drug	Guideline advice[b]		Age for licensed prescribing in bipolar disorder/mania/hypomania, years	
	NICE	AACAP	UK	USA
Risperidone	First-line	First-line	≥18 (mania)	≥10 (mania/mixed)
Valproate semisodium	Second-line for augmentation (first-line if previously successful); maintenance. Not to be used in girls <18 years and avoid in women of child-bearing potential	First-line	≥18 (mania)	≥18 (mania: extended-release tablets also approved)
Ziprasidone	–	First-line	Not licensed	≥18 (adjunct maintenance treatment – under review for children and adolescents)
Asenapine	–	–	≥18 (acute manic/mixed episodes)	≥18 (acute manic/mixed episodes)
Olanzapine/fluoxetine combination	–	Bipolar depression	Not licensed	≥18 (bipolar depression)

AACAP, American Academy of Child and Adolescent Psychiatry; NICE, National Institute for Health and Care Excellence; EMA, European Medicines Agency; NICE, National Institute for Health and Care Excellence's Clinical Guideline 38 (National Collaborating Centre for Mental Health, 2006).

a. For up-to-date licensing information in the UK with specific details of indications, refer to the summaries of product characteristics on the electronic medicines compendium (www.medicines.org.uk/EMC/default.aspx). The information here may differ from that listed in the *British National Formulary*.

b. Note that the evidence base is rapidly changing and guideline information may quickly become out of date; clinicians therefore need to also consider the latest evidence.

c. National Institute for Health and Care Excellence (2013).

d. Guidelines from the Child Psychiatric Workgroup on Bipolar Disorder (Kowatch *et al*, 2005).

this should be withdrawn abruptly or gradually, depending on clinical need and risk of discontinuation/withdrawal symptoms. In the UK, only lithium carbonate and aripiprazole are licensed for adolescents with bipolar disorder, although risperidone, quetiapine and olanzapine have also been approved in the USA.

Lithium or valproate are suggested as a first-line treatment if either has been previously successful with the patient, although lithium is not recommended for acute mania if symptoms are severe, in view of its slower onset of action. The NICE guidelines advise that valproate should not be prescribed to girls, owing to its possible association with polycystic ovary syndrome. Lithium or valproate can also be used as an augmentation strategy, if an antipsychotic alone is ineffective. The NICE guidelines recommend that carbamazepine, gabapentin, lamotrigine and topiramate should not be routinely used for acute mania. For long-term treatment, NICE advises the use of lithium, olanzapine or valproate, and either switching medications or using a second agent in the event of an inadequate response. Carbamazepine and lamotrigine should be considered if a trial of combined agents proves ineffective.

Principles of prescribing

In view of the paucity of the evidence base and concerns regarding potentially serious adverse effects, the risks and benefits of medication need careful consideration with the family and young person. If medication is commenced, the principle is to 'start low and go slow', with closer monitoring than in adults, including close monitoring of suicide risk. Medication should be prescribed in a psychosocial therapeutic framework with an emphasis on managing overactivity, sleep hygiene, diet and structured activities. Bipolar disorder affects numerous developmental processes, including academic, social and family functioning, and therefore treatment needs to be multimodal, including liaison with appropriate agencies and targeting relapse prevention (American Academy of Child and Adolescent Psychiatry, 2007b).

Adverse effects

All mood stabilisers and antipsychotics are associated with potentially harmful adverse effects, and should therefore be used judiciously, with careful monitoring of physical parameters (Pfeifer et al, 2010).

Children and adolescents are at higher risk than adults for antipsychotic-induced weight gain (Correll et al, 2010) and, possibly, extrapyramidal side-effects (EPSEs). Although adverse events have usually been minor in trials of second-generation antipsychotics, longer-term open-label studies have indicated that some adverse events, such as the metabolic effects, may be severe and potentially life-threatening in the long term (Zuddas et al, 2011). Data for adults with schizophrenia who have received long-term antipsychotic treatment demonstrate that these drugs have a subtle but measurable influence on brain tissue loss over time, suggesting the importance of careful risk–benefit review of dosage and duration of treatment as well as off-label use (Ho *et al*, 2011). Olanzapine is associated with the greatest degree of weight gain and, after risperidone, is most likely to induce hyperprolactinaemia. Aripiprazole seems least likely to induce hyperprolactinaemia and weight gain, and quetiapine appears to confer an intermediate risk for weight gain, with little effect on prolactin levels or EPSEs (Correll *et al*, 2010; Fraguas *et al*, 2011). Tardive dyskinesia is an important rarer adverse effect, thought to occur less frequently with second- than with first-generation antipsychotics. However, it may be more common in children and adolescents than in adults. One report found that the 1-year incidence of tardive dyskinesia in paediatric populations was <1% (Pfeifer *et al*, 2010). Neuroleptic malignant syndrome is similarly a serious rare adverse effect thought to be less common with second-generation antipsychotics. It typically presents with rigidity, autonomic instability and hyperthermia, and clinicians should be alert to its early signs.

Lithium can cause a range of adverse effects, including nausea, headache, acne, weight gain, diabetes insipidus, tremor, hypothyroidism and renal impairment. Lithium intoxication occurs at blood levels >1.5 mmol/l, and can be caused by intentional overdose, drug interactions, an increase in dose, a decrease in renal excretion, medical illness and excessive fluid loss. Maternal use in the first trimester is also associated with Ebstein's anomaly, a congenital cardiac valve defect. Valproate has been associated with sedation, headache, gastrointestinal symptoms, weight gain, pancreatitis, hepatotoxicity, alopecia, thrombocytopenia, high levels of teratogenicity and, controversially, polycystic ovary syndrome. Rapid titration of lamotrigine has been associated with a rare but serious rash and subsequent progression to Stevens–Johnson syndrome (generally agreed to be a form of toxic epidermal necrolysis). Adverse effects of carbamazepine include rash, sedation, nausea, dizziness, agranulocytosis, aplastic anaemia, and an increased risk of Stevens–Johnson syndrome in patients of Asian ancestry (Pfeifer *et al*, 2010).

Additional treatment strategies

The use of antidepressants in bipolar disorder is a controversial option; adult guidelines do not recommend their use without anti-manic medication and generally tend to favour quetiapine monotherapy for first-line treatment (Fountoulakis *et al*, 2012). The NICE guidelines (National Collaborating Centre for Mental Health, 2006) do not recommended antidepressants for rapid-cycling or mixed affective states.

Attention-deficit hyperactivity disorder occurs commonly with bipolar disorder and caution is necessary when treating child and adolescent bipolar disorder with stimulants as this medication may exacerbate manic symptoms. Young people with bipolar disorder and ADHD may also be less responsive to anti-manic treatment (Pfeifer *et al*, 2010).

As with depression, medication for bipolar disorder should always be prescribed within a psychosocial framework. Functional family therapy (psychoeducation, medication adherence sessions, communication training, problem-solving and relapse prevention) seems to be an effective adjunct to medication for reducing depressive symptoms in adolescents with bipolar disorder over the longer term (Miklowitz *et al*, 2008). Brief adjunctive psycho-educational group psychotherapy involving parents and children is associated with improved outcome for children with major mood disorders, including bipolar disorder (Fristad *et al*, 2009). Healthy eating and exercise should be emphasised throughout treatment to prevent excessive weight gain.

Conclusion

Major depression and bipolar disorder in children and adolescents are serious disabling conditions associated with considerable morbidity as well as increased risk of suicide. Depression in young people is associated with high levels of persistence and recurrence into adult life, and the majority of children and adolescents with bipolar I disorder will continue to experience persistent disorder throughout adolescence, together with high levels of morbidity and disability (Wozniak *et al*, 2011). Although the implications of subthreshold bipolar disorder remain unclear, studies indicate that young people with bipolar symptoms also suffer from high levels of morbidity, and therefore treatments need to be developed for these young people to reduce the likelihood of progression to fully syndromal bipolar disorder.

Although the treatment of major depression and the diagnosis of bipolar disorder in young people remain controversial, antidepressants are an important therapeutic option for moderate to severe depression, and medication is the first-line treatment of choice in cases of bipolar disorder that meet diagnostic criteria. However, the risks and benefits of pharmacological treatment require careful consideration with families and young people before prescribing, and medication should always be given within a psychosocial treatment framework, with close monitoring of mental state, suicidality and physical parameters, and addition of specific psychological therapies as indicated. In particular, the risk of suicide from an untreated mood disorder needs to be carefully evaluated and considered when weighing up the potential risks and benefits of commencing medication. The evidence base for pharmacological treatment remains limited, and future studies need to focus on the most impaired adolescents for whom the potential benefits of medication are more likely to outweigh the associated risks.

References

American Academy of Child and Adolescent Psychiatry (2007*a*) Practice parameter for the assessment and treatment of children and adolescents with depressive disorders. *Journal of the American Academy of Child & Adolescent Psychiatry*, **46**, 1503–1526.

American Academy of Child and Adolescent Psychiatry (2007*b*) Practice parameter for the assessment and treatment of children and adolescents with bipolar disorder. *Journal of the American Academy of Child & Adolescent Psychiatry*, **46**, 107–25.

American Psychiatric Association (2013) *Diagnostic and Statistical Manual of Mental Disorders (5th edn) (DSM-5)*. APA.

Anderson IM, Ferrier IN, Baldwin RC, *et al* (2008) Evidence-based guidelines for treating depressive disorders with antidepressants: a revision of the 2000 British Association for Psychopharmacology guidelines. *Journal of Psychopharmacology*, **22**, 343–396.

Axelson DA, Birmaher B, Strober MA, *et al* (2011) Course of subthreshold bipolar disorder in youth: diagnostic progression from bipolar disorder not otherwise specified. *Journal of the American Academy of Child & Adolescent Psychiatry*, **50**, 1001–1016.

Baldessarini RJ, Tondo L, Strombom IM, *et al* (2007) Ecological studies of antidepressant treatment and suicidal risks. *Harvard Review of Psychiatry*, **15**, 133–145.

Barbui C, Esposito E, Cipriani A (2009) Selective serotonin reuptake inhibitors and risk of suicide: a systematic review of observational studies. *CMAJ*, **180**, 291–297.

Biederman J, Joshi G, Mick E, *et al* (2010) A prospective open-label trial of lamotrigine monotherapy in children and adolescents with bipolar disorder. *CNS Neuroscience and Therapeutics*, **16**, 91–102.

Birmaher B, Axelson D, Goldstein B, *et al* (2009) Four-year longitudinal course of children and adolescents with bipolar spectrum disorders: the Course and Outcome of Bipolar Youth (COBY) study. *American Journal of Psychiatry*, **166**, 795–804.

Brent D, Emslie G, Clarke G, *et al* (2008) Switching to another SSRI or to venlafaxine with or without cognitive behavioral therapy for adolescents with SSRI-resistant depression: the TORDIA randomized controlled trial. *JAMA*, **299**, 901–913.

Bridge JA, Iyengar S, Salary CB, *et al* (2007) Clinical response and risk for reported suicidal ideation and suicide attempts in pediatric antidepressant treatment: a meta-analysis of randomized controlled trials. *JAMA*, **297**, 1683–1696.

Bridge JA, Birmaher B, Iyengar S, *et al* (2009) Placebo response in randomized controlled trials of antidepressants for pediatric major depressive disorder. *American Journal of Psychiatry*, **166**, 42–49.

Committee on Safety of Medicines (2003) *Use of Selective Serotonin Reuptake Inhibitors (SSRIs) in Children and Adolescents with Major Depressive Disorder (MDD)*. Medicines and Healthcare products Regulatory Agency.

Correll CU, Sheridan EM, DelBello MP (2010) Antipsychotic and mood stabilizer efficacy and tolerability in pediatric and adult patients with bipolar I mania: a comparative analysis of acute, randomized, placebo-controlled trials. *Bipolar Disorders*, **12**, 116–141.

Cortes E, Cubano A, Lewis JE, *et al* (2011) Antidepressants at autopsy in Hispanic suicidal youth in Miami-Dade County, Florida. *Journal of Forensic Sciences*, **56**, 155–160.

Cox GR, Callahan P, Churchill R, *et al* (2012) Psychological therapies versus antidepressant medication, alone and in combination for depression in children and adolescents. *Cochrane Database of Systematic Reviews*, 11, CD008324.

Curry J, Rodhe P, Simons A, *et al* (2006) Predictors and moderators of acute outcome in the Treatment for Adolescents with Depression Study (TADS). *Journal of the American Academy of Child & Adolescent Psychiatry*, **45**, 1427–1438.

DelBello MP, Schwiers ML, Rosenberg HL, *et al* (2002) A double-blind, randomized, placebo-controlled study of quetiapine as adjunct treatment for adolescent mania. *Journal of the American Academy of Child & Adolescent Psychiatry*, **41**, 1216–1223.

DelBello, MP, Findling RL, Kushner S, *et al* (2005) A pilot controlled trial of topiramate for mania in children and adolescents with bipolar disorder. *Journal of the American Academy of Child & Adolescent Psychiatry*, **44**, 539–547.

DelBello MP, Kowatch RA, Adler CM, *et al* (2006) A double-blind randomized pilot study comparing quetiapine and divalproex for adolescent mania. *Journal of the American Academy of Child & Adolescent Psychiatry*, **45**, 305–313.

DelBello MP, Chang K, Welge JA, *et al* (2009) A double-blind, placebo-controlled pilot study of quetiapine for depressed adolescents with bipolar disorder. *Bipolar Disorders*, **11**, 483–493.

Dubicka B, Hadley S, Roberts C (2006) Suicidal behaviour in youths with depression treated with new-generation antidepressants: meta-analysis. *British Journal of Psychiatry*, **189**, 393–398.

Dubicka B, Elvins B, Roberts C, *et al* (2010) Combined treatment with cognitive–behavioural therapy in adolescent depression: meta-analysis. *British Journal of Psychiatry*, **197**, 433–440.

Dudley M, Goldney R, Hadzi-Pavlovic D (2010) Are adolescents dying by suicide taking SSRI antidepressants? A review of observational studies. *Australasian Psychiatry*, **18**, 242–245.

Emslie G, Kratochvil C, Vitiello B, *et al* (2006) Treatment for Adolescents with Depression Study (TADS): safety results. *Journal of the American Academy of Child & Adolescent Psychiatry*, **45**, 1440–1455.

Emslie GJ, Kennard BD, Mayes TL, *et al* (2008) Fluoxetine versus placebo in preventing relapse of major depression in children and adolescents. *American Journal of Psychiatry*, **165**, 459–467.

Emslie GJ, Mayes T, Porta G, *et al* (2010) Treatment of Resistant Depression in Adolescents (TORDIA): week 24 outcomes. *American Journal of Psychiatry*, **167**, 782–791.

Findling RL, Nyilas M, Forbes RA, *et al* (2009) Acute treatment of pediatric bipolar I disorder, manic or mixed episode, with aripiprazole: a randomized, double-blind, placebo-controlled study. *Journal of Clinical Psychiatry*, **70**, 1441–1451.

Fountoulakis KN, Kasper S, Andreassen O, *et al* (2012) Efficacy of pharmacotherapy in bipolar disorder: a report by the WPA section on pharmacopsychiatry. *European Archives of Psychiatry and Clinical Neuroscience*, **262** (suppl. 1), 1–48.

Fraguas D, Correll CU, Merchán-Naranjo J, *et al* (2011) Efficacy and safety of second-generation antipsychotics in children and adolescents with psychotic and bipolar spectrum disorders: comprehensive review of prospective head-to-head and placebo-controlled comparisons. *European Neuropsychopharmacology*, **21**, 621–645.

Fristad MA, Verducci JS, Walters K, *et al* (2009) Impact of multifamily psychoeducational psychotherapy in treating children aged 8 to 12 years with mood disorders. *Archives of General Psychiatry*, **66**, 1013–1021.

Geller B, Luby JL, Joshi P, *et al* (2012) A randomized controlled trial of risperidone, lithium, or divalproex sodium for initial treatment of bipolar I disorder, manic or mixed phase, in children and adolescents. *Archives of General Psychiatry*, **69**, 515–528.

Gibbons RD, Brown CH, Hur K, *et al* (2007) Relationship between antidepressants and suicide attempts: an analysis of the Veterans Health Administration data sets. *American Journal of Psychiatry*, **164**, 1044–1049.

Goodyer I, Dubicka B, Wilkinson P, *et al* (2007) Selective serotonin reuptake inhibitors (SSRIs) and routine specialist care with and without cognitive behaviour therapy in adolescents with major depression: randomised controlled trial. *BMJ*, **335**, 142–146.

Haas M, DelBello MP, Pandina G, *et al* (2009) Risperidone for the treatment of acute mania in children and adolescents with bipolar disorder: a randomized, double-blind, placebo-controlled study. *Bipolar Disorders*, **11**, 687–700.

Hetrick SE, McKenzie JE, Cox GR, *et al* (2012) Newer generation antidepressants for depressive disorders in children and adolescents. *Cochrane Database of Systematic Reviews*, **11**, CD004851.

Ho B-C, Andreasen NC, Ziebell S, *et al* (2011) Long-term antipsychotic treatment and brain volumes: a longitudinal study of first-episode schizophrenia. *Archives of General Psychiatry*, **68**, 128–137.

Hughes CW, Emslie GJ, Crismon L, *et al* (2007) Texas Children's Medication Algorithm Project: update from Texas Consensus Conference Panel on Medication Treatment of

Childhood Major Depressive Disorder. *Journal of the American Academy of Child & Adolescent Psychiatry*, **46**, 667–686.

Jerrell JM (2010) Neuroendocrine-related adverse events associated with antidepressant treatment in children and adolescents. *CNS Neuroscience and Therapeutics*, **16**, 83–90.

Kirsch I, Deacon BJ, Huedo-Medina TB, *et al* (2008) Initial severity and antidepressant benefits: a meta-analysis of data submitted to the Food and Drug Administration. *PLoS Medicine*, **5**, e45.

Kowatch RA, Fristad M, Birmaher B, *et al* (2005) Treatment guidelines for children and adolescents with bipolar disorder. *Journal of the American Academy of Child & Adolescent Psychiatry*, **44**, 213–235.

Kronenberg S, Apter A, Brent D, *et al* (2007) Serotonin transporter polymorphism (5-HTTLPR) and citalopram effectiveness and side effects in children with depression and/or anxiety disorders. *Journal of Child and Adolescent Psychopharmacology*, **17**, 741–750.

Liu HY, Potter MP, Woodworth KY, *et al* (2011) Pharmacologic treatments for pediatric bipolar disorder: a review and meta-analysis. *Journal of the American Academy of Child & Adolescent Psychiatry*, **50**, 749–762.

Maalouf FT, Atwi M, Brent DA (2011) Treatment-resistant depression in adolescents: review and updates on clinical management. *Depression and Anxiety*, **28**, 946–954.

March J, Silva S, Petrycki S, *et al* (2004) Fluoxetine, cognitive–behavioral therapy, and their combination for adolescents with depression. Treatment for Adolescents With Depression Study (TADS) Randomized Controlled Trial. *JAMA*, **292**, 807–820.

March J, Silva S, Petrycki, S, *et al* (2007) The Treatment for Adolescents with Depression Study (TADS): long-term effectiveness and safety outcomes. *Archives of General Psychiatry*, **64**, 1132–1143.

Medicines and Healthcare Products Regulatory Agency (2011) Citalopram and escitalopram: QT interval prolongation – new maximum daily dose restrictions (including in elderly patients), contraindications, and warnings. *Drug Safety Update*, **5** (5), A1.

Miklowitz DJ, Axelson DA, Birmaher B, *et al* (2008) Family-focused treatment for adolescents with bipolar disorder: results of a 2-year randomized trial. *Archives of General Psychiatry*, **65**, 1053–1061.

Moskos MA, Olson L, Halbern SR, *et al* (2007) Utah youth suicide study: barriers to mental health treatment for adolescents. *Suicide and Life-Threatening Behavior*, **37**, 179–186.

National Collaborating Centre for Mental Health (2005) *Depression in Children and Young People: Identification and Management in Primary, Community and Secondary Care* (Clinical Guideline 28). National Institute for Health and Clinical Excellence.

National Collaborating Centre for Mental Health (2006) *Bipolar Disorder: The Management of Bipolar Disorder in Adults, Children and Adolescents, in Primary and Secondary Care* (Clinical Guideline 38). National Institute for Health and Clinical Excellence.

National Institute for Health and Care Excellence (2013) *Aripiprazole for treating moderate to severe manic episodes in adolescents with bipolar I disorder* (NICE Technology Appraisal Guidance 292). NICE.

Pavuluri MN, Henry DB, Findling RL, *et al* (2010) Double-blind randomized trial of risperidone versus divalproex in pediatric bipolar disorder. *Bipolar Disorders*, **12**, 593–605.

Pfeifer JC, Kowatch RA, DelBello MP (2010) Pharmacotherapy of bipolar disorder in children and adolescents: recent progress. *CNS Drugs*, **24**, 575–593.

Posternak MA, Zimmerman M (2005) Is there a delay in the anti-depressant effect? A meta-analysis. *Journal of Clinical Psychiatry*, **66**, 148–158.

Rongrong T, Emslie G, Mayes T, *et al* (2009) Early prediction of acute antidepressant treatment response and remission in pediatric major depressive disorder. *Journal of the American Academy of Child & Adolescent Psychiatry*, **48**, 71–78.

Simon GE, Savarino J, Operskalski B, *et al* (2006) Suicide risk during antidepressant treatment. *American Journal of Psychiatry*, **163**, 41–47.

Tohen M, Kryzhanovskaya L, Carlson G, *et al* (2007) Olanzapine versus placebo in the treatment of adolescents with bipolar mania. *American Journal of Psychiatry*, **164**, 1547–1556.

Valuck RJ, Libby AM, Sills MR, *et al* (2004) Antidepressant treatment and risk of suicide attempt by adolescents with major depressive disorder: a propensity-adjusted retrospective cohort study. *CNS Drugs*, **18**, 1119–1132.

Vitiello B, Riddle MA, Yenokyan G, *et al* (2012) Treatment moderators and predictors of outcome in the Treatment of Early Age Mania (TEAM) study. *Journal of the American Academy of Child & Adolescent Psychiatry*, **51**, 867–878.

Wagner KD, Kowatch RA, Emslie GJ, *et al* (2006) A double-blind, randomized, placebo-controlled trial of oxcarbazepine in the treatment of bipolar disorder in children and adolescents. *American Journal of Psychiatry*, **163**, 1179–1186.

Wagner KD, Redden L, Kowatch R, *et al* (2009) A double-blind, randomized, placebo-controlled trial of divalproex extended-release in the treatment of bipolar disorder in children and adolescents. *Journal of the American Academy of Child & Adolescent Psychiatry*, **48**, 519–532.

Wilkinson P, Dubicka B, Kelvin R, *et al* (2009) Treated depression in adolescents: predictors of outcome at 28 weeks. *British Journal of Psychiatry*, **194**, 334–341.

Windfuhr K, While D, Hunt I, *et al* (2008) Suicide in juveniles and adolescents in the United Kingdom. *Journal of Child Psychology and Psychiatry*, **49**, 1155–1165.

World Health Organization (1992) *The ICD-10 Classification of Mental and Behavioural Disorders: Clinical Descriptions and Diagnostic Guidelines*. WHO.

Wozniak J, Petty CR, Schreck M, *et al* (2011) High level of persistence of pediatric bipolar-I disorder from childhood onto adolescent years: a four year prospective longitudinal follow-up study. *Journal of Psychiatric Research*, **45**, 1273–1282.

Zuddas A, Zanni R, Usala T (2011) Second generation antipsychotics (SGAs) for non-psychotic disorders in children and adolescents: a review of the randomized controlled studies. *European Neuropsychopharmacology*, **21**, 600–620.

CHAPTER 10

Cognitive–behavioural therapy with children, young people and families: from individual to systemic therapy

Nicky Dummett and Roger Lakin

Cognitive–behavioural therapy (CBT) is fundamentally a collaborative, empirical process of shared discovery (Salkovskis, 2002) in which client and therapist together derive a hypothesis, the 'formulation' (Persons, 1989), about the aetiology and maintenance of the client's problem. This formulation encompasses the unique predicament and response of the client in their particular present and past life contexts. This hypothesis is continuously refined in therapy as the client tests its validity against their experience and uses it to select cognitive and behavioural interventions. Instead of giving solutions, the therapist's emphasis is on guided discovery using Socratic dialogue (Padesky & Greenberger, 1995) and systematic use of case-specific and standardised ratings to promote self-help and problem-solving. Failure to appreciate that therapy is explicitly based on a shared formulation, rather than being a collection of techniques, has resulted in a disparate range of interventions being used as 'CBT for children' (Stallard, 2002). There is now widespread appreciation of the need to define CBT for children, young people and families and, in particular, to ensure that interventions are formulation based (an opinion confirmed at the inaugural meeting of the Child and Adolescent Special Interest Branch of the British Association for Behavioural and Cognitive Psychotherapies (BABCP) in 2001).

By 'children and young people' we mean individuals up to the age of 18. For conciseness in this chapter we refer to them simply as children.

The evidence base

A significant body of evidence supports the use of CBT to treat a wide range of child and adolescent mental health problems such as depression (Harrington *et al*, 1998; March *et al*, 2004), generalised anxiety (Barrett *et al*, 2001), conduct disorder (White *et al*, 2003), interpersonal problems (Spence & Donovan, 1998), phobias (Silverman *et al*, 1999), social phobia

(Spence *et al*, 2000), school refusal (King *et al*, 1998), sexual abuse (Jones & Ramchandani, 1999), pain management (Sanders *et al*, 1994), eating disorders (Schmidt, 1998), post-traumatic stress disorder (Smith *et al*, 1998) and obsessive–compulsive disorder (Barrett *et al*, 2005). Alongside other treatments, CBT has been specifically recommended in National Institute for Health and Care Excellence (NICE) guidance for children and young people with depression (National Collaborating Centre for Mental Health, 2005*a*), attention-deficit hyperactivity disorder (National Institute for Health and Clinical Excellence, 2008), post-traumatic stress disorder (National Collaborating Centre for Mental Health, 2005*b*), obsessive–compulsive disorder (National Collaborating Centre for Mental Health, 2005*c*) and bipolar disorder (National Collaborating Centre for Mental Health, 2006),

There is also evidence in favour of using family cognitive–behavioural interventions on their own or to augment standard treatments for childhood behavioural and emotional disorders (Northey *et al*, 2003). More detailed process research is needed, however, to identify active components, individual or systemic, of CBT and indications for or against its use with specific disorders in younger populations. In adult work, limitations of CBT are becoming more well-defined (for example, it is appropriate only if problematic behavioural and cognitive responses are occurring frequently in the present), but it is less clear what the limitations of CBT may be in working with younger age groups or on a systemic basis. Drinkwater (2005) has highlighted the need for empirical research comparing formulation-based with manualised CBT. For reviews, see Stallard (2002) and Drinkwater & Stewart (2002).

A fuller evidence base is, of course, also emerging for use of longer-established psychotherapeutic approaches with children and families (Roth *et al*, 2006).

Incorporating systemic and developmental perspectives

A key difficulty in CBT with children and families has been the absence of both a generic template for formulation and a process that can incorporate not only wider interpersonal and systemic factors but also developmental perspectives and insights more commonly associated with other psychotherapies. A systemic perspective is specifically required to look at major maintaining factors outside of the child. To this end, Tarrier & Calam (2002) have called for explicit incorporation of systems theory and epidemiological and social context into cognitive–behavioural case formulation for all age groups. It is simply not appropriate to extrapolate from adult models, since children are in a process of developing cognitive and other dimensions of functioning; they exist in and are dependent on the context of their families and carers and physical and cultural environments;

Box 10.1 Core features of cognitive–behavioural therapy

- Formulation based, empirical
- Collaborative therapeutic relationship promoted through guided discovery using Socratic questioning, with appropriate sharing of responsibility for change
- Structured and problem focused, teaches problem-solving
- Integrates cognitive and behavioural strategies
- Assumes that cognitions (not simply events) determine outcomes

---

and they are learning to meet their needs within the context of their major attachment relationships.

There is growing clinical experience indicating that systemic cognitive–behavioural formulation (Dattilio, 2005; Dummett, 2006) can be used with children and their families to explore developmental, attachment, interpersonal, family and wider-system processes. In addition, psychological phenomena such as repression, projection and transference, more traditionally the currency of other psychotherapeutic approaches, can be explicitly used within the systemic formulation by expressing them in cognitive–behavioural terms.

Concepts and processes fundamental to CBT

Cognitive–behavioural therapy aims to promote self-help by helping clients learn to find and evaluate their own solutions to both present and future problems (Box 10.1). Formulation is a dynamic process undertaken jointly by therapist and client that promotes a collaborative, rather than expert-led therapeutic relationship with sharing of the responsibility for change (Box 10.2).

Box 10.2 The cognitive–behavioural formulation

- A hypothesis or working model/representation of the major processes of cause and effect linking cognitions, thoughts, behaviours, moods and bodily symptoms in causing and maintaining problems
- Usually written, but can be visual (imagery) or verbal – whichever has most relevance and utility for the client
- Collaboratively derived on a case-by-case basis through guided discovery
- Testable, so that the client/family can confirm that this is an accurate reflection of their difficulties
- A template from which to derive interventions and predict consequences, positive and negative, of any change
- Helpful in refocusing therapy and for exploring difficulties during therapy

---

The template for a cognitive–behavioural formulation for an individual client is based on the Beckian cognitive model and the premise that in any problem situation associated with dysphoric mood there will be four functionally distinct components of response: the affective, cognitive, physiological and behavioural (Fig. 10.1). These four systems of response are interdependent, and also interact with the social and physical environment through many mechanisms of cause and effect (Rachman, 1978). The latter include operant and classical conditioning, physiology, social learning and attachment processes.

The Beckian cognitive model (Beck, 1979) postulates three levels of cognition. Relatively unconscious core beliefs, which derive from early life experiences, lead to more consciously held conditional assumptions and negative automatic thoughts, the latter being active at the so-called four systems of response level. Core beliefs and conditional assumptions are then reinforced, largely through social learning, within the context of the attachment relationships and family and cultural contexts of early life. They are therefore strongly influenced by dominant family and cultural narratives.

Core beliefs

Core beliefs are fairly absolute statements about the self (e.g. 'I am strong/ weak/unlovable'), about the world (e.g. 'it is a dangerous place') and about others (e.g. 'they are stronger than me/will reject me') that constitute an internal working model of reality. Since core beliefs may be positive or negative evaluations of the self, environment and others, they can serve both adaptive and maladaptive purpose, but reactions to negative core beliefs tend to be associated with problem situations.

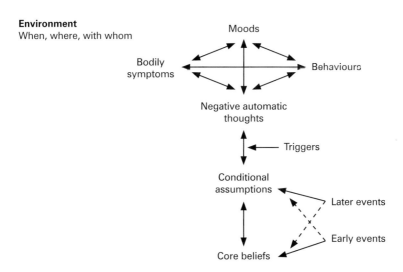

Fig. 10.1 A template for an individual cognitive–behavioural formulation.

Conditional assumptions

Conditional assumptions are expectations of the self or 'rules to live by'. They have a defensive function in relation to negative core beliefs and have often had an adaptive function at an earlier stage of life, for example, in leading to submissive behaviours that have reduced persecutory attack but are less suited to present circumstances. They are expressed in 'if ..., then ...' terms, for example: 'If I always keep other people happy, then I am lovable'. In day-to-day problem episodes, certain triggers activate conditional assumptions, resulting in situation-specific negative automatic thoughts.

Vignette 1

A young person grew up with one parent who usually shouted when upset and one parent who, owing to underlying but unacknowledged mental health difficulties of their own, became rapidly overwhelmed by any upset in the family. She developed difficulties when, in adolescence, she was unable to advocate for her needs, particularly in peer relations. She discovered in therapy that she had unconsciously adopted the conditional assumption 'never get anyone upset, even if it means I don't get what I need'. She was able to make changes to this once she had consciously considered the origin and present functionality of this rule for living.

Collaborative development of cognitive–behavioural case formulation

The case formulation is started at the very beginning of therapy. It is developed and refined collaboratively by client and therapist as assessment and therapy progress. It is achieved by means of recent-event analysis. This is a fundamental technique in CBT that uses Socratic dialogue (see below) to explore the client's affective, cognitive, physiological and behavioural reactions during problem episodes and also, as therapy progresses, their less conscious underlying core cognitions. In recent-event analysis, clients are encouraged to identify and separate their responses to recent typical examples of the problem and to explore whether and how these responses are causally linked. This is a powerful tool for engaging with children, since it allows them to relive recent problems in session and to feel 'heard' by the therapist.

Vignette 2

A young person in care questioned following overdose initially gave blocking 'Fine' or 'Don't know' answers, since in her experience 'Adults usually don't really want to know what it's been like for me'. However, when asked to go through in detail the sequence of what she had been thinking and feeling about her situation at the time of the overdose, she felt more inclined to speak. She felt further encouraged as she and her interviewer shared an overt acknowledgement that her behaviour might be in some way understandable. She also reported that she was surprised that her interviewer 'kept checking with me that they'd understood what I really meant rather than just assuming they knew'.

The formulation needs to be represented in a way that has most salience for the client. It is usually diagrammatic, but it may be narrative or expressed in symbols or imagery. The client's own language, images and experiences are used to represent elements of the formulation (Fig. 10.2). The degree of complexity reflects the shared understanding at the time and does not go beyond what is meaningful for the client (according to their developmental level and emotional state). Amplifying and maintaining cycles are collaboratively identified and predictions made about the possible consequences of change in any of the components.

Routine and regular use of case-based ratings of belief and affect intensity can greatly clarify which maintaining cycles predominate and regularly refocus collaborative attention. Specific links are made with past experience and these are integrated into the formulation. Helpful historical questions include 'Can you remember the first time in your life this ever happened?' and 'Have there been other times in your life that remind you of this?'. Therapy thus promotes the skills of self-observation and monitoring. Change can occur relatively rapidly at the level of negative automatic thoughts, but usually takes weeks or months at the deeper levels of conditional assumptions or core beliefs. Behavioural interventions include graded exposure to feared situations and identification and targeting of escape, avoidance and safety behaviours.

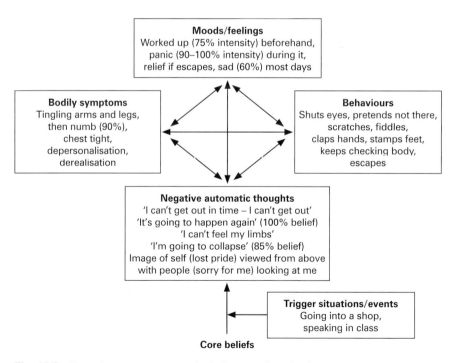

Fig. 10.2 Sample recent event-analysis for a panic episode.

Box 10.3 The basics of Socratic questioning

Questions are asked that:

- the client has the knowledge to answer
- draw attention to relevant information outside the client's present focus
- generally move between concrete/specific and more abstract/general
- apply new information to the client's beliefs so that the client can:
  - evaluate a previous conclusion
  - construct a new idea.

Socratic questioning

The Socratic questioning style (Box 10.3) is not unique to CBT, but it is fundamental in the practice of this intervention. As a therapist skill, Socratic questioning needs time, training and reflective practice to develop. It is based on the observation that people change their thinking more readily if the rationale for change comes from their own insights, rather than from the therapist's (Dattilio & Padesky, 1990).

Systemic cognitive–behavioural formulation

In CBT with children, the formulation must encompass not only a four-systems perspective and the Beckian cognitive model, but also interpersonal and family factors, including attachment issues and systemic and cultural influences (Box 10.4). Furthermore, it must take into account developmental and biological factors and the hierarchy of children's needs (primacy of physical and emotional security and nurturance, for example)

Box 10.4 Additional criteria for formulation with children

- Incorporating interpersonal, family, attachment, systemic, cultural and developmental factors and intrinsic difficulties
- Being simple and understandable as a basis for communication between child, family, therapist and other key people or bodies, while still being comprehensive enough to include and make understandable all major processes of cause and effect that trigger and maintain difficulties
- Testable, so that the child/family can confirm that this is an accurate reflection of their difficulties
- A template from which to derive and select interventions and predict consequences, positive and negative, of any change (i.e. also predicts difficulties in treatment and likely timescales for change)
- Helpful in refocusing therapy and for exploring difficulties during therapy

---

that need to be satisfied before higher-order therapeutic interventions are attempted. The formulation must be comprehensive but sufficiently succinct to be meaningful to the child.

Although specific models incorporating systemic factors have been suggested in cases of eating disorders (Fairburn *et al*, 1999), application beyond these disorders has not been widely described. There were a number of early attempts at predominantly cognitively based family formulation models (Schwebel & Fine, 1992; Smith & Schwebel, 1995; Dattilio, 2005), but these have not explicitly incorporated affective, physiological and behavioural components.

Structure for systemic cognitive–behavioural formulation

Figure 10.3 shows a structure for systemic cognitive–behavioural formulation that can be used in clinical practice.

Maintaining cycles are identified collaboratively in sessions through repeated Socratic recent-event analysis of both problematic and positive events. All the key people involved in maintaining the child's problem are represented by slowly developing the picture to include as many of the elements illustrated in Fig. 10.3 as is clinically appropriate.

The child's individual formulation, complete to the degree they have agreed in advance to share it, is central to the systemic case formulation. Also key is a chronology (from bottom upwards, to allow linking with appropriate levels of cognition) of major life events from age 0–5 years, over 5 years, since onset of symptoms or distress, and as present day-to-day situational triggers of acute difficulties. Surrounding this is a structure long valued in child and adolescent mental health service practice – a genogram representing the key family relationships around the child. In addition, all other relationships involved in and possibly maintaining the child's problems are represented. These might include peers, other helping agencies and maybe even the therapist. Ideas of proximity are incorporated, since the child, and family if relevant, will be asked to decide on the positioning of individuals in deriving this initial sculpting of key relationships.

Often, family influences need to be labelled in the formulation as carer core beliefs, commonly reflecting dominant family or cultural narratives and relating to their life experience. Major life events are therefore listed for the individuals most involved in maintaining the child's problem or most critical to the child for support. Each individual is asked early in therapy to give a prioritised problem list (of the key difficulties they think need to be addressed through therapy), with their perception of severity for each item, and to say which specific changes or aims they wish for. These are noted in the shared formulation (as shown in Fig. 10.3). Cultural influences such as illness models are also listed in the formulation, either in the surrounding environment or as cognitions of key individuals.

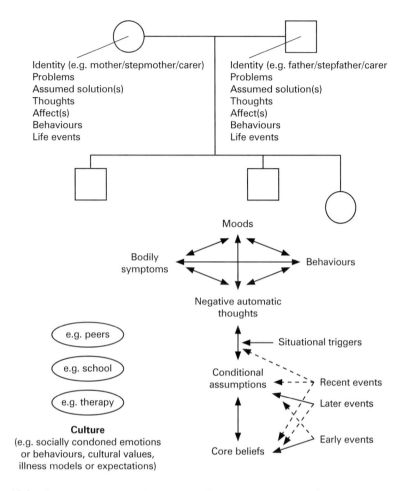

Culture
(e.g. socially condoned emotions
or behaviours, cultural values,
illness models or expectations)

Fig. 10.3 Systemic cognitive–behavioural formulation template for clinical use.

Use of systemic cognitive–behavioural formulation in practice

The location and nature of major maintaining processes in the formulation will help prioritise interventions and will also have prognostic importance. Where key maintaining processes involve core beliefs, longer-term working will be required, since change at this level of cognition is much slower, often taking months or even years. For this reason, family sessions are usually offered every 3 or 4 weeks over several months, much as with more traditional forms of family therapy.

Where individual maintaining factors predominate, individual CBT will be the treatment of choice. However, in many cases, systemic CBT will need to be offered in parallel with individual therapy.

Rating of belief levels (e.g. 'I believed this 75% at the time', on a 0–100% scale from 'not believed at all' to 'believed with 100% certainty') and affect-level ratings (e.g. 0–100% or 0–10, from 'feeling not present' to 'the strongest I've ever felt it') are very helpful in clarifying which processes are most active in problem situations.

Vignette 3

In a family recent-event analysis of difficult family times, a teenager and her parents were individually asked to rate their emotional distress and belief levels for the thoughts that had most upset them during times they had identified as difficult.

What emerged was that the parental levels of distress had been consistently very high during times of difficulty. The parents' most intensely believed cognitions did include worry that their daughter was getting upset, but far more consistent and intensely experienced than these worries were parental perceptions that their partner was misunderstanding their intentions or criticising their behaviour. In contrast, the teenager's distress in situations had been low, but she was chronically irritated by her parents' arguing.

The rating of cognitions and affect enabled the parents to see which distressing thoughts (of the wide variety of cognitions active in the problem situation) had been most instrumental in leading to their emotional responses in the situation. Instead of being linked to accurate perception of their daughter's emotional state, they were most intensely linked to relationship difficulties, which they subsequently chose to address in marital therapy.

The formulation can be developed in a greatly simplified form, starting with a blank piece of paper or simple self-statement, with the child and/or family slowly building it up from reflections on their own experience. Ideally, it should be revisited and repeatedly re-derived through recent-event analysis for subsequent similar problem situations over time to clarify which processes usually predominate. For example, in an individual session with a child who has come to understand 'I shout because I'm afraid', further exploration might be restricted to adding 'Dad gets cross if I shout'. More insightful wider work around this basic formulation can then be explored with the wider family or, for older children, with the children themselves, to yield more complex systemic processes of cause and effect and inform an evolving systemic formulation.

Vignette 4

A boy had been labelled by himself and his family as 'a liar'. There were indeed concrete examples of times when 'things he had told his father' had led to intense family distress. Faced with this partial picture of the family situation, he and his family had concluded that he was indeed 'responsible for all upset at home'.

In individual sessions, the boy was encouraged to describe the wider family situation in four-systems terms, highlighting the behaviour, apparent feelings and (where known) thoughts not only of himself but of those around him. It was also suggested that he consider the helpfulness (or otherwise) not only of his own responses but of the responses of other family members too. This revealed that his father had moved out of the family home and that the older children and the mother now believed themselves to be a fully independent family unit. All the others had chosen to no longer communicate directly with the father, but the boy had chosen to still see him.

He recounted times he had 'lied' to his father and acknowledged that what was actually happening was that he was not daring to contradict distorted beliefs his father held about his mother. He identified active intense beliefs at these times that 'Dad might have a breakdown if he's upset too much' and that 'Dad might fly off the handle if I upset him'. It was acknowledged that it would have been very difficult for him to have behaved differently because of these circumstances.

After considering the contributions of other family members together with his own, he was asked to complete a 'responsibility pie' for upset in the family. He then rated his own contribution (originally seen as 'nearly 100%') as much smaller, 'possibly smaller' than that of other key players. He was subsequently better able to articulate this perspective to his family.

In family working, the construction of new meaning that occurs in shared recent-event analysis is emphasised. Family members are encouraged to consider initially their individual perspectives at times of difficulty but then, working together, to derive a script that reflects the fuller family experience. Family members need to feel sufficiently comfortable and safe with sessions and with the relationships in the room to drop their habitual defences and reflect not only on the experiences and reactions of others but also on their own, and at times to voice extreme personal reactions. For this reason, positive events are usually considered first.

Vignette 5

The parents of a teenage boy who had a history of extreme refusal to attend school identified a particular Sunday night as having been 'very difficult'. The boy and his parents were invited to carry out four-systems analyses of the episode, first as individuals and then as a family.

The parents reported that their son had come to them on the evening in question in an apparently distressed state. The mother reported having had an immediate surge of terror and fear (95% belief level) that he might self-harm. She had consequently avoided further conversation and 'spent the evening on egg-shells to avoid any further distress'. The father reported an immediate feeling of frustration and impotence and the belief that he would be the person expected to ensure school attendance the next day and that his wife would blame him when he could not do so. He described 'going into a rage' and leaving the house. In contrast, their son (who had gone to school on the Monday morning without a problem) initially failed to recall the incident at all, but then remembered that he had actually gone to ask his parents where to find something in the house and that he had in the end gone to find it unaided as they had seemed to be arguing about something.

As the family gradually shared their experiences, all in the room (including the therapist) were surprised to hear the expectations each had had of each other on that occasion. Both parents acknowledged surprise and perplexity but then relief to find that the beliefs about the evening that had had coloured their emotional state for days had had no basis in fact. Further exploration revealed individual historical reasons underlying both parents' reactions on this and other occasions.

Clinicians and therapists assess families to consider the best treatment approach in light of the available evidence base. Some families will benefit more from this systemic CBT, and others from more individualised CBT. Although a significant proportion of children do benefit from CBT, a significant minority do not do well or drop out of treatment. Rey *et al* (2011) reviewed treatment failures in CBT with young people. They concluded that severity of symptoms and comorbid disorders, parental psychopathology and marital conflict, and minimal engagement with therapy on the part of both the young person and the parents, were contributing factors. Helping families engage with therapy is a key concern of therapists. The ideas outlined above may help clinicians communicate with children and families in a different way than with individualised CBT, and this could help forge the strong alliance that has shown to be so important in all therapies.

Incorporating development, attachment and insights from other psychotherapies

Recent-event analysis and wider-system cognitive–behavioural formulation allow children and families to explore processes more commonly investigated through other psychotherapeutic modalities. The projective processes of object relations theory may, for example, be represented as cognitions at core belief level (e.g. 'She always criticises me') or negative automatic thoughts in the acute problem situation (e.g. 'She is criticising me again'). Similarly, the experience of the paranoid–schizoid and depressive positions can be expressed in four-systems terms. Transference and countertransference processes may be located in the formulation as relationship-focused cognitions and consequent affect(s) and behaviour(s), and cultural influences may be represented in the formulation as articulated cognitions of key individuals. Figure 9.4 illustrates how sequences of interacting attachment-related behaviours and affects can be observed.

Developmental and biological factors are accommodated and represented in the systemic template by starting with the clinically observed 'primary' functional deficit in a system of response or cognitive level for the individual concerned. For example, with attention-deficit disorder, the primary deficit may be noted to be a cognitive deficit in planning, in consequential thinking or in both, or to be impulsive behaviour or general lack of attention to social cues. By working through the formulation with the child and/or family, the consequences of this (poor self-esteem, peer rejection, etc.) can be identified, together with other, possibly maintaining or exacerbating, factors such as parental cognitions (overanticipation of maladaptive behaviour) or behaviours (overcontrol). This can similarly be carried out for pervasive developmental disorders, specific intellectual and physical difficulties or simply to accommodate the child's present developmental level.

161

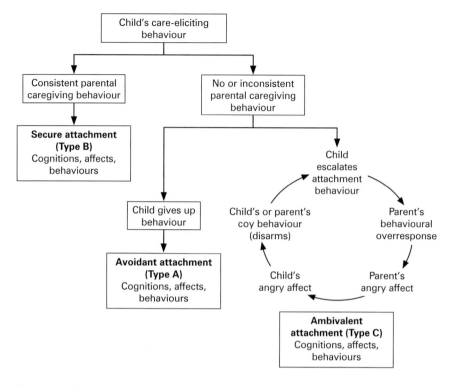

Fig. 10.4 The major attachment patterns, expressed in four-systems terms.

Examples of inaccurate or rigid cognitive responses (e.g. in some intellectual disabilities) or motor responses (e.g. in dyspraxia) are noted in the formulation under the appropriate system of response. Their effects in terms of other people's perceptions, expectations and behavioural responses can then be traced through the systemic formulation.

Conclusion

Formulation is the foundation of empirical therapy and is a core feature of CBT. Growing clinical experience reveals that formulation-based cognitive–behavioural working can be extended to systemic process working that incorporates developmental level, attachment processes and insights from other psychotherapies. The approach described in this chapter has been derived from empirical application of core cognitive–behavioural theory and processes to working on a systemic basis. It appears to offer a comprehensive systemic framework that can be used with individuals, carer–dependant dyads, families and wider systems. It provides a structure that has been useful in supervision and therapist training. Although this approach has yet to be formally evaluated, in clinical practice there is growing experience that it opens up new ways of understanding and opportunities for change.

References

Barrett PM, Duffy AL, Dadds MR, *et al* (2001) Cognitive–behavioural treatment of anxiety disorders in children: long-term (6-year) follow-up. *Journal of Consulting and Clinical Psychology*, **69**, 135–141.

Barrett P, Farrell L, Dadds M, *et al* (2005) Cognitive–behavioral family treatment of childhood obsessive–compulsive disorder: long-term follow-up and predictors of outcome. *Journal of the American Academy of Child & Adolescent Psychiatry*, **44**, 1005–1014.

Beck AT (1979) *Cognitive Therapy for Depression*. Guilford Press.

Dattilio FM (2005) Restructuring of family schemas: a cognitive–behavior perspective. *Journal of Marital and Family Therapy*, **31**, 15–29.

Dattilio FM, Padesky CA (1990) *Cognitive Therapy with Couples*. Professional Resource Exchange.

Drinkwater J (2005) Cognitive case formulation. In *Cognitive Behaviour Therapy for Children and Families* (2nd edn) (ed P Graham), pp. 84–99. Cambridge University Press.

Drinkwater J, Stewart DA (2002) Cognitive therapy in children and young people. *Current Opinion in Psychiatry*, **15**, 377–381.

Dummett N (2006) Processes for systemic cognitive behavioural therapy with children, young people and families. *Behavioural and Cognitive Psychotherapy*, **34**, 179–189.

Fairburn CG, Shafran R, Cooper PJ (1999) A cognitive behavioural theory of anorexia nervosa. *Behaviour Research and Therapy*, **37**, 1–13.

Harrington R, Whittaker J, Shoebridge P, *et al* (1998) Systematic review of efficacy of cognitive behaviour therapies in childhood and adolescent depressive disorder. *BMJ*, **316**, 1559–1563.

Jones DPH, Ramchandani P (1999) *Child Sexual Abuse: Informing Practice from Research*. Blackwell.

King NJ, Tonge BJ, Heyne D, *et al* (1998) Cognitive–behavioral treatment of school-refusing children: a controlled evaluation. *Journal of the American Academy of Child & Adolescent Psychiatry*, **37**, 395–403.

March J, Silva S, Petrycki S, *et al* (2004) Fluoxetine, cognitive-behavioral therapy, and their combination for adolescents with depression: Treatment for Adolescents with Depression Study (TADS) randomized controlled trial. *JAMA*, **292**, 807–820.

National Collaborating Centre for Mental Health (2005a) *Depression in Children and Young People: Identification and Management in Primary, Community and Secondary Care* (Clinical Guideline 28). National Institute for Health and Clinical Excellence.

National Collaborating Centre for Mental Health (2005b) *Post-Traumatic Stress Disorder (PTSD): The Management of PTSD in Adults and Children in Primary and Secondary Care* (Clinical Guideline 26). National Institute for Health and Clinical Excellence.

National Collaborating Centre for Mental Health (2005c) *Obsessive-Compulsive Disorder: Core Interventions in the Treatment of Obsessive-Compulsive Disorder and Body Dysmorphic Disorder* (Clinical Guideline 31). National Institute for Health and Clinical Excellence.

National Collaborating Centre for Mental Health (2006) *Bipolar Disorder: The Management of Bipolar Disorder in Adults, Children and Adolescents, in Primary and Secondary Care* (Clinical Guideline 38). National Institute for Health and Clinical Excellence.

National Institute for Health and Clinical Excellence (2008) *Attention Deficit Hyperactivity Disorder: Diagnosis and Management of ADHD in Children, Young People and Adults* (NICE Clinical Guideline 72). NICE.

Northey WF, Wells KC, Silverman WK, *et al* (2003) Childhood behavioural and emotional disorders. *Journal of Marital and Family Therapy*, **29**, 523–542.

Padesky CA, Greenberger D (1995) *Clinician's Guide to Mind Over Mood*. Guilford Press.

Persons JB (1989) *Cognitive Therapy in Practice: A Case Formulation Approach*. WW Norton.

Rachman S (1978) Human fears: a three systems approach. *Scandinavian Journal of Behaviour Therapy*, **7**, 237–245.

Rey Y, Marin CE, Silverman WK (2011) Failures in cognitive-behavior therapy for children. *Journal of Clinical Psychology*, **67**, 1140–1150.

Roth A, Pilling S (2008) Using an evidence-based methodology to identify competencies required to deliver effective cognitive behavioural therapy for depression and anxiety disorders. *Behavioural and Cognitive Psychotherapy*, **36**, 129–147.

Roth A, Fonagy P, Parry G, et al (2006) *What Works for Whom? A Critical Review of Psychotherapy Research* (2nd edn). Guilford Press.

Salkovskis PM (2002) Empirically grounded clinical interventions: cognitive–behavioural therapy progresses through a multi-dimensional approach to clinical science. *Behavioural and Cognitive Psychotherapy*, **30**, 3–9.

Sanders MR, Shepherd RW, Cleghorn G, et al (1994) The treatment of recurrent abdominal pain in children: a controlled evaluation of cognitive–behavioral family intervention and standard pediatric care. *Journal of Consulting and Clinical Psychology*, **62**, 306–314.

Schmidt U (1998) Eating disorders and obesity. In *Cognitive-Behaviour Therapy for Children and Families* (ed P Graham), pp. 262–281. Cambridge University Press.

Schwebel AI, Fine MA (1992) Cognitive–behavioural family therapy. *Journal of Family Psychotherapy*, **3**, 73–91.

Silverman WK, Kurtinees WM, Ginsburg GS, et al (1999) Contingency management, self-control, and education support in the treatment of childhood phobic disorders: a randomized clinical trial. *Journal of Consulting and Clinical Psychology*, **67**, 675–687.

Smith GB, Schwebel AI (1995) Using a cognitive–behavioural family model in conjunction with systems and behavioural family therapy models. *American Journal of Family Therapy*, **23**, 203–212.

Smith P, Perrin S, Yule W (1998) Post-traumatic stress disorders. In *Cognitive-Behaviour Therapy for Children and Families* (ed P Graham), pp. 127–142. Cambridge University Press.

Spence SH, Donovan C (1998) Interpersonal problems. In *Cognitive-Behaviour Therapy for Children and Families* (ed P Graham), pp. 217–245. Cambridge University Press.

Spence SH, Donovan C, Brechman-Toussaint M (2000) The treatment of childhood social phobia: the effectiveness of a social skills training-based cognitive–behavioural intervention with and without parental involvement. *Journal of Child Psychology and Psychiatry*, **41**, 713–726.

Stallard P (2002) Cognitive behaviour therapy with children and young people: a selective review of key issues. *Behavioural and Cognitive Psychotherapy*, **30**, 297–309.

Tarrier, N, Calam, R (2002) New developments in cognitive–behavioural case formulation. *Epidemiological, systemic and social context: an integrative approach. Behavioural and Cognitive Psychotherapy*, **30**, 311–328.

White C, McNally D, Cartwright-Hatton S (2003) Cognitively enhanced parent training. *Behavioural and Cognitive Psychotherapy*, **31**, 99–102.

CHAPTER 11

Anxiety disorders

Aaron K. Vallance and Victoria Fernandez

Anxiety is an uncomfortable experience characterised by emotional (e.g. unease, distress), cognitive (e.g. fears, worries, helplessness), physiological (e.g. muscle tension) and behavioural (e.g. avoidance) changes. The anxious child commonly focuses on the future, fearful of danger, either specific or undefined. Anxiety that is excessive or contextually or developmentally inappropriate, causing significant distress and/or functional impairment, can be classified as an anxiety disorder. Although rarely recognised, too little anxiety might also be considered 'disordered': callous unemotional traits may be such a manifestation (Frick *et al*, 1999).

In ICD-10, anxiety disorders are classified into a cluster of related conditions: separation anxiety, generalised anxiety, social phobia, panic disorder and simple phobias (World Health Organization, 1992). Although beyond the remit of this chapter, anxiety can feature in other psychiatric conditions. In obsessive–compulsive disorder (OCD), obsessions generate anxiety which the individual then tries to neutralise through compulsions. Indeed, DSM-5 defines and differentiates obsessions and compulsions through their causal relationships with anxiety (American Psychiatric Association, 2013). This may be a simplification: although compulsions may initially relieve anxiety, they can aggravate it as the disorder progresses (Heyman *et al*, 2006). Swedo *et al* (1998) describe separation anxiety as a characteristic feature of the proposed 'paediatric autoimmune neuro-psychiatric disorders associated with streptococcal infections' (PANDAS) subset of OCD, although recent research disputes this (Murphy *et al*, 2012). Anxiety also occurs in post-traumatic stress disorder (PTSD), particularly when traumatic memories are triggered. Avoidance behaviour and hypervigilance are common and can be seen as an adaptive response to avoid further dangers, albeit one that is excessive, distressing and/or impairing. Anxiety in PTSD may relate to dysfunction of the hypothalamic–pituitary–adrenal (HPA) axis.

From an evolutionary perspective, anxiety is an emotional response intrinsically shaped by natural selection: its very purpose is to ensure safety, avoid danger and keep the individual alive (at least long enough to pass on their genes). Anxiety is therefore a normal and important facet of human experience and functioning.

The various subtypes of anxiety disorder probably evolved to give a selective advantage of superior protection against particular kinds of danger

165

Table 11.1 Evolutionary protective roles associated with anxiety-related behaviours

Behaviour	Protective role
Escape or avoidance	Distances an individual from certain threats
Aggressive defence	Harms the source of danger
Freezing/immobility	Helps to locate and assess the danger Concealment Inhibits the predator's attack reflex
Submission/appeasement	Protects the individual when the threat comes from their own group Submission to group leaders and to group norms prevents dangerous expulsion from the group Mild shyness may promote acceptance Separation anxiety can help promote the attachment of the child to the mother

After Marks & Nesse (1994).

(Marks & Nesse, 1994). Commonalities, however, exist between these subtypes, for example in their shared behavioural responses (Table 11.1). Again, this may be evolutionarily driven, reflecting a need for flexibility in dealing with uncertain or indefinable threats. Furthermore, physiological and behavioural responses useful against one type of danger are likely to protect against other types as well. Indeed, our hunter-gatherer ancestors would have faced multiple threats: predators, starvation, climate, falls and exposure.

The shifting manifestation of anxiety through different developmental stages may also have an evolutionary basis (Table 11.2). Fears tend to occur at the age they become adaptive: for example, fear of animals occurs from 2 to 3 years old, when there is increased exploration, and this may have a protective value. In adolescents, developing cognitive maturity endows individuals with a growing capacity to imagine and ruminate on abstract

Table 11.2 Fear and its typical developmental stages

Age	Typical fears
9 months to 3 years	Sudden movements or loud noises, separation from caregivers, strangers
3–6 years	Animals, the dark, 'monsters/ghosts'
6–12 years	Performance anxiety
12–18 years	Social anxiety, fear of failure/rejection
Adulthood	Illness, death

threats. The developmental aspect of anxiety is an important consideration: what is seen as normal for a young child may be considered a disorder in an older child. So, for example, screaming when separated from a mother may be quite normative in a preschool child, but in an 11-year-old it would be unusual.

Epidemiology

Anxiety disorders are some of the most prevalent psychiatric disorders in children and adolescents, particularly among girls (Table 11.3). They also frequently co-occur: at least one-third of children presenting with an anxiety disorder meet the criteria for two or more subtypes. Moreover, general comorbidity with other psychiatric disorders – including oppositional defiant disorder and attention-deficit hyperactivity disorder (ADHD), substance misuse and depression – is approximately 40%; comorbidity with depressive disorder is about 28%. Anxiety disorders are frequently found in autism spectrum disorders, with rates as high as 84% (Muris *et al*, 1998).

Clinical features of anxiety disorders

The ICD-10 diagnostic criteria for all types of anxiety disorder stipulate the presence of both emotional and physiological symptoms, either in a specific feared situation or for a specific duration.

Separation anxiety disorder

Separation anxiety disorder is an excessive and/or developmentally inappropriate anxiety about separation from attachment figures. Excessive worrying about the figure's welfare may also occur. Impairment might include school refusal (possibly exacerbated by specific school anxiety), avoidance of visiting friends' homes or difficulty sleeping alone. The ICD-10 criteria include onset before 6 years of age and duration of at least 4 weeks.

Table 11.3 Epidemiological characteristics of anxiety disorders in children and adolescents

Disorder	Prevalence, %	Typical age at onset
Separation anxiety disorder	2–4	Prepuberty; peaks at 7 years
Generalised anxiety disorder	3	Increased incidence in adolescence
Panic disorder	5	Late teens
Social phobia	1–7	11–15 years
Specific phobia	2–4	>5 years

Source: Vallance & Garralda (2011).

Generalised anxiety disorder

Generalised anxiety disorder encompasses multiple and persistent worries (e.g. regarding family, friendships, school or appearance) not restricted to any one situation or object, lasting at least 6 months. Comorbidity (e.g. with depression) is particularly common. In ICD-10, diagnostic criteria for children and adolescents are differentiated from those for adults. The former include an additional 'difficult-to-control worries' criterion, and requires three or more physical symptoms from six, a condensed list to reflect the reduced prominence of autonomic arousal in children.

It is not clear yet what modifications will be made in the revised version, ICD-11, although Shear (2012) proposes various changes for the adult criteria, including a requirement that worry must occur frequently and/or excessively, focusing the somatic criteria on restlessness and muscle tension, and permitting the diagnosis even in the presence of other anxiety disorders. Interestingly, these criteria are already present in the ICD-10 children's diagnosis.

Social phobia and social anxiety disorder of childhood

Social phobia is accompanied by an excessive fear of embarrassment or scrutiny. Avoidance of particular social situations reinforces the associated anxiety and could eventually impede social skills development and, at the most extreme, result in debilitating social isolation. In DSM-5, 'social phobia' is a single category, but in ICD-10 it is differentiated from 'social anxiety disorder of childhood' (American Psychiatric Association, 2013). Social anxiety disorder of childhood occurs at a developmental stage at which social anxiety reactions are appropriate – diagnostically, it must manifest before 6 years of age – but in an affected child they involve significant severity, persistence or impairment lasting for at least 4 weeks. In contrast, social phobia reflects social anxiety later in life, and includes blushing, shaking, or fear of vomiting, micturition or defecation; no minimum duration of symptoms is given.

Emmelkamp (2012) argues that ICD-11 should also include a minimum symptom duration for social phobia, following the new inclusion of a minimum 6 months' duration in DSM-5. Wittchen *et al* (1999) distinguish between generalised social phobia (across multiple settings) and non-generalised: the former is associated with greater chronicity, impairment and comorbidity. Autism spectrum disorder is a differential (particularly where social isolation is a function of impaired social communication and/or lack of social interest rather than frank anxiety) or occasionally comorbid diagnosis.

Specific or simple phobias

Specific or simple phobias are defined by excessive fear of specific objects or situations that provoke an immediate anxiety response on exposure, causing significant distress and/or functional impairment, for example because of avoidance. Fyer (1998) describes subtypes relating to: animals, specific situations, nature/environment (e.g. water, heights) and blood injury. Not only do they differ in their triggers, they may also vary with respect to symptomatology, age at onset and heritability. Blood injury phobia, for example, has a distinct biphasic physiological response. Some typical fears held by children and adolescents are described in Table 11.2. The DSM-5 criteria no longer require the individual to recognise that their anxiety is excessive or unreasonable: instead, the onus is on the clinician to determine whether anxiety is disproportionate to the situation.

This particular DSM-5 criterion of due proportion also relates to agoraphobia, which encompasses an often overlapping cluster of phobias relating to at least two of crowds, public places, leaving home and travelling alone. Various specific worries may reinforce the anxiety, including fears of collapsing, being left helpless in public and being unable to escape. Persistent avoidance may result in the experience of minimal anxiety, so that the agoraphobia escalates until the individual becomes housebound.

Panic disorder

Panic disorder involves repeated and unexpected attacks of severe anxiety not restricted to any particular situation, accompanied by multiple physical symptoms. It often originates from the occasional panic attack in adolescence, although only a small proportion of young people who have such attacks subsequently develop the disorder. Anticipatory anxiety about future attacks or their perceived implications (e.g. losing control, being judged, etc.) is common. In keeping with ICD-10, DSM-5 has now separated agoraphobia and panic disorder into distinct entities, particularly as many individuals with agoraphobia do not experience panic symptoms.

Assessment

Children and young people with anxiety disorders may not present to services overtly complaining of anxiety. They may also have difficulty articulating their experiences or be confused or embarrassed by them. Nevertheless, making an early diagnosis is important, as many anxiety disorders remain untreated in the community, causing distress and impeding academic and social functioning.

Assessment should differentiate between developmentally appropriate fears and anxiety disorders. It should also consider potential aetiological factors and developmental influences. Differential and comorbid diagnoses include autism spectrum disorder, oppositional defiant disorder, ADHD, depression and PTSD. Differentiating between diagnoses can be challenging given the overlapping symptoms. For example, fatigue, irritability, and sleep and concentration problems occur in both generalised anxiety and depression.

169

History-taking should aim to exclude medical disorders and drugs that can mimic or provoke anxiety states (Table 11.4). If an organic disorder suggests itself, it can be followed up through physical examination and targeted investigations (BMJ Evidence Centre, 2012). Liaison with general practitioners and/or paediatricians may be indicated.

Validated self-report scales such as the Multidimensional Anxiety Scale for Children (MASC; March *et al*, 1997) and the Screen for Child Anxiety Related Disorders (SCARED; Birmaher *et al*, 1997) have shown correlation with anxiety severity and treatment effects. Clinician scales include the Pediatric Anxiety Rating Scale (PARS; Research Unit on

Table 11.4 Medical conditions and drugs that can mimic anxiety symptoms, with potential further investigations

	Notes	Possible further investigations
Medical conditions		
Hyperthyroidism	Characteristic symptoms include goitre, weight loss, warm moist skin, heat intolerance and ophthalmopathy The most common cause is the autoimmune Grave's disease, which is not uncommon in adolescents	Thyroid function tests
Arrhythmias	Sinus tachycardia is a normal increase in heart rate (e.g. exercise, excitement) The most common childhood abnormal tachycardia is supraventricular	Electrocardiogram and echocardiogram
Epilepsy	'Ictal fear' can accompany focal seizures Anxiety symptoms may occur as a seizure prodromal symptom	Electroencephalogram
Pheochromocytoma	Characteristic symptoms include tachycardia and hypertension Mostly presents in young adulthood, but can occur earlier if hereditary	24-hour urine test for vanillylmandelic acid and metadrenaline
Asthma	Characteristic symptoms include wheezing, cough, chest-tightness Asthma is common in childhood, and is associated with an increased risk of panic disorder (where it is also a differential diagnosis) and separation anxiety	Pulmonary function tests
Drugs		
Street drugs	For example, amphetamines, cocaine	Urine drug screen
Sympathomimetics	For example, pseudoephedrine for nasal congestion	
Caffeine	From tea, coffee, caffeinated drinks	

Pediatric Psychopharmacology Anxiety Study Group, 2003). Assessment should also focus on the distress and impairment to the individual and their family. This would include suicidality, which is increased in anxiety disorders. Adolescents may also resort to alcohol and other substances as ways of coping.

Aetiology

Despite their symptomatic variation, anxiety disorders may share some common aetiological or pathophysiological characteristics.

Temperament

Research suggests a relationship between pre-existing personality traits and later anxiety disorders. One such trait is inhibited temperament, or behavioural inhibition, defined by Kagan and colleagues as a tendency to show apprehension to novel or unfamiliar situations, together with raised reactivity of the sympathetic nervous system (Kagan & Snidman, 1999). Such behavioural inhibition in early childhood is a risk factor for anxiety, particularly social phobia, later in childhood and adolescence (Perez-Edgar & Fox, 2005). Similar associations have been reported for shyness and an anxious-resistant attachment style. The 21-year longitudinal study by Goodwin et al (2004) showed that anxious/withdrawn behaviour at 8 years of age increased the risk of anxiety disorders and depression in adolescence and young adulthood.

However, the relationship is complex, it varies according to the study (Degnan et al, 2010) and much of the association may lie at the extremes of temperament (Kagan et al, 2002). Furthermore, other moderating factors (e.g. peer rejection, exclusion and victimisation) play a significant role as the child develops.

Genetics

Family studies indicate an association between parental anxiety and depression and anxiety disorders in offspring. The association appears to be largely non-specific (in terms of anxiety subcategory), except for a particular relationship between parental panic disorder and offspring separation anxiety disorder (Biederman et al, 2004).

Twin studies in adults suggest that generational transmission is primarily accounted for by non-shared environmental and genetic factors, with a heritability of about 40% for panic, generalised and agoraphobic anxiety, and specific phobias (Hettema et al, 2001). Such studies in children show more variation. For example, Bolton et al (2006) reported a heritability of 60% for specific phobias and 73% for separation anxiety disorder, whereas Eley et al (2008) found the figures to be 46% and 14% respectively. Both studies show significant influence of non-shared environmental factors.

171

However, the latter study also shows a significant shared environmental contribution for specific phobia (at 0.27, as for non-shared factors), which suggests that familial factors (such as parental overprotection or control) may be as influential as non-shared factors (e.g. conditioning) for this disorder.

Furthermore, research indicates both common and distinct genetic aetiologies across some types of anxiety and affective disorder. For example, generalised anxiety and major depressive disorders appear to share a common genetic aetiology, but diverge in their non-shared environmental factors. Twin studies in adults indicate a similar genetic substrate underlying panic disorder and generalised anxiety disorder, but a distinct one for specific phobias (Hettema et al, 2005). Another twin study showed a shared genetic diathesis between adult-onset panic attacks and earlier separation anxiety disorder, but not for what was previously called childhood overanxious disorder (Roberson-Nay et al, 2012). The paediatric anxiety twin study by Eley et al (2008), however, showed no significant genetic covariation between specific phobias, separation anxiety and social phobia, implying distinct biological substrates for each.

Twin studies therefore indicate that genetic factors endow a broad susceptibility to anxiety in general as opposed to a specific disorder. This again may reflect an evolutionary 'balancing act' between specialisation (to deal potently with specific threats) and generalisation (necessary for protection against several types of danger arising from the evolutionary coexistence of multiple threats). There is probably a stronger relationship between genetic factors and various neuropsychological processes (including behavioural inhibition) or traits (e.g. neuroticism), rather than specific psychiatric disorders.

Finally, adult molecular genetic studies suggest serotonin transporter dysfunction, although paediatric studies are few. Fox et al (2005) explored gene–environment interaction and showed that children with a combination of the short 5-HTT allele and low social support had increased risk for behavioural inhibition.

Neuroimaging and neuropsychology

The few neuroimaging studies conducted with children have shown some interesting structural findings. Replicating results in adults, Koolschijn et al (2013) found an association between reduced left hippocampal volume and higher scores for anxiety and depression on the Child Behavior Checklist. Milham et al (2005) found reduced left amygdala grey matter volume associated with anxiety disorders. Intriguingly, a pilot follow-up study showed recoveries in amygdala grey matter volume after successful 8-week intervention with selective serotonin reuptake inhibitors (SSRIs) or psychotherapy.

Various studies have explored relationships between early temperament and neuroanatomy or neurophysiology. Schwartz et al (2003) used functional magnetic resonance imaging (MRI) to show that adults who had had an inhibited (compared with uninhibited) temperament at 2 years old showed greater amygdala signal response to novel faces. Schwartz *et al* (2010) subsequently used structural MRI to show that adults who had had a low-reactive temperament in infancy showed greater left orbitofrontal cortex thickness, whereas those who had had high reactivity showed greater right ventromedial prefrontal cortex thickness. Functional MRI research in young people with generalised anxiety disorder has shown that variations in state anxiety modulate associations between attention and activation in a 'fear circuit' encompassing the amygdala, ventral prefrontal cortex and the anterior cingulate cortex (McClure *et al*, 2007).

Pine (2007) has attempted to unify neuroimaging research (e.g. amygdala–prefrontal circuitry abnormalities) with affective and cognitive research (e.g. memory, learning, emotional regulation and fear conditioning) in a single neuropsychological model. This describes various information-processing biases in anxiety disorder: for example, the tendency to direct attention towards environmental threats, and appraise such threats as particularly meaningful and dangerous. The development of neural substrates underlying the fear response and anxiety is likely to involve complex gene–environment interplay, including the influence of early life experiences (Fox *et al*, 2005).

Parent–child interactions and the family environment

Retrospective and observational studies have found that parental over-control, rejection and modelling of anxious behaviours are consistently and significantly associated with childhood shyness and paediatric anxiety disorders (Degnan *et al*, 2010). Specifically, aspects of parenting behaviour (e.g. oversolicitous, intrusive or controlling parenting), style (e.g. authoritarian, permissive, low-proactive and low-supportive parenting as perceived by children, or overprotective parenting as reported by parents), psychopathology (e.g. parents diagnosed with panic disorder and/or depression), personality (e.g. maternal neuroticism) and the parent–child relationship (e.g. insecure attachment) have been linked with heightened behavioural inhibition and/or anxiety in children. Parenting factors are therefore likely moderators of the relationship between behavioural inhibition and the development of childhood anxiety. However, the degree to which the child's anxiety has a reverse influence on parenting is unclear. These parenting styles are also implicated in other child psychiatric disorders.

Such parenting may hinder the development of autonomy, resulting in a child who experiences the environment as more threatening and less safe. Lack of parental emotional availability, for example as a result of social adversities such as overcrowding, poverty and marital discord, may impede parents' ability to help contain their children's anxieties; children living in families where there are such chronic stressors are more likely to experience insecurity and to feel anxious and fearful. Also, parents who themselves have increased trait anxiety and sense of threat may exacerbate the perception of threat in these children and obstruct the development of coping skills; modelling may therefore be a significant contributing factor.

Parent–child interaction also, of course, occurs *in utero*, and research shows that maternal stress or anxiety in pregnancy can influence psychopathology in the offspring (Glover, 2011). Bergman *et al* (2007) showed that prenatal stress predicts observed fearfulness in the offspring. Van den Bergh & Marcoen (2004) used multiple regression analysis to show that maternal state anxiety in the second (but not the third) trimester correlates with anxiety in 8- and 9-year-olds. O'Connor *et al* (2002) showed that antenatal anxiety (but not depression) in late pregnancy is independently associated with behavioural/emotional problems in 4-year-olds.

Prenatal stress may also lead to neuroanatomical changes in offspring, such as reduced hippocampal and grey matter volume (Glover, 2011), consistent with neuroimaging data discussed above. From an evolutionary perspective, the effects of prenatal stress on fetal neurodevelopment may allow offspring to readily adapt to the same potentially stress-inducing environment as experienced by the mother. Glover (2011) also suggests that outcomes become non-adaptive if the manifesting anxiety is excessively extreme for the respective environment.

Traumatic life events

Traumatic events predispose not only to PTSD, but also to various anxiety disorders, particularly specific phobia and social phobia (McLaughlin *et al*, 2012). Pine *et al*'s (2002) longitudinal study found that adverse life events in adolescence were associated with symptoms of generalised anxiety disorder in adulthood, but only in females.

Respiratory dysregulation

Recurrent dyspnoea, particularly in asthma, is a risk factor for paediatric anxiety disorders such as panic and separation anxiety (Goodwin *et al*, 2003). Sensitivity to carbon dioxide, a respiratory stimulant, has also been found in children with anxiety disorders, particularly separation anxiety disorder (Pine *et al*, 2005).

Interventions

The National Institute for Health and Care Excellence (NICE) guideline on generalised anxiety and panic disorders in adults covers principles that can be extrapolated to children and adolescents (National Institute for Health and Clinical Excellence, 2011). For example, early psychoeducation can help families understand the condition and provide reassurance, and self-help may encompass written and electronic materials. Interventions with a significant evidence base include cognitive–behavioural therapy (CBT) and SSRI medication. It is important to ascertain the expectations and preferences of the young people and their families and to make treatments developmentally appropriate.

CBT and psychological therapy

As already mentioned, the NICE guideline recommends CBT for anxiety disorders. It incorporates both cognitive (e.g. reframing, positive self-talk, challenging unhelpful thoughts, and weighing up evidence for and against expected events) and behavioural processes (e.g. systematic desensitisation, exposure and response prevention for specific phobias, relaxation training, modelling and rewarding wanted behaviour, and role-play).

Depending on the anxiety disorder and the child's age, either cognitive or behavioural strategies can be emphasised. Various manuals (e.g. Stallard, 2002) provide accessible material for both clinician and patient. Family and school can support the child and help with graded exposure tasks and experiments such as those described by Kendall *et al* (2005).

Table 11.5 A comparison of two meta-analyses of the efficacy of psychological therapies for anxiety disorders

	Mean effect size	
Factor	Ishikawa *et al* (2007) 20 studies	Reynolds *et al* (2012) 55 studies (48 on CBT)
CBT (overall *v.* control)	n.a.	0.66*
CBT (pre- *v.* post-)	0.94*	n.a.
CBT *v.* passive control	0.68*	0.77*
CBT *v.* active control	0.61*	0.39*
Individual CBT	0.66*	0.85*
Group CBT	0.59*	0.58*
Fewer sessions	<11 sessions: 0.54*	<9h: 0.02–0.35*
Many sessions	≥11 sessions: 0.70*	≥9h: 0.65*–0.77*
Parental involvement *v.* no parental involvement	0.03*	0.57*
Parental involvement		0.63*–0.69*
Child <14 years	n.a.	0.63*
Adolescent ≥14 years	n.a.	1.38*
University clinics	0.77*	n.a.
Non-university clinics	0.37*	n.a.

CBT, cognitive–behavioural therapy; n.a., not available.
*$P<0.05$.

Two relatively recent meta-analyses of psychological therapies for anxiety disorders in children and young people (Ishikawa *et al*, 2007; Reynolds *et al*, 2012) also included a few trials relating to PTSD and OCD (Table 11.5). Both meta-analyses showed significant effect sizes for CBT, which remained significant but attenuated when analysis was limited to studies with an active control methodology (as opposed to waiting-list or treatment-as-usual groups). Both reported that involving parents had a positive but, perhaps surprisingly, relatively minor effect.

These two meta-analyses also yielded some divergent data, possibly because of their differing inclusion criteria, number of studies included, date of publication and outcome measures. While the Ishikawa team found little difference in effect size between delivering fewer versus many sessions, the Reynolds team showed that having less than 9 hours of therapy reduced the effect size and less than 4 hours had minimal therapeutic effect. And whereas the Ishikawa team demonstrated little difference in effect size between group and individual CBT, the Reynolds team showed a particularly high effect size for individual CBT. However, delivering CBT to a group may arguably enhance efficiency and provide peer support and reassurance. An open trial has recently shown evidence supporting a novel CBT package (Emotion Detectives Treatment Protocol) delivered to a group of children with various anxiety and depressive disorders (Bilek & Ehrenreich-May, 2012).

Computerised CBT packages such as Stressbusters (Abeles *et al*, 2009) have now been developed for childhood anxiety disorders. Their advantages and disadvantages are listed in Box 11.1 (Richardson *et al*, 2010). Two

---

Box 11.1   Advantages and disadvantages of delivering CBT online

Potential advantages	*Potential disadvantages*
Reduces potential stigma of attending mental health service	Evaluation often shows high drop-out rate
May be easier to share personal information with a computer than face to face	Problematic if difficulties with internet access
Young people are a 'digital native' generation, at ease with technology	Needs significant self-motivation to complete all modules
Useful if there are problems accessing face-to-face CBT (e.g. availability and waiting lists)	Difficulty re-creating all the specific and complex elements of face-to-face therapy, as well as therapeutic rapport
Packages accessible anytime, anywhere	
Standardised outcome measures can be built into software packages	After Richardson *et al* (2010)

randomised controlled trials, each with over 70 participants, showed significant differences between CBT (using the BRAVE-ONLINE package) and control groups. Furthermore, remission rates in the treatment groups were approximately 75% at 6 months (March *et al*, 2009) and at 12 months (Spence *et al*, 2006). Spence *et al*'s study also included a clinic-based CBT arm; overall results showed no significant difference between internet- and clinic-delivered CBT.

The evidence base for other forms of psychological therapy is less robust. Family therapy may help where dysfunctional patterns of family interaction influence the child's anxiety symptoms. Parents may also need support for their own difficulties with anxiety and/or separation to prevent them from exacerbating their child's symptoms.

Pharmacotherapy

The NICE guidelines for adults advise that medication or CBT be tried if self-help or psychoeducational groups are unsuccessful, or if there is significant impairment. However, in children, research has shown added efficacy of combining medication with CBT (Walkup *et al*, 2008). In practice, medication tends to be used in combination with psychological therapy where possible, and is perhaps most considered in older children with more severe symptoms, taking into account side-effect profiles and comorbid conditions.

Pharmacotherapy practice has shifted away from tricyclic antidepressants towards SSRIs for childhood anxiety disorders. These have a stronger evidence base and safer side-effect profiles, including relative safety in overdose. Research has demonstrated the efficacy of fluoxetine and fluvoxamine for paediatric social phobia, generalised anxiety disorder and separation anxiety disorder (Research Unit on Pediatric Psychopharmacology Anxiety Study Group, 2001; Birmaher *et al*, 2003). Two studies support efficacy and tolerability of sertraline for childhood generalised anxiety disorder (Rynn *et al*, 2001; Walkup *et al*, 2008); the Walkup *et al* study also included participants with social phobia and separation anxiety.

In studies of children and adolescents, the therapeutic use of SSRIs has been associated with suicidal ideation and non-fatal suicidal acts (of the order of 4%, *v.* about 2% in placebo groups), although the benefit of using them might outweigh the risk of emergent suicidal behaviour (Hawton *et al*, 2012). This risk appears to relate to other diagnoses as well as depression. For depressive disorder, the Medicines and Healthcare products Regulatory Agency (MHRA; 2003) and NICE advise that only fluoxetine has a favourable risk/benefit profile, making it the first-line SSRI for depression. The situation regarding anxiety disorders is less clear and NICE (National Collaborating Centre for Mental Health, 2005) does not comment specifically on medication for children with these conditions: in the UK, no antidepressants are currently licensed for paediatric anxiety disorders, although sertraline and fluvoxamine are licensed for paediatric OCD.

There is little evidence to support the use of non-antidepressant medication. Studies have failed to show significant efficacy of benzodiazepines, and their side-effects, for example behavioural disinhibition, are a risk. Such side-effects can also occur for buspirone, although case reports and open studies have shown some efficacy. There have been few studies of beta blockers. Further information on pharmacotherapy in paediatric anxiety disorder can be found in Chapter 7.

Prognosis

Studies evaluating longitudinal outcomes indicate that childhood anxiety disorders generally remit. For example, the prospective study by Last *et al* (1996) on children with a mean age of 12 years found that recovery rates over 3–4 years were 96% for separation anxiety disorder, 86% for social anxiety disorder, 80% for overanxious disorder, and about 70% for specific phobia and panic disorder. The prognosis for anxiety disorders depends on type of disorder, comorbidity, age at onset and severity at baseline. The 2-year longitudinal study by Broeren *et al* (2013), exploring developmental trajectories for various types of childhood anxiety symptoms, also showed that high levels of initial behavioural inhibition correlated with 2-year trajectories of higher anxiety.

Weems' review (2008) describes some inconsistencies across different research studies. For example, prospective longitudinal studies of childhood anxiety disorders have reported estimates of stability from 4 to 80%. These studies may show wide variability for many reasons (e.g. disorder type, age at onset, the informant, the sample, and the method and duration of assessment). Age at onset may be a significant factor, since there are specific age differences in the predominant expression of the symptoms of childhood anxiety: epidemiological data on the age at onset of anxiety disorders are generally consistent with the normative trajectories of fear development (Tables 11.2 and 11.3).

Concerning the prediction of adult-onset anxiety disorders, studies often point to little specificity. The community epidemiological study by Bittner *et al* (2007) showed that various anxiety disorders in childhood predicted anxiety and other psychiatric disorders in adolescence; the only exception was that generalised anxiety disorder specifically predicted only conduct disorder. In contrast, the longitudinal study by Pine *et al* (1998) showed that adolescent social phobia predicted primarily social phobia in adulthood, whereas simple phobias predicted primarily simple phobias. They also found broad associations between generalised anxiety, panic and major depressive disorders, with a particularly strong association between adolescent depression and adult generalised anxiety disorder. The 7-year longitudinal study by Aschenbrand *et al* (2003) explored whether childhood separation anxiety specifically constitutes a precursor for later panic disorder and agoraphobia, but found no evidence of this. Overall, adolescent anxiety or depression predicts an approximate two- to threefold increase in risk for adult anxiety disorders (and for suicide attempts, psychiatric admissions, and alcohol and substance misuse).

Weems (2008) argues for heterotypical continuity in anxiety disorder: although an individual's anxiety disorder may remit and return, often as a different disorder type, underneath lies a core maladaptive anxiety emotion that exhibits a larger degree of continuity. Various aetiological factors (e.g. genetic, temperamental, neuropsychological, interpersonal and environmental) may influence the emergence and course of anxiety disorders; normative developmental changes may also affect their trajectory and expression into specific disorders.

Conclusion

Paediatric anxiety disorders are relatively common and often disabling. They increase the risk of psychopathology in adult life, especially anxiety and depressive disorders. This chapter has necessarily presented a succinct review of a vast topic. The changing classifications require clinicians to be familiar with diagnostic criteria in order to detect these disorders, which are so often comorbid with other childhood psychiatric presentations. Research evidence is accumulating about the aetiology of these conditions, the contribution of genetics and environmental events, and the influence of parent and family interactions. Insights into the neuroimaging and neuropsychological findings are intriguing. Increasing our understanding of evidence-based interventions, including the role of psychopharmacology, is essential so that targeted interventions can be used to inform and support families and improve children's symptoms.

References

Abeles P, Verduyn C, Robinson A, *et al* (2009) Computerized CBT for adolescent depression ('Stressbusters') and its initial evaluation through an extended case series. *Behavioural and Cognitive Psychotherapy*, **37**, 151–165.

American Psychiatric Association (2013) *Diagnostic and Statistical Manual of Mental Disorders (5th edn) (DSM-5)*. APA.

Aschenbrand SG, Kendall PC, Webb A, *et al* (2003) Is childhood separation anxiety disorder a predictor of adult panic disorder and agoraphobia? A seven-year longitudinal study. *Journal of the American Academy of Child & Adolescent Psychiatry*, **42**, 1478–1485.

Bergman K, Sarkar P, O'Connor TG, *et al* (2007) Maternal stress during pregnancy predicts cognitive ability and fearfulness in infancy. *Journal of the American Academy of Child & Adolescent Psychiatry*, **46**, 1454–1463.

Biederman J, Monuteaux MC, Faraone SV, *et al* (2004) Does referral bias impact findings in high-risk offspring for anxiety disorders? A controlled study of high-risk children of non-referred parents with panic disorder/agoraphobia and major depression. *Journal of Affective Disorders*, **82**, 209–216.

Bilek EL, Ehrenreich-May J (2012) An open trial investigation of a transdiagnostic group treatment for children with anxiety and depressive symptoms. *Behavior Therapy*, **43**, 887–897.

Birmaher B, Khetarpal S, Brent D, *et al* (1997) The Screen for Child Anxiety Related Emotional Disorders (SCARED): scale construction and psychometric characteristics. *Journal of the American Academy of Child & Adolescent Psychiatry*, **36**, 545–553.

Birmaher B, Axelson DA, Monk K, *et al* (2003) Fluoxetine for the treatment of childhood anxiety disorders. *Journal of the American Academy of Child & Adolescent Psychiatry*, **42**, 415–423.

Bittner A, Egger HL, Erkanli A, *et al* (2007) What do childhood anxiety disorders predict? *Journal of Child Psychology and Psychiatry*, **48**, 1174–1183.

BMJ Evidence Centre (2012) Generalised Anxiety Disorder. *Best Practice*. BMJ Evidence Centre (http://bestpractice.bmj.com/best-practice/monograph/120/diagnosis/step-by-step.html). Accessed 1 Oct 2013.

Bolton D, Eley T, O'Connor TG, *et al* (2006) Prevalence and genetic and environmental influences on anxiety disorders in 6-year-old twins. *Psychological Medicine*, **36**, 335–344.

Broeren S, Muris P, Diamantopoulou S, *et al* (2013) The course of childhood anxiety symptoms: developmental trajectories and child-related factors in normal children. *Journal of Abnormal Child Psychology*, **41**, 81–95.

Degnan KA, Almas AN, Fox NA (2010) Temperament and the environment in the etiology of childhood anxiety. *Journal of Child Psychology and Psychiatry*, **51**, 497–517.

Eley TC, Rijsdijk F, Perrin S, *et al* (2008) A multivariate genetic analysis of specific phobia, separation anxiety and social phobia in early childhood. *Journal of Abnormal Child Psychology*, **36**, 839–848.

Emmelkamp PMG (2012) Specific and social phobias in ICD-11. *World Psychiatry*, **11** (suppl 1), 94–99.

Fox NA, Nichols KE, Henderson HA, *et al* (2005) Evidence for a gene–environment interaction in predicting behavioral inhibition in middle childhood. *Psychological Science*, **16**, 921–926.

Frick PJ, Lilienfeld SO, Ellis M, *et al* (1999) The association between anxiety and psychopathic traits dimensions in children. *Journal of Abnormal Child Psychology*, **27**, 383–392.

Fyer AJ (1998) Current approaches to etiology and pathophysiology of specific phobia. *Biological Psychiatry*, **44**, 1295–1304.

Glover V (2011) Annual Research Review: Prenatal stress and the origins of psychopathology: an evolutionary perspective. *Journal of Child Psychology and Psychiatry*, **52**, 356–367.

Goodwin RD, Pine DS, Hoven CW (2003) Asthma and panic attacks among youth in the community. *Journal of Asthma*, **40**, 139–145.

Goodwin RD, Fergusson DM, Horwood LJ (2004) Early anxious/withdrawn behaviours predict later internalising disorders. *Journal of Child Psychology and Psychiatry*, **45**, 874–883.

Hawton K, Saunders KE, O'Connor RC (2012) Self-harm and suicide in adolescents. *Lancet*, **379**, 2373–2382.

Hettema JM, Neale MC, Kendler KS (2001) A review and meta-analysis of the genetic epidemiology of anxiety disorders. *American Journal of Psychiatry*, **158**, 1568–1578.

Hettema JM, Prescott CA, Myers JM, *et al* (2005) The structure of genetic and environmental risk factors for anxiety disorders in men and women. *Archives of General Psychiatry*, **62**, 182–189.

Heyman I, Mataix-Cols D, Fineberg NA (2006) Obsessive–compulsive disorder. *BMJ*, **333**, 424–429.

Ishikawa S, Okajima I, Matsuoka H, *et al* (2007) Cognitive behavioural therapy for anxiety disorders in children and adolescents: a metaanalysis. *Child and Adolescent Mental Health*, **12**, 164–172.

Kagan J, Snidman N (1999) Early childhood predictors of adult anxiety disorders. *Biological Psychiatry*, **46**, 1536–1541.

Kagan J, Snidman N, McManis M, *et al* (2002) One measure, one meaning: multiple measures, clearer meaning. *Development and Psychopathology*, **14**, 463–475.

Kendall PC, Robin JA, Hedtke KA, *et al* (2005) Considering CBT with anxious Youth? Think exposures. *Cognitive and Behavioral Practice*, **12**, 136–150.

Koolschijn PCMP, van IJzendoorn MH, Bakermans-Kranenburg MJ, *et al* (2013) Hippocampal volume and internalizing behavior problems in adolescence. *European Neuropsychopharmacology*, **23**, 622–628.

Last CG, Perrin S, Hersen M, *et al* (1996) A prospective study of childhood anxiety disorders. *Journal of the American Academy of Child & Adolescent Psychiatry*, **35**, 1502–1510.

March JS, Parker JD, Sullivan K, *et al* (1997) The Multidimensional Anxiety Scale for Children (MASC): factor structure, reliability, and validity. *Journal of the American Academy of Child & Adolescent Psychiatry*, **36**, 554–565.

March S, Spence SH, Donovan CL (2009) The efficacy of an internet-based cognitive–behavioural therapy intervention for child anxiety disorders. *Journal of Pediatric Psychology*, **34**, 474–487.

Marks I, Nesse R (1994) Fear and fitness: an evolutionary analysis of anxiety disorders. *Ethology and Sociobiology*, **15**, 247–261.

McClure EB, Monk CS, Nelson EE, *et al* (2007) Abnormal attention modulation of fear circuit function in pediatric generalized anxiety disorder. *Archives of General Psychiatry*, **64**, 97–106.

McLaughlin KA, Greif Green J, Gruber MJ, *et al* (2012) Childhood adversities and first onset of psychiatric disorders in a national sample of US adolescents. *Archives of General Psychiatry*, **69**, 1151–1160.

Medicines and Healthcare products Regulatory Agency (2003) Safety review of anti-depressants used by children completed (press release). MHRA (http://www.mhra.gov.uk/NewsCentre/Pressreleases/CON002045). Accessed 9 Dec 2013.

Milham MP, Nugent AC, Drevets WC, *et al* (2005) Selective reduction in amygdala volume in pediatric generalized anxiety disorder: a voxel-based morphometry investigation. *Biological Psychiatry*, **57**, 961–966.

Muris P, Steerneman P, Merckelbach H, *et al* (1998) Comorbid anxiety symptoms in children with pervasive developmental disorders. *Journal of Anxiety Disorders*, **12**, 387–393.

Murphy TK, Storch EA, Lewin AB (2012) Clinical factors associated with pediatric auto-immune neuropsychiatric disorders associated with streptococcal infections. *Journal of Pediatrics*, **160**, 314–319.

National Collaborating Centre for Mental Health (2005) *Depression in Children and Young People: Identification and Management in Primary, Community and Secondary Care* (Clinical Guideline 28). National Institute for Health and Clinical Excellence.

National Institute for Health and Clinical Excellence (2011) *Generalised Anxiety Disorder and Panic Disorder (with or without Agoraphobia) in Adults: Management in Primary, Secondary and Community Care* (NICE Clinical Guideline 113). NICE.

O'Connor TG, Heron J, Glover V (2002) Antenatal anxiety predicts child behavioral/emotional problems independently of postnatal depression. *Journal of the American Academy of Child & Adolescent Psychiatry*, **41**, 1470–1477.

Perez-Edgar K, Fox NA (2005) Temperament and anxiety disorders. *Child and Adolescent Psychiatric Clinics of North America*, **14**, 681–706.

Pine D (2007) Research review: a neuroscience framework for pediatric anxiety disorders. *Journal of Child Psychology and Psychiatry*, **48**, 631–648.

Pine DS, Cohen P, Gurley D, *et al* (1998) The risk for early-adulthood anxiety and depressive disorders in adolescents with anxiety and depressive disorders. *Archives of General Psychiatry*, **55**, 56–64.

Pine DS, Cohen P, Johnson JG, *et al* (2002) Adolescent life events as predictors of adult depression. *Journal of Affective Disorders*, **68**, 49–57.

Pine DS, Klein RG, Roberson-Nay R, *et al* (2005) Response to 5% carbon dioxide in children and adolescents: relationship to panic disorder in parents and anxiety disorders in subjects. *Archives of General Psychiatry*, **62**, 73–80.

Research Unit on Pediatric Psychopharmacology Anxiety Study Group (2001) Fluvoxamine for the treatment of anxiety disorders in children and adolescents. *New England Journal of Medicine*, **344**, 1279–1285.

Research Unit on Pediatric Psychopharmacology Anxiety Study Group (2003) The Pediatric Anxiety Rating Scale (PARS): development and psychometric properties. *Journal of the American Academy of Child & Adolescent Psychiatry*, **42**, 13–21.

Reynolds S, Wilson C, Austin J, *et al* (2012) Effects of psychotherapy for anxiety in children and adolescents: a meta-analytic review. *Clinical Psychology Review*, **32**, 251–262.

Richardson T, Stallard P, Velleman S (2010) Computerised cognitive behavioural therapy for the prevention and treatment of depression and anxiety in children and adolescents: a systematic review. *Clinical Child and Family Psychology Review*, **13**, 275–290.

Roberson-Nay R, Eaves LJ, Hettema JM, *et al* (2012) Childhood separation anxiety disorder and adult onset panic attacks share a common genetic diathesis. *Depression and Anxiety*, **29**, 320–327.

Rynn MA, Siqueland L, Rickels K (2001) Placebo-controlled trial of sertraline in the treatment of children with generalized anxiety disorder. *American Journal of Psychiatry*, **158**, 2008–2014.

Schwartz CE, Wright CI, Shin LM, *et al* (2003) Inhibited and uninhibited infants 'grown up': adult amygdalar response to novelty. *Science*, **300**, 1952–1953.

Schwartz CE, Kunwar PS, Greve DN, *et al* (2010) Structural differences in adult orbital and ventromedial prefrontal cortex predicted by infant temperament at 4 months of age. *Archives of General Psychiatry*, **67**, 78-84.

Shear MK (2012) Generalized anxiety disorder in ICD-11. *World Psychiatry*, **11** (suppl 1), 82–88.

Spence SH, Holmes JM, March, S, *et al* (2006) The feasibility and outcome of clinic plus internet delivery of cognitive-behaviour therapy. *Journal of Consulting and Clinical Psychology*, **74**, 614–621.

Stallard P (2002) *Think Good, Feel Good: A Cognitive Behaviour Therapy Workbook for Children and Young People*. John Wiley & Sons.

Swedo SE, Leonard HL, Garvey M, *et al* (1998) Pediatric autoimmune neuropsychiatric disorders associated with streptococcal infections: clinical description of the first 50 cases. *American Journal of Psychiatry*, **155**, 264–271.

Vallance AK, Garralda ME (2011) Anxiety disorders in children and adolescents. In *Child Psychology and Psychiatry: Frameworks for Practice* (eds D Skuse, H Bruce, L Dowdney), pp. 169–174. Blackwell.

Van den Bergh BR, Marcoen A (2004) High antenatal maternal anxiety is related to ADHD symptoms, externalizing problems, and anxiety in 8- and 9-year-olds. *Child Development*, **75**, 1085–1097.

Walkup JT, Albano AM, Piacentini J, *et al* (2008) Cognitive behavioral therapy, sertraline, or a combination in childhood anxiety. *New England Journal of Medicine*, **359**, 2753–2766.

Weems CF (2008) Developmental trajectories of childhood anxiety: identifying continuity and change in anxious emotion. *Developmental Review*, **28**, 488–502.

Wittchen HU, Stein MB, Kessler RC (1999) Social fears and social phobia in a community sample of adolescents and young adults: prevalence, risk factors and co-morbidity. *Psychological Medicine*, **29**, 309–323.

World Health Organization (1992) *The ICD-10 Classification of Mental and Behavioural Disorders: Clinical Descriptions and Diagnostic Guidelines*. WHO.

CHAPTER 12

Somatising: clinical presentations and aetiological factors

Olivia Fiertag and Mary Eminson

Psychological and physical (somatic) symptoms are closely interconnected, and somatisation (Box 12.1) is commonly seen in both primary and secondary care settings. Somatic symptoms are extremely common in children and adolescents, a population who often find it difficult to express their feelings and emotions through language. It is understood that 2–10% of children in the general population complain of bodily aches and pains (stomach aches, joint pains and headaches) that are likely to be medically unexplained (Garralda, 2005). Sometimes, these symptoms lead to significant distress, impairment in functioning and healthcare-seeking behaviour. Somatising disorders can have a significant impact not only on the children themselves but also on their families and healthcare resources. If somatising continues into adulthood it can lead to wide-ranging distress and impairment.

Developmental factors have an important influence on the presentation of disorders. One such factor is that children and adolescents are dependants, largely reliant on adults for significant aspects of 'illness behaviour' (Mechanic, 1962). Illness behaviour includes the way in which symptoms are responded to, and the extent to which medical consultation and lifestyle alterations are undertaken. Parents and carers have a powerful impact when they respond to (or ignore) children's physical complaints, attribute

---

Box 12.1 Definitions

Medically unexplained symptoms All bothersome or recurrent bodily symptoms that are not due to a recognised medical illness.

Somatisation A constellation of clinical and behavioural features indicating that a person is experiencing and communicating psychological distress through physical symptoms not accounted for by pathological findings; the person attributes these symptoms to a physical illness and seeks medical help. The production of symptoms is usually not under conscious control, although in children and adolescents it is particularly difficult to establish the level of conscious control.

significance to (or give reassurance about) these complaints, facilitate (or otherwise) the children's use of healthcare facilities and involve them in (or withdraw them from) normal life activities.

Other developmental factors, especially the level of cognitive and verbal competence, have long been recognised as important determinants of the ability to express emotional distress directly by speech. In young children, a variety of primitive and regressive behaviours are commonly recognised as signalling emotional discomfort of various kinds. Similarly, early in development, those who are less sophisticated in their understanding and less skilled in their verbal expression of psychological distress are more likely to express their feelings in other, more indirect ways. As psychological distress inevitably has somatic components, somatic symptoms may therefore be one way in which emotional distress is both experienced and communicated by young people. However, just being a child is not in itself sufficient to explain the extent of somatising disorders. A variety of other explanations are relevant and must be sought, including temperamental, psychosocial, cultural, environmental and family factors.

In this chapter we will examine the classification, epidemiology, aetiology and clinical presentations of somatising disorders in children and adolescents. For the purpose of this chapter, we are defining somatising disorders to include only those conditions in young people in which somatic symptoms are complained of, these symptoms cannot be explained sufficiently in terms of a physical disorder, and impairment is being caused. Disorders such as enuresis, encopresis and eating disorders, which may be somatic expressions of emotional distress, are not included. We address the assessment process, management and prognosis in Chapter 13.

Classification

The clinical patterns of somatising disorders that occur in childhood and adolescence vary and, unsurprisingly, presentations in adolescence often have a closer resemblance to adult disorders than is the case in earlier childhood. Box 12.2 summarises the disorders as defined by the current ICD-10 (World Health Organization, 1996). The recently released DSM-5 (American Psychiatric Association, 2013) replaces the DSM-IV category of somatoform disorders with somatic symptom disorders. These are characterised by somatic symptoms associated with distress/dysfunction. This category (Box 12.3) includes 'somatic symptom disorder', 'illness anxiety disorder', 'conversion disorder (functional neurological symptom disorder)', 'psychological factors affecting other medical conditions', 'factitious disorder' and 'other specified somatic symptom and related disorder'. Chronic fatigue syndrome is not described separately in DSM-5, although in ICD-10 it is classified as neurasthenia (in the neurotic, stress related and somatoform disorders section that follows the somatoform category). It has sufficient features in common with the DSM-5 somatic

Box 12.2 Major diagnostic categories for somatising disorders in children and adolescents, based on ICD-10

Adjustment disorders

Mixtures of psychological symptoms (anxiety, temper and irritability) and regressive behaviours such as thumb-sucking and bedwetting (which may include physical symptoms) arising in response to life events or stresses. The physical symptoms are typically headaches, stomach and joint pains, but may be multiple and in any system.

Dissociative (conversion) disorders (includes transient dissociative disorders)

Loss of function, mainly movement or sensation: blindness, deafness, paroxysmal non-epileptic events (formerly pseudoseizures), paralysis and loss of sensation are the most common presentations in childhood and adolescence.

Somatoform disorders

Various presentations in which different symptoms predominate. Common characteristics are repeated presentation of physical symptoms with requests for medical investigations, despite doctors' failure to find clinical symptoms and consequent reassurances that the symptoms have no physical basis. Any physical findings do not explain the nature and extent of the symptoms and distress.

Categories include:

- somatisation disorder – 2 years of multiple, variable symptoms
- undifferentiated somatoform disorder – 6 months of multiple, variable symptoms with less severity and handicap than somatisation disorder
- hypochondriacal disorder – persistent preoccupation with, and belief in, the presence of at least one serious physical illness
- persistent somatoform pain disorder – severe, distressing pain that is more persistent and dominant than the multiple aches and pains of other categories
- other somatoform disorders – physical complaints limited to specific systems or parts of the body, and disorders of sensation such as tingling and numbness; there is no minimum timescale for the complaints.

Chronic fatigue syndrome (CFS) (neurasthenia)

Criteria adopted by the Association for Child Psychology and Psychiatry Working Group (and adapted from those for adults) have largely replaced the ICD-10 neurasthenia categories.

Criteria include:

- disabling fatigue, affecting physical and mental functioning (the cardinal symptom)
- other symptoms, including aches and pains, headaches, sleep disturbance and concentration difficulties
- a definite onset, which may or may not occur after a viral illness
- a minimum duration of 6 months, although treatment may need to begin sooner.

Anxiety and/or depressive symptoms may be present and do not preclude a CFS diagnosis. Other psychiatric disorders, such as anorexia nervosa or a depressive disorder, should be distinguished from CFS.

(After World Health Organization, 1996)

Box 12.3   DSM-5: somatic symptom and related disorders

Somatic symptom disorder

Where significant somatic symptoms are present and causing significant distress

Illness anxiety disorder

The individual has extensive worries about health but no or minimal somatic symptoms

Conversion disorder (functional neurological symptom disorder)

Presenting symptom is neurological in nature but incompatible with neurological pathophysiology

Psychological factors affecting other medical conditions

Presence of one or more clinically significant psychological or behavioural factors that adversely affect the medical condition by increasing the risk of suffering, death or disability

Factitious disorder

Falsification of physical or psychological signs or symptoms

Other specified somatic symptom and related disorder

Unspecified somatic symptom and related disorder

Note that 75% of cases previously diagnosed as hypochondriasis are subsumed under the diagnosis of somatic symptom disorder; 25% of patients previously diagnosed with hypochondriasis have high health anxiety in the absence of somatic symptoms and would not meet the criteria for an anxiety disorder – these are classified under illness anxiety disorder. Chronic fatigue syndrome or neurasthenia (as classified in ICD-10) was not in DSM-IV, and in DSM-5 would be subsumed under the diagnosis of somatic symptom disorder.

---

symptom and conversion disorders to be included when discussing the other DSM-5 somatising conditions.

In ICD-10 the term dissociative disorder is used to describe presentations with a partial or complete loss of normal integration between memories, awareness of identity, sensations and control of bodily movements. In children with somatising, the type of dissociation usually seen involves an abnormality in bodily movements/sensations (i.e. dissociative disorder of movement and sensation). Although classified under dissociative disorders in ICD-10, conversion disorders share many features with the other somatoform disorders and therefore are appropriate to be included when focusing on somatising. By contrast, in DSM-5 this type of presentation with loss of mobility or sensation would be classed as a conversion disorder (functional neurological symptom disorder) within the somatic symptoms disorder category (rather than within the DSM category of dissociation, which includes only dissociative amnesia/depersonalisation/derealisation/

other dissociative disorders). The term conversion disorder suggests that emotional distress is being converted into physical symptoms, whereas the term dissociation assumes a detachment rather than a conversion as the mechanism underpinning the symptoms. In DSM-5, the depersonalisation/derealisation type of dissociative presentations is separated from the functional neurological presentations, perhaps because the functional neurological type are much more 'somatic' than the depersonalisation type. Therefore children presenting with loss of movement/sensation are categorised under somatic symptom disorders, not dissociative disorders. However in ICD-10, disorders of sensation and movement are classified under the dissociative category. These disorders can be explained as both a conversion and a dissociative experience.

Differences between the classification systems thus persist, continuing to cause confusion clinically and difficulties in epidemiological studies and research. In the current ICD-10 classification (World Health Organization, 1996), only two categories of somatising disorder are specific to developmental stage: adjustment reactions and transient dissociative disorders of childhood. If not placed in either of these categories, children and adolescents must be accommodated within the adult categories, even though the terminology and symptom descriptions are usually ill-suited to a childhood population.

Out of all the somatising disorders, the most commonly seen in children and adolescents are persistent somatoform pain disorders, dissociative disorders and chronic fatigue syndrome (neurasthenia). We focus on these three, including somatoform disorders as a whole (not just persistent somatoform pain disorders). For completeness, adjustment disorder is also included because it describes many short-lived, single- or multiple-symptom presentations. Additionally, we describe factitious disorders, which have many similarities to somatisation in presentation and management, and indeed are included by DSM-5 within somatic symptom disorders. Factitious disorders similarly present with somatic symptoms that have no acknowledged physical cause and may result in significant impairment. In clinical practice it is often hard to make a distinction between what is conscious manipulation and what is a psychosomatic presentation. We have also included a brief description of pervasive withdrawal (also referred to as pervasive refusal syndrome) as, although not a distinct condition in current diagnostic manuals, clinical reports suggest particular features which in some presentations mark this out as a very severe form of somatising disorder.

Epidemiological studies

Children (studies generally begin around 3 years of age) report more somatic symptoms such as stomach ache and headaches as they get older, rates continuing to increase right through adolescence. There is not much known about the exact incidence or prevalence of the different somatising disorders. However, the epidemiology of recurrent somatic complaints, medically unexplained symptoms and specific psychosomatic factors (i.e. physical or psychological factors that, alone or in combination, increase the likelihood that emotional distress is expressed through somatic symptoms) is better documented. Recurrent and troublesome somatic symptoms occur in 2–10% of children and adolescents in the general population; about 10% attending primary care or paediatric services have medically unexplained symptoms; and identifiable associated or contributing psychological factors are present in 25–50% of all children presenting with physical symptoms (Garralda, 2005).

Overall, girls experience more somatic symptoms and somatising disorders than boys (Egger *et al*, 1999), and girls report more symptoms as puberty and adolescence proceed (LeResche *et al*, 2005). In the majority of studies, girls have been found to report symptoms at increasing rates during adolescence, whereas reporting levels by boys of some somatic symptoms, for example abdominal pain, fall during this time (LeResche *et al*, 2005). Although this is the general age and gender pattern, there are some variations across different types of somatising. Puberty has also been found to be a more important marker than age alone. Janssens *et al* (2011) found that pubertal status was associated with some, but not all, functional somatic symptoms, suggesting that biological factors are differentially involved in the aetiology of somatising.

Although this is the general age and gender pattern, there are some variations across different types of somatising. The Early Developmental Stages of Psychopathology (EDSP) study reports that most pain and undifferentiated disorders start in childhood and early adolescence. However, dissociative (conversion) disorder tends to arise later, with a median age at onset of 16 years (Lieb *et al*, 2000).

The EDSP study also found that 12% of 14 - to 24-year-olds had suffered from a somatoform disorder at some point during their life. Somatoform disorders were linked to low socioeconomic status, except for pain disorder, which was linked to higher educational status (Lieb *et al*, 2000; Garralda, 2005). Chronic fatigue-like symptoms occur in 2% of children and young people (Jordan *et al*, 2000), but the full syndrome is rare, occurring in only 0.19% of children in the UK (Chalder *et al*, 2003; Garralda & Chalder, 2005). The prevalence of conversion disorder across the world is not known, but a national surveillance study of children seen by paediatricians in Australia found rates of 2.3–4.2 per 100 000 children under 16 years (Kozlowska *et al*, 2007). A national surveillance study in the UK has found a 12-month incidence of 1.3 per 100 000 children under 16 (Ani *et al*, 2013).

Aetiology

Childhood somatising disorders are likely to be caused by a combination of wide-ranging predisposing, precipitating and maintaining factors relating to the child, family and environment (Box 12.4). These factors may influence the child's experience and complaint of physical symptoms. In addition, illness behaviour may influence the child's vulnerability and/or resilience

---

Box 12.4 Factors affecting the presentation and persistence of somatising disorders in children and adolescents

Predisposing factors

Family

- Many somatic symptoms experienced, with possible genetic predisposition
- Limited in verbal communication about emotional matters
- Parental history of physical health problems, somatising illness, anxiety or depression
- Difficulties in setting boundaries for the children
- Parental overinvolvement
- Beliefs contrary to considering psychological explanations of illness

Child

- Temperament, including conscientiousness, emotional lability, vulnerability, feelings of worthlessness and high-achieving orientation
- Earlier emotional abuse
- Difficulties in social relating
- Difficulty expressing emotions because of lower IQ

Precipitating factors

Child

- Anxiety, depression
- Life stresses of all types – overt and covert
- Physical illness
- Problems with peer group
- Academic problems and cognitive limitations
- Low self-esteem

Parent

- Life events/crises

Environment

- Life stressors on the child, e.g. teasing or bullying
- Academic pressure on the child (external or self-imposed)

Maintaining factors

Child,* parent and professional

- Current family relationship difficulties
- *Predicament is resolved by symptoms (Taylor, 1982)
- Family model of serious illness
- Current parental mental ill health, particularly anxiety and somatisation
- *Problems at school
- Models of sickness and conflict avoidance
- Benefits of sick role
- Professional behaviour that reinforces anxieties and sick role

---

to developing somatisation. Biological, psychological, individual, family and environmental factors are relevant to both the complaints and the illness-behaviour responses to them. It is important to note, however, that none of these factors is, on its own, either necessary or sufficient for such a presentation: a combination of vulnerability and trigger factors will be unique to each child and family. This point is emphasised because in the past there was often an incorrect assumption that all children or families with a particular presentation 'must' possess certain risk factors, for example that major family dysfunction must be a feature of somatoform presentations in a child with severe somatic symptoms. However, the aetiology may be very different for two children with similar symptoms.

Genetics

Genetic factors can play an important role in sensitivity to pain and other bodily sensations. For example, a heritable polymorphism in the gene for catecholamine-O-methyltransferase (COMT) influences the experience of pain (Diatchenko et al, 2005). Associations between anxiety and depression (which are common in people with somatising disorders) have been shown to be related to a common genetic predisposition (e.g. Kessler, 2000) as well as genetic pleiotropy (Kendler et al, 2007). Hariri et al (2002) found a specific functional polymorphism in the promoter region of the serotonin transporter gene to be associated with anxiety and exaggerated amygdala responses to novelty. A genetic basis linking depression with life adversity (Caspi et al, 2003) and with functional somatic symptoms has also been suggested (Yeo et al, 2004; Campo, 2012).

Cultural factors

Somatising occurs worldwide and a World Health Organization (WHO) study found that somatisation presentations were common in primary care in Brazil, Chile, China, France, Germany, Greece, India, Italy, Japan, Nigeria, The Netherlands, Turkey, the UK and the USA (Gureje et al, 1997). Somatisation was frequently associated with comorbid depressive and anxiety disorders. Although this study was conduced some time ago, there is nothing to suggest that the situation is any different today. Headaches, musculoskeletal pains and abdominal pains are the most common symptoms of somatisation, but there are additional symptoms specific to certain cultures and geographical regions. For example, numbness and feelings of heat are reported in certain populations in Africa, burning hands and feet in some peoples in India, and fatigue in Western countries (Fiertag et al, 2012).

There is a wide range of health beliefs and conventions about illnesses and of ways in which psychological distress may be expressed across different families and different ethnic and other cultural groups. In particular, cultural factors will affect beliefs about symptoms and the seriousness attached to them, as will currently topical illnesses and concerns. Attitudes to the medical profession, to health and to the benefits or otherwise of normal school and social activities vary widely across cultures and may have powerful shaping effects on parents and children.

Factors associated with physical symptoms

Psychological conditions, in particular anxiety and depression, are common comorbidities that have an influence on the presence of physical symptoms. Strong associations are reported between functional somatic symptoms, anxiety and depression across the lifespan (Campo, 2012). Young children of nursery age who have frequent somatic complaints are more likely to have concurrent behavioural and emotional problems (Domenech-Llaberia et al, 2004). Temperamental factors such as anxiety traits, perfectionism, sensitivity and conscientiousness have been reported in many clinical studies as being relevant to vulnerability to developing somatisation (Garralda, 2010). Those who perceived their self-competence as low were more likely to have high levels of symptoms. Biological factors are also important. Children with recurrent abdominal pain, for example, report greater increases in symptoms than other children after a water-load challenge, suggesting enhanced gastrointestinal sensitivity (Walker et al, 2006). In addition to its neurological role in mood disorders, serotonin has been highlighted as an important neurotransmitter in the gastrointestinal tract, influencing peristaltic activity (Campo et al, 2003). In chronic fatigue, infections such as mononucleosis have been implicated in some cases, but the research remains conflicting and is not universally supported (Lombardi et al, 2009; Erlwein et al, 2010).

Early-life experiences with many care disruptions and poor parental care are also associated with increased symptom reports and are found in the histories of adults with excessive unexplained symptoms (Craig et al, 1993). Such factors may include abuse, neglect and conditional care-taking, by which is meant attending to children when they complain of physical symptoms, but not when they make other types of request, for example, for affection. A consistent finding of these studies is that questionnaires identify those with a general tendency to report symptoms in adolescence. It is this trend to report physical symptoms that is consistently associated with other markers of disturbance and distress. Family factors have an influence on the level of children's symptoms – if parents have physical symptoms they are more likely to have children with increased rates of symptoms.

Both poor general school performance and poor attainment relative to teachers' perceptions of the individual's ability are associated with more symptoms (Eminson et al, 1996). Chronically stressful social and family situations such as parental disharmony also increase symptoms, as do acute life stresses (change of school, acute family problems).

191

Factors that affect illness behaviour

Children themselves, even at a young age, make a significant contribution to illness behaviour, despite the relative importance of parents in decisions about how their children's complaints are managed. In descriptive studies, children as young as 3 or 4 years display an understanding of illness behaviour. They can appreciate that expectations of behaviour are different in those who are sick and that, by displaying certain behaviour, they can adopt a sick role and subsequently be relieved of normal activities (Wilkinson, 1988). Thus, an understanding of the sick role is readily acquired at an early stage, as part of family life, although this will be heavily influenced by parental models. As would be expected, older children are able to display independently a wide range of illness behaviours.

Parents or caregivers are the ultimate decision makers about the responses made to children's symptoms and illness behaviour. These adults decide whether a child's complaints are sufficiently severe to allow them to be judged to be sick, and if so, whether they should be treated as sick, for example by missing school, being given medicine or being taken to a health professional. Most parents find it relatively easy to decide when a physical illness has come to an end and when to support and encourage the child to resume a normal life by going back to school. Such parents will explore and resolve with the child and teachers the reasons behind any reluctance to return to school. But for some parents, who are conscientious, caring and have no other parenting problems, these decision-making processes become difficult, and they find it hard to encourage their child to ignore any residual symptoms and return to ordinary activities. The reasons for this difficulty in encouraging a return to normal life are often related to early parenting experiences, parental anxiety or aspects of the parent–child relationship. It has been demonstrated (McGrath, 1995) that the mother's attitude to pain has an effect on the length of time their child is away from school following illness. Parents' belief in a physical cause for a child's chronic fatigue symptoms is associated with a poorer prognosis (Rangel & Garralda, 2000).

Parental ill health (mental or physical) may be associated with difficulty in believing that a child is healthy or has only minor illness, and with anxiety about the child's health and a distorted or pessimistic analysis of the situation. Parental depression and anxiety have been associated with somatising in children (Craig et al, 2002; Campo et al, 2007). Studies have shown that parents with more physical and mental health problems are more likely to have children with functional somatic symptoms than are parents without such complaints (Hotopf et al, 1998).

It has been suggested that, independent of the other cognitive, social, cultural and psychological factors, individuals differ in their capacity to express emotions directly, and that to some extent this is learnt within families. This is the basis of concepts such as psychological mindedness and alexithymia, which means having no word for feelings (Sifneos, 1973). This may help to explain why physical complaints are an easier route to expressing distress in some families. Another way these ideas have been expressed has been in the notion of conditional care-taking, as described above.

Early emotional and physical abuse have also been linked with limited emotional expression combined with functional somatic complaints (Craig *et al*, 1993). Certainly, in clinical practice children and adolescents with multiple symptoms who come from emotionally deprived and neglectful backgrounds are commonplace, and the function of symptoms as primitive markers of distress is often recognisable. Dissociation from painful emotional experiences in early life, retaining only an awareness of physical distress, is one possible explanatory mechanism.

Clinical presentations

In this section we outline the main presentations of the somatising disorders seen most frequently in children and adolescents. However, the following features are usually common to all somatising disorders: first, a temporal relationship between psychosocial stressors and development of physical symptoms; second, symptoms and impairment of a nature and persistence out of keeping with the pathophysiology; third, the frequent presence of a concurrent psychiatric disorder, typically anxiety or depression. The key diagnostic definitions for somatising disorders in children and adolescents according to ICD-10 are outlined in Box 12.2. These are likely to be modified when the ICD-11 criteria are formalised (publication of ICD-11 is expected by 2015).

Adjustment reactions

Adjustment reaction is probably the most accurate psychiatric label for the common, short-lived but sometimes recurrent symptoms presented to general practitioners or paediatricians. Developmentally, these are the first disorders to be seen and are as common in boys as in girls. Characteristically beginning in early or middle childhood, stomach aches, headaches, joint pains or tiredness are the focus of recurrent complaints that cause parents to seek medical advice. They result in the child missing school and limiting social activities. Although these presentations are so common that to make generalisations about background causes is only broadly applicable, anxiety is often a contributing factor. In younger children, oppositional behaviours and behavioural disturbance are more common in those presenting with frequent somatic symptoms (Domenech-Llaberia *et al*, 2004). These children are often shy and compliant outside the home and they use somatic complaints to express distress, usually in a long-standing pattern, often with family traits of anxiety, protectiveness and somatisation.

Dissociative (conversion) disorders

In ICD-10, these are described as disorders characterised by partial or complete loss of bodily sensations or movements. In DSM-5 they are referred to as conversion disorder (functional neurological symptom disorder) (see 'Classification' section above for more details). Loss or disturbance of motor function in any modality and paroxysmal non-epileptic events (previously known as pseudoseizures) are the most common, appearing from middle childhood (Goodyer & Taylor, 1985; Grattan-Smith *et al*, 1988). Less commonly, children and young people present with loss of sight, hearing or sensation or with fugue (extremely rare in children) or mutism. Sometimes, transient disorders do not come to the attention of medical services or, if the child is taken to an accident and emergency department or other clinic, symptoms remit quickly with reassurance. Only those with prolonged reactions are likely to present in a mental health arena. Symptoms are often brought on by a stressful traumatic event and usually remit after a few weeks or months. Although *la belle indifférence* – a lack of concern about symptoms – is frequently seen in adult presentations of dissociation, it is rarely present in children.

In typical paroxysmal non-epileptic events, clinical features of an epileptic seizure will be present but with no accompanying electroencephalogram (EEG) changes, resulting in potential diagnostic delays. In a review of 883 patients in a paediatric epilepsy clinic (Kotagal *et al*, 2002), 15% had paroxysmal non-epileptic events. Of these, 3% occurred in preschool children, 43% in 5- to 12-year-olds and 87% in 12- to 18-year-olds. Epilepsy and paroxysmal non-epileptic events can coexist, but those with both conditions account for a small proportion of patients with epilepsy. Paroxysmal non-epileptic events occurred in 1.5% of children with epilepsy.

The capacity for experiencing unexplained symptoms or losses of function is extremely widespread in young people and in girls in particular. Lieb *et al* (2000) demonstrated higher rates of somatising, including somatoform, pain and dissociative (conversion) symptoms, in females than in males. Indeed, females predominate in epidemic presentations generally known as mass hysteria or mass sociogenic illness (Roach, 2013). These phenomena can occur in schools or workplaces and are usually focused on topical fears. Most sufferers make a speedy recovery. Those whose symptoms persist beyond the few days of the epidemic will usually be found to be more vulnerable, and more of the risk factors for somatoform disorders will be found in their background histories.

Somatoform disorders

This category, which includes somatisation disorder, hypochondriacal disorder (see below) and persistent somatoform pain disorder (see below), includes uncommon, but far from rare, disorders usually seen in paediatric clinics. The most common type to occur in childhood is persistent somatoform pain disorder. Unfortunately, the clinical examples in ICD-10 (World Health Organization, 1996) are atypical of childhood and adolescence, an age at which genitourinary symptoms, for example, are rare. These patients will be found attending most paediatric specialties, often with gastrointestinal complaints, joint pain, abdominal pain (typically a diffuse or intense periumbilical pain), and other pains and neurological symptoms. More girls than boys present in this way and, even by mid-adolescence, there may be a severe picture of increasingly poor school attendance and attainment and social withdrawal. Even the milder forms include young people with a range of personal and family-background vulnerabilities, and may also include body image symptoms, with self-harm and eating problems. There may be accompanying altered bowel habit, vomiting and lethargy. The child may look pale, which can reinforce the family's belief in an organic pathology.

In the more severe and chronic adolescent presentations, a proportion of individuals will also show disturbances of conduct. Predisposing factors include more severe and earlier emotional and behavioural problems, attachment difficulties and sometimes emotional, physical or sexual abuse. Major family dysfunction may be present, with recent obvious psychosocial stresses. Family disorganisation may include breakdown and criminality. There may be a long history of intermittent milder physical complaints and abnormal illness behaviour, usually with patchy school attendance, together with a family history of both organic physical illness and marked illness behaviour. The extent to which lifestyles are altered by the somatising disorder varies widely, as does the tendency to consult doctors and seek investigations. It may also vary in an individual at different times. Often the young person and their family demonstrate indifference or antagonism to psychological or psychiatric help, and they neglect concurrent organic physical conditions and fail to attend follow-up for them. Educational failure almost invariably follows.

Hypochondriacal disorder

Virtually unknown before adolescence, and uncommon during it, hypochondriasis appears to be the last somatoform disorder to develop clinically. It is characterised by an unshakeable belief in the presence of an illness or disease based on a misinterpretation or misunderstanding of physical symptoms. However, body dysmorphic disorder, included in this category for ICD-10 (but categorised with obsessive–compulsive and related disorders in DSM-5), is more common, making its mark from mid-adolescence onwards, but with much overlap with eating disorders. Adolescents are particularly vulnerable to developing preoccupations with the skin and acne. There is some evidence to suggest that adolescent preoccupation with acquiring illnesses such as cancer may represent subclinical forms of hypochondriasis (Fritz *et al*, 1997; Dell & Campo, 2011). Patients who have hypochondriasis are at risk of iatrogenic harm

195

from seeking medical and surgical interventions for their symptoms. Lack of standardised assessment instruments or operationally defined criteria for hypochondriasis are likely to slow the identification of any such disorders in adolescent medicine.

Pain disorders (persistent somatoform pain disorders)

There is substantial overlap with the other categories of somatising disorders outlined above and occurring in middle childhood and adolescence, usually presenting through secondary paediatric or orthopaedic care. Some children who initially present as having adjustment disorders (e.g. with headaches or abdominal pain) reach criteria for pain disorder later. Pain clinics may contain a number of sufferers (and incidentally may also provide an acceptable way to involve mental health professionals through focusing initially on symptom relief). As in other somatising disorders, a proportion of patients have frank psychological symptoms (usually depression, often thought by the patient to be secondary to their pain and somatic complaints). A typical example of a patient is an adolescent girl with pain in her arm, which is therefore unused and may show secondary physical changes as a result. Rheumatologists and orthopaedic surgeons often use the term 'reflex sympathetic dystrophy' to describe a condition of uncertain aetiology, sometimes with organic components, where psychological factors play a significant role in the illness (Murray et al, 2000). Careful enquiry can uncover many other symptoms, including fatigue.

Chronic fatigue syndrome (neurasthenia)

Disabling fatigue has long been recognised as a troublesome condition that affects girls more than boys from middle childhood onwards and has many different diagnostic labels. There is wide speculation about possible aetiologies, including immunological, nutritional and other hypotheses. Although fatigue is by definition the most prominent among the physical symptoms (Box 12.2), there are usually many others, and sleep disturbance and eating problems are common. The fatigue can result in inactivity and subsequent loss of muscle bulk.

In most studies girls predominate, a finding common to all adolescent somatising disorders. Family factors associated with the condition include family illness, both physical and psychological, protectiveness and difficulty with boundary setting. In one study of children and adolescents with chronic fatigue syndrome (Rangel et al, 2000), standardised measures comparing sufferers with controls revealed that sufferers were more likely to have personality difficulty or disorder, and the common personality features were emotional lability and a tendency to be high achieving, conscientious, perfectionist, sensitive, vulnerable and to feel worthless. Depressive disorder is found in more than a third of young people with chronic fatigue syndrome, and comorbid anxiety is also common. Garralda

& Rangel (2005), studying chronic fatigue syndrome sufferers, found that 44% had had depressive disorders and 24% anxiety disorders in the previous year.

Pervasive withdrawal (pervasive refusal syndrome)

Pervasive withdrawal is a rare but potentially life-threatening state, in which children withdraw from the world and stop walking, talking, eating, drinking and taking part in any activity. While in this state, these children often avoid taking part in any treatment aimed at returning them to normal functioning. Also described as a pervasive refusal syndrome (Thompson & Nunn, 1997; Lask, 2004), it includes children with a variety of problems, not just somatisation. However, in the children with somatisation, withdrawal seems to be behind the refusal, perhaps as a type of highly dysfunctional coping mechanism. Although not a validated syndrome or recognised diagnosis in the current diagnostic manuals, it is increasingly being reported in the literature (Jaspers *et al*, 2009; McNicholas *et al*, 2013). In many cases it represents an extreme state of somatisation, but in some it may be an extreme manifestation of various disorders, one of which is as depression.

Pervasive withdrawal affects females more than males and occurs across all ages. It is thought to be rare but the incidence is unknown. Case reports and reviews (Von Folsach & Montgomery, 2006; Jaspers *et al*, 2009; McNicholas *et al*, 2013) suggest that a number of personal, familial and environmental characteristics, similar to those occurring in the other somatising disorders, are contributory factors: traumatic life events and/ or mental illness, for example. Marked improvement and recovery from the disorder have been described, but the duration is long, ranging from 3 months to 3 years, with many patients requiring psychiatric hospital admission for more than a year.

Factitious disorders

Factitious disorders, when physical symptoms are produced by the patient but the origin is denied, are unusual in young people, but present to all paediatric specialists from middle childhood onwards (Libow, 2000). Presentations commonly involve existing lesions such as skin rashes or sutures, which have been interfered with to produce more pathology, or lesions being created by picking at the skin or the eye. Some children have a single symptom; many seem to have an intense desire for medical attention, in active pursuit of a sick role. Some presentations, both acute and chronic, are accompanied by other somatic symptoms or somatising disorders, with which there is substantial overlap. The more elaborate and extensively pursued fabrications are more likely to indicate significant major difficulties in personal relationships, often with a superficial and immature relating style but without overt psychiatric symptoms. In these most severe cases, difficult temperamental traits may be traced to very early disturbance in relationships, with disrupted attachments, sometimes including extensive physical, emotional and sexual abuse, very similar to the picture described earlier in some severe somatoform disorders. Others in intact families may not have a background of abuse, but may have few personal resources and a predicament or dilemma (e.g. major school failure or unpopularity; current sexual abuse outside the family) that is resolved by the results of the fabrication, or to which attention is drawn by the fabrication.

Conclusion

Despite the ubiquity of medically unexplained physical symptoms in childhood and adolescence, and the chronicity and impairment of the more severe illnesses seen by paediatric liaison mental health services, this remains a neglected area in research terms. Clinical series and broad-brush epidemiological studies, some from many years ago, have been supplemented only relatively recently by more up-to-date work on clinical presentations of fatigue, recurrent abdominal pain and dissociative presentations. Biological, psychological and social factors are relevant to both the experience and report of unexplained somatic complaints, and to the ways in which the individuals and their carers respond to them. Further rigorous research on these factors is needed, and robust collaborations between mental health and paediatrics are required.

References

American Psychiatric Association (2013) *Diagnostic and Statistical Manual of Mental Disorders (5th edn) (DSM-5)*. APA.

Ani C, Reading R, Lynn R, *et al* (2013) Incidence and 12-month outcome of non-transient childhood conversion disorder in the UK and Ireland. *British Journal of Psychiatry*, **202**, 413–418.

Campo JV (2012) Annual Research Review: Functional somatic symptoms and associated anxiety and depression – developmental psychology in paediatric practice. *Journal of Child Psychology and Psychiatry*, **53**, 575–592.

Campo JV, Dahl RE, Williamson DE, *et al* (2003) Gastrointestinal distress to serotonergic challenge: a risk marker for emotional disorder? *Journal of the American Academy of Child Adolescent Psychiatry*, **42**, 1221–1226.

Campo JV, Bridge J, Lucas A, *et al* (2007) Physical and emotional health of mothers of youth with functional abdominal pain. *Archives of Pediatrics & Adolescent Medicine*, **161**, 131–137.

Caspi A, Sugden K, Moffitt TE, *et al* (2003) Influence of life stress on depression: moderation by a polymorphism in the 5-HTT gene. *Science*, **301**, 386–389.

Chalder T, Goodman R, Hotopf M, *et al* (2003) Epidemiology of chronic fatigue syndrome and self reported myalgic encephalomyelitis in 5–15 year olds: cross sectional study. *BMJ*, **327**, 654–655.

Craig TKJ, Boardman AP, Mills K, *et al* (1993) The South London somatisation study. I: Longitudinal course and the influence of early life experiences. *British Journal of Psychiatry*, **163**, 579–588.

Craig TK, Cox AD, Klein K (2002) Intergenerational transmission of somatisation behaviour: a study of chronic somatisers and their children. *Psychological Medicine*, **32**, 805–816.

Dell ML, Campo JV (2011) Somatoform disorders in children and adolescents. *Psychiatric Clinics of North America*, **34**, 643–660.

Diatchenko L, Slade GD, Nackley AG, *et al* (2005) Genetic basis for individual variations in pain perception and the development of a chronic pain condition. *Human Molecular Genetics*, **14**, 135–143.

Domenech-Llaberia E, Jané C, Canals J, *et al* (2004) Parental reports of somatic symptoms in preschool children: prevalence and associations in a Spanish sample. *Journal of the American Academy of Child & Adolescent Psychiatry*, **43**, 598–604.

Egger HL, Costello EJ, Erkanli A, *et al* (1999) Somatic complaints and psychopathology in children and adolescents: stomach aches, muscular-skeletal pains and headaches. *Journal of the American Academy of Child & Adolescent Psychiatry*, **38**, 852–860.

Erlwein O, Kaye S, McClure MO, *et al* (2010) Failure to detect the novel retrovirus XMRV in chronic fatigue syndrome. *PLoS ONE*, **5**, e8519.

Eminson DM, Benjamin S, Shortall A, *et al* (1996) Physical symptoms and illness attitudes in adolescents: an epidemiological study. *Journal of Child Psychology and Psychiatry*, **37**, 519–527.

Fiertag O, Taylor S, Tareen A, *et al* (2012) Somatoform disorders. In *IACAPAP e-Textbook of Child and Adolescent Mental Health* (ed JM Rey), sect. I, ch.1. International Association for Child and Adolescent Psychiatry and Allied Professions.

Fritz GK, Fritsh S, Hagino O (1997) Somatization disorders in children and adolescence: A review of the past 10 years. *Journal of the American Academy of Child & Adolescent Psychiatry*, **36**, 1329–1338.

Garralda ME (2005) Functional somatic symptoms and somatoform disorders in children. In *A Clinician's Handbook of Child and Adolescent Psychiatry* (eds C Gillberg, R Harrington, HC Steinshausen), pp. 246–268. Cambridge University Press.

Garralda ME (2010) Unexplained physical complaints. *Child and Adolescent Psychiatric Clinics of North America*, **19**, 199–209.

Garralda ME, Chalder T (2005) Chronic fatigue syndrome in childhood. *Journal of Child Psychology and Psychiatry*, **46**, 1143–1151.

Garralda ME, Rangel L (2005) Chronic fatigue syndrome: comparative study with emotional disorders. *European Journal of Child and Adolescent Psychiatry*, **14**, 424–430.

Goodyer I, Taylor DC (1985) Hysteria. *Archives of Disease in Childhood*, **60**, 680–681.

Grattan-Smith P, Fairley M, Procopis P (1988) Clinical features of conversion disorder. *Archives of Disease in Childhood*, **63**, 408–414.

Gureje O, Simon GE, Ustun TB, *et al* (1997) Somatization in cross-cultural perspective: a World Health Organization study in primary care. *American Journal of Psychiatry*, **154**, 989–995.

Hariri AR, Mattay VS, Tessitore A, *et al* (2002) Serotonin transporter genetic variation and the response of the human amygdala. *Science*, **297**, 400–403.

Hotopf M, Carr S, Mayou R, *et al* (1998) Why do children have chronic abdominal pain, and what happens to them when they grow up? *BMJ*, **316**, 1196–1200.

Janssens KAM, Rosmalen JGM, Ormel J, *et al* (2011) Pubertal status predicts back pain, overtiredness, and dizziness in American and Dutch adolescents. *Pediatrics*, **128** (3), 553–559.

Jaspers T, Hanssen GMJ, Van der Valk JA, *et al* (2009) Pervasive refusal syndrome as part of the refusal–withdrawal–regression spectrum: critical review of the literature illustrated by a case report. *European Child and Adolescent Psychiatry*, **18**, 645–651.

Jordan KM, Ayers PM, Jahn SC, *et al* (2000) Prevalence of fatigue and chronic fatigue syndrome-like illness in children and adolescents. *Journal of Chronic Fatigue Syndrome*, **6**, 3–21.

Kendler KS, Gardner CO, Gatz M, *et al* (2007) The sources of comorbidity between major depression and generalized anxiety disorder in a Swedish national twin sample. *Psychological Medicine*, **37**, 453–462.

Kessler RC (2000) The epidemiology of pure and comorbid generalized anxiety disorder: a review and revaluation of recent research. *Acta Paediatrica*, **102**, 7–13.

Kotagal P, Cota M, Wyllie E, *et al* (2002) Paroxysmal nonepileptic events in children and adolescents. *Pediatrics*, **110**, e46.

Kozlowska K, Nunn KP, Rose D, *et al* (2007) Conversion disorder in Australian pediatric practice. *Journal of the American Academy of Child & Adolescent Psychiatry*, **46**, 68–75.

Lask B (2004) Pervasive refusal syndrome. *Advances in Psychiatric Treatment*, **10**, 153–159.

LeResche L, Mancl LA, Drangsholt MT, *et al* (2005) Relationship of pain and symptoms to pubertal development in adolescents. *Pain*, **118**, 201–209.

Libow JA (2000) Child and adolescent illness falsification. *Pediatrics*, **105**, 336–342.

Lieb R, Pfister H, Mastaler M, *et al* (2000) Somatoform syndromes and disorders in a representative population sample of adolescents and young adults: prevalence, comorbidity and impairments. *Acta Psychiatrica Scandinavica*, **101**, 194–208.

Lombardi VC, Ruscetti FW, Das Gupta J, *et al* (2009) Detection of an infectious retrovirus in blood cells of patients with chronic fatigue syndrome. *Science*, **326**, 585–589.

McGrath PJ (1995) Aspects of pain in children and adolescents. *Journal of Child Psychology and Psychiatry*, **36**, 717–730.

McNicholas F, Prio C, Bates G (2013) A case of pervasive refusal syndrome: a diagnostic conundrum. *Clinical Child Psychology and Psychiatry*, **18**, 137–150.

Mechanic D (1962) The concept of illness behaviour. *Journal of Chronic Disorders*, **15**, 189–194.

Murray CS, Cohen A, Perkins T, *et al* (2000) Morbidity in reflex sympathetic dystrophy. *Archives of Disease in Childhood*, **82**, 231–233.

Rangel L, Garralda E (2000) Personality in adolescents with chronic fatigue syndrome. *European Child and Adolescent Psychiatry*, **9**, 39–45.

Rangel L, Garralda E, Levin M, *et al* (2000) Personality in adolescents with chronic fatigue syndrome. *European Child and Adolescent Psychiatry*, **9**, 39–45.

Roach S (2013) Mass hysteria and the media: *Folie à Troupeau. Pediatric Neurology*, **49**, 6–7.

Sifneos P (1973) The prevalence of 'alexithymic' characteristics in psychosomatic patients. *Psychotherapy and Psychosomatics*, **22**, 255–262,

Taylor DC (1982) The components of sickness: disease, illnesses and predicament. In *One Child* (eds J Apley, C Ounsted), pp. 1–13. Spastics International Medical Publications.

Thompson SL, Nunn KP (1997) The pervasive refusal syndrome: the RAHC experience. *Clinical Child Psychology and Psychiatry*, **2**, 145–165.

Von Folsach, LL, Montgomery E (2006) Pervasive refusal syndrome among asylum-seeking children. *Clinical Child Psychology and Psychiatry*, **11**, 457–473.

Walker LS, Williams SE, Smith CA, *et al* (2006) Parent attention versus distraction: impact on symptom complaints by children with and without chronic functional abdominal pain. *Pain*, **122**, 43–52.

Wilkinson SR (1988) *The Child's World of Illness: The Development of Health and Illness Behaviour.* Cambridge University Press.

World Health Organization (1996) *Multiaxial Classification of Child and Adolescent Psychiatric Disorders: The ICD-10 Classification of Mental and Behavioural Disorders in Children and Adolescents.* WHO.

Yeo A, Boyd D, Lumsden S, *et al* (2004) Association between a functional polymorphism in the serotonin transporter gene and diarrhea predominant irritable bowel syndrome in women. *Gut*, **53**, 1452–1458.

CHAPTER 13

Somatising: management and outcomes

Olivia Fiertag and Mary Eminson

In this chapter we outline the treatment of children and adolescents with somatising conditions. The major diagnostic groups for these conditions (according to ICD-10; World Health Organization, 1992), in approximate descending order of prevalence, are adjustment, dissociative (conversion), somatoform and factitious disorders, and neurasthenia (chronic fatigue syndrome). The aetiology and clinical presentations of these disorders are discussed in Chapter 12, together with descriptions of the corresponding disorders in DSM-5 (American Psychiatric Association, 2013). Despite work in the past decade on the treatment of recurrent abdominal pain (Campo *et al*, 2004; Walker *et al*, 2006) and chronic fatigue (Rangel *et al*, 2000a; Garralda & Chalder, 2005), somatising conditions remain an area in which there is little systematic treatment research. Epidemiological studies give us a broad description of outcomes (Lieb *et al*, 2000; Kozlowska, 2001; Chalder *et al*, 2003; Ani *et al*, 2013) and there are many useful clinical accounts of the management of these disorders (Wright *et al*, 2000; Kozlowska *et al*, 2007; Fiertag *et al*, 2012).

Which professional should manage somatising disorders?

The decision about the appropriate clinician to manage a somatising disorder should depend on who has the skills to maximise the chances of recovery to normal functioning. This depends on the severity of the presentation, its impact on the young person's current functioning and how long symptoms have lasted.

Paediatricians and general practitioners (GPs) undertake the management of many adjustment, dissociative (conversion) and factitious disorders, and mild relapses of any somatising conditions. The presentations they manage are most likely to be of single or multiple physical symptoms (abdominal pain, joint pains, headaches), fatigue associated with obvious stresses of any kind, recent-onset losses of function, and unexplained symptoms after a clear physical illness. Their management forms a routine part of primary

Box 13.1 Key elements of initial management by primary care or paediatric professionals

- Take a good history, within a biopsychosocial framework, which identifies stresses and recent life events
- Provide clear reassurance about negative physical findings when the appropriate investigations have been completed
- Examine family beliefs about illness in order to prepare for the step of encouraging a return to a normal lifestyle
- Provide a model to explain psychosomatic symptoms to the family

care and paediatric practice. Key elements of management in paediatric and primary care are listed in Box 13.1.

Child and adolescent mental health services (CAMHS), preferably in the form of a paediatric liaison mental health service, should become involved if initial management has been unsuccessful, if there is diagnostic uncertainty involving possible somatisation, if there are significant psychiatric symptoms at the outset, or if the young person is already severely impaired. For this involvement to be successfully achieved, paediatric medical, surgical and associated specialists (e.g. physiotherapists) must recognise the nature of the presentation, be aware of the different kinds of somatising disorder, acknowledge the importance of a biopsychosocial formulation and be alert to likely psychiatric symptoms in the patients. Continued joint management by physical and mental health clinicians is helpful, especially where there is an element of organic illness. The skills of several different CAMHS professionals may often be required in the management of somatising conditions that are severe, handicapping and chronic.

Whether this referral (to CAMHS or a paediatric liaison CAMHS service) is made early or after a period of paediatric management, the way this crucial task is performed may encourage successful rehabilitation and treatment or, conversely, could leave the family continuing a search for physical explanations for the symptoms. A tendency to look for physical as opposed to psychological explanations is often a prominent feature of the family's response to somatising conditions, and reluctance to accept the involvement of any mental health professional or service may be persistent and strong. Engaging the family and stressing that all of the professionals believe in the child's experience of the symptoms is essential, including acknowledging that the child is not 'putting it on'. A positive, unapologetic attitude to the referral by the paediatrician or GP will maximise the chances of successful engagement and conveys a clear message that the CAMHS service is uniquely well placed to deliver a set of effective treatments to speed the young person's recovery.

For patients and families who meet criteria for CAMHS referral, but who reject such involvement, management may rely on liaison between CAMHS and other medical and non-medical staff. This is addressed later in this chapter, in the section 'When CAMHS referral is not taken up by the family'.

Assessment

Although comprehensive assessment of somatising disorders involves assessment processes similar to those used for other child and adolescent disorders, the level of attention that must be paid to engagement of these patients and their families sets them apart from more routine referrals. Establishing engagement is necessary from the outset. It is often best achieved through careful attention to the history of the illness, its impact and management so far. Understanding the family's illness beliefs, the level of conviction that the illness has a physical cause, the level of satisfaction with physical investigations and explanations, and views about the psychiatric referral are critical components for success in this engagement process. It is important to explore what physical examinations and investigations have been done already and to ensure that all physical interventions are complete.

After this has been established, the normal personal and family histories are obtained. Attention should be paid to the predisposing, precipitating and maintaining factors in the child, the family and the environment within a biopsychosocial framework (see Box 12.4 in Chapter 12). A detailed family medical history is necessary to establish whether other family members have had similar physical symptoms, whether serious illness was the cause or the symptoms remained unexplained, and the extent to which family members have been affected by ill health (physical and mental) of all kinds. The apparent failure of doctors to find the cause of a family member's complaints (sometimes with serious consequences) may undermine parents' confidence in medical opinions and become a source of repeated uncertainty.

The assessment of the child or adolescent is relatively routine, taking into account current physical symptoms, physical state and functional mobility, mental state and ability to relate and engage. Current functioning in terms of sleep, appetite, peer relationships, school attendance and ability to perform academic work is reviewed. It is important to find the young person's views of the cause of the illness, although these usually mirror parental views quite closely. Screening for comorbid psychiatric disorders needs to be carried out: in particular, anxiety and depression may be present.

Establishing an explanation of psychosomatic relationships that both the young person and the family can understand is crucial: how physical symptoms, including fatigue, may genuinely be present, even when

203

currently there is no physical abnormality. Analogies are useful, for example the tension headache experienced at some time by most adults and acknowledged by the sufferer to have a psychological cause but to be extremely physically painful. If other examples of physical discomfort affected by psychosocial factors can be found from within the family's own experience (e.g. asthma worsened by emotional distress) these usually carry the most weight.

During the assessment the clinician should establish a formulation of the illness that incorporates pre-existing vulnerabilities, precipitating events or illness and maintaining factors within a biopsychosocial framework. The formulation will rarely be complete after the initial assessment. Sometimes this is because the family's view of the pre-illness functioning is so positive, compared with the present, that earlier difficulties are hard to see. Any suggestion of earlier problems may be perceived as criticism and rejected. Sometimes, especially in perfectionist, striving children who have achieved highly but at significant personal cost (Lask, 1986), the premorbid functioning really did appear to be effortlessly successful, until a physical illness supervened and it became clear that resuming previous activities was too demanding. Nevertheless, tentative hypotheses will be established at this initial stage, with a need to clarify areas of uncertainty in future and to revisit the potential biopsychosocial contributory factors throughout the assessment and management process.

It is usually helpful to share the 'predisposing, precipitating, maintaining' approach with the family and to stress that recovery through rehabilitation can be achieved without an initial understanding of all the aetiological factors. This is a helpful step in counteracting 'either/or', 'physical v. psychological' thinking. Parents may begin to think of triggers themselves. Families may assume that the final precipitant for a somatising disorder must be a substantial stress in its own right. However, in a young person with extensive predisposing factors, an apparently trivial physical or psychological stress may be sufficient to provoke a conversion (dissociative) disorder or the beginning of an episode of severe fatigue.

The final stage of the assessment is to engage the patient and family with further therapeutic work via CAMHS follow up. This may be facilitated by providing details of evidence that the service has successfully treated other young people with similar conditions. For some families, greater clarification of physical investigations and their meaning must be undertaken because significant doubts remain and will resurface unless addressed. Such clarification interviews are often best conducted in a joint paediatric/psychiatric/family session: this leaves less room for confusion or different nuances in interpretation. A dedicated paediatric liaison CAMHS service or group of professionals is the least stigmatised option for assessment and treatment and will also facilitate confident joint working between paediatric and mental health professionals. In the absence of such provision, the child mental health professional must do what they can to address family anxieties and beliefs and provide a platform for a collaborative treatment programme. If engagement is very difficult to achieve, for example if the family believe in a physical cause for their child's illness, or are fearful of the implications of CAMHS involvement, such difficulties are best acknowledged openly, allowing families to return to CAMHS at a later juncture if they wish. This challenging group of families may be best managed by continued liaison with paediatricians.

Questionnaires and interview schedules

Instruments to measure physical symptoms and functional impairment are useful at the assessment stage and to monitor progress during treatment. Symptom diaries may be helpful to document severity and frequency of symptoms over time. A visual representation may demonstrate progress even before it is noticed subjectively and therefore may help to encourage therapeutic optimism and motivation to engage. Questionnaires that may help with engagement at the assessment and throughout treatment include those that measure somatic symptoms, such as the Somatic Symptom Checklist (Eminson *et al*, 1996) and the Children's Somatization Inventory (Garber *et al*, 1991), and those that measure function, such as the Functional Disability Inventory (Walker & Greene, 1991). In chronic fatigue syndrome, the Chalder Fatigue Self-report scale (Chalder *et al*, 1993) is helpful. In all of the somatising disorders, depression and anxiety symptoms are useful baseline measurements, and scales specific to these conditions can be used together with a global functioning measure such as HoNOSCA (Gowers *et al*, 1999). Questionnaires to screen for other comorbid disorders may also be helpful. Psychometric testing may be of benefit, especially in determining whether there is a difference between the educational expectations of the child and their actual abilities.

Comorbid psychiatric conditions

Comorbid psychiatric conditions may precede the development of the somatising disorder or may develop during its course. A recent review by Campo (2012) highlights the relationship between functional somatic symptoms, anxiety and depression and suggests that across the lifespan there is little evidence to support natural boundaries between these three phenomena. The Early Developmental Stages of Psychopathology (EDSP) study (Lieb *et al*, 2000) reported that dissociative (conversion) disorders were associated with eating disorders, and pain disorders were associated with depression, panic and post-traumatic stress disorder in older adolescents. Somatising disorders can also, of course, coexist with organic illnesses. It is important to identify and treat comorbid psychiatric conditions where they are present, although establishing comorbidity and distinguishing between potential diagnoses can be difficult, especially when biological and psychological symptoms coexist, such as in a child with epileptic seizures and paroxysmal non-epileptic events.

Management

Treatment setting

The setting for the work (out-patient, day or in-patient) will depend on the degree of chronicity, level of impairment and previous progress, especially the extent and nature of family difficulties, as will the decision about the appropriate professional to undertake the intervention. It is evident that for severe and complex cases, and depending on the relative importance of individual and family factors in each case, input will be needed from more than one person and that a team approach will be required to integrate the interventions. This is particularly true where day or in-patient treatment is undertaken. The issue of engagement does not, of course, disappear after the initial assessment, and family concerns need to be addressed throughout the treatment, as interventions are rarely successful if the patient or family are not on board with the approach.

The length of treatment also varies a great deal. A series of out-patient appointments over 4–6 months may be sufficient. The more chronic and incapacitating sicknesses may require input over 1–2 years, several months of which may be in-patient or day-patient care. Even longer support may occasionally be necessary to maintain relatively healthy functioning.

Principles of treatment

The principles of treatment (Box 13.2) are similar for all the somatising disorders. The main aim is to help the young person and their family to gradually resume a lifestyle dedicated less to illness and more to normal activities, while simultaneously attending to factors in the child, family and environment which have made that difficult. This involves understanding all the stresses and factors that were identified in the assessment and helping the child and family to remediate them.

The variety of techniques and approaches used will depend on the young person's age and developmental stage and the symptoms and severity of the disorder. The emphasis that needs to be placed on the different aspects, including the extent to which the child requires individual treatment away from joint sessions and the pace of progress that can be achieved, will depend on the nature and chronicity of the presentation. If the young person is deeply regressed and withdrawn, the pace of work is of necessity much slower and adapted carefully to the functional developmental level.

A team approach is needed because working with the young person might demand different skills and techniques from working with their parents, with or without the young person. The team approach also needs

---

Box 13.2   Principles of managing somatising disorders in children and adolescents

- Understand the family's beliefs about the illness, level of conviction for physical cause, satisfaction with investigations and views about involvement of mental health services
- Explore the child's expectations of the ultimate goals (as they may be unrealistically high)
- Acknowledge that the child has a real illness affecting their life and do not convey embarrassment when communicating the diagnosis
- Make the family aware of the high prevalence of somatisation (2–10%), as this may reassure parents about the absence of an organic cause
- Emphasise that it may take time but the majority of patients recover well
- Focus on helping the family and child develop ways of coping with the symptoms, rather than on reducing functional impairment
- Encourage expression of feelings, emotional distress, underlying worries or fears through direct, verbal means rather than through physical complaints
- Manage the physical symptom(s) with a variety of methods, depending on type and illness stage: monitoring using diaries or pain charts; distraction with activity; cognitive–behavioural techniques
- Find strategies to resume gradually, rather than avoid, activities normal for the developmental stage
- Pay attention to areas of functioning that have become disrupted, such as sleep patterns, exercise and study
- Set modest initial goals and continue setting achievable, consistent, agreed goals for change in activities
- Treat concurrent psychiatric symptoms such as depression or anxiety: this may include medication or other psychological approaches
- Consider physiological mechanisms contributing to symptoms, e.g. contracture secondary to immobilisation
- Consider all possible maintaining factors in the child or family: problems of learning, temperament, peer relations, family relationships
- Consider parental capacity to encourage recovery through activity, and if there is continued persistent pursuit of abnormal illness behaviour by parents, explore the reasons so that these can be addressed
- Prevent unnecessary medical investigation and interventions through paediatric and primary care liaison, with agreement about gate-keeping of referrals to other medical and surgical specialists
- Maintain a systemic perspective throughout, so that the pace of change in the child, family and professional network does not become unsynchronised. Other professionals involved with the family (e.g. from health and educational services, self-help groups) may have very different beliefs about management and outcome, and unless the family (and professionals) are helped to resolve conflicting advice, through clarification and discussion, they may find it difficult to maintain their support of an active rehabilitation programme

to include liaison with professionals across agencies, including education, paediatrics and sometimes Social Services. Effective communication between the professionals is needed to ensure that the interventions from different agencies or professionals are mutually consistent and there is a clear, understandable management strategy for the young person and their family. The treatment should aim to develop a partnership between child, family and professionals.

Cultural considerations

Throughout the treatment process it is important to explore and address culture-specific family attitudes and beliefs about the symptoms and the treatments. In addition, it is important to find out what interventions have already been tried or what the family is concurrently using, including culture-specific interventions such as spiritual healers. Spending time with the family discussing alternative explanations will enhance engagement and deter them from solely seeking help from practitioners of alternative medicine (Fiertag *et al*, 2012).

Specific treatments

Specific management strategies may involve individual psychological work, family work and liaison with Social Services and schools. As already mentioned, coordination of all the professionals is vital to ensure that everyone is working towards the same goals. A wide range of techniques can be used, but it is important to individualise the treatment package and define the reasons why a particular approach is chosen. Progress towards goals relevant to the treatment approach and the target symptom should be measured regularly. Not all target symptoms are physical, and functional goals such as better peer relations and school attendance may be more important than reduction of physical complaints and curing of symptoms. Motivational techniques may be helpful in engaging the young person and family in the treatment.

Box 13.3 Elements of cognitive–behavioural family treatment

- Discuss investigations and rationale for pain management
- Encourage self-monitoring of pain
- Help parents to reinforce normal 'good health' or 'well' behaviour (and reduce attention to symptoms), promote distraction, ignore non-verbal pain behaviours, avoid modelling the sick role, discriminate seriousness of symptoms
- Help young person to develop healthy coping skills: relaxation, positive self-talk, distraction, positive imagery
- Teach problem-solving skills
- Encourage participation in everyday activities
- Increase attention when symptom free by instituting pleasant joint activities

(Adapted from Garralda, 2008)

Cognitive–behavioural therapy

The best evidence for effectiveness in treating somatisation comes from family cognitive–behavioural therapy for recurrent abdominal pain (Box 13.3). Randomised controlled studies have shown that, compared with standard medical care, this approach results in greater pain reduction, lower relapse rates, lower interference with daily activities and increased parental satisfaction (Sanders et al, 1994; Robins et al, 2005). After controlling for pre-treatment levels of pain, the mother's caregiving strategies and the child's coping strategies were significant independent predictors of pain behaviour after the treatment. Avoiding repeatedly reassuring children about their symptoms is part of the treatment. Parents and children are encouraged to spend activity time together in symptom-free periods.

In chronic fatigue, several adult trials have shown cognitive–behavioural therapy and graded exercise therapy to be beneficial (Whiting et al, 2001). Cognitive approaches are also effective for those with other symptoms, pains and hypochondriacal concerns (Garralda, 2010; Dell & Campo, 2011).

Modifications may need to be made to enable parts of the cognitive approach to be used with younger and less able children and to be combined with behavioural approaches to integrate work with parents and child. Examples of specific cognitive–behavioural techniques that may be used include symptom diaries, limiting the attention given to the symptom, relaxation techniques, graded exposure to activities and psychoeducation on the links between physical and psychological pain.

Behavioural therapy

In relatively well-functioning children and families where the level of impairment is limited, behavioural management of specific single or multiple symptoms has been shown to be successful in both children and adolescents (Larsson, 1992; McGrath & Reid, 1995). Behavioural approaches can be particularly useful in dissociative (conversion) disorders. In adjustment disorders and somatoform disorders with minor levels of impairment this may be the only treatment required and can be delivered on an out-patient basis. Behavioural therapy is used to minimise maladaptive behaviours, reinforce healthy behaviours, and address illness behaviour and behaviours that have secondary gains.

Sleep hygiene

Careful attention to sleep hygiene is the first step in treating many chronic or severe illnesses. This uses routine techniques to ensure that the young person is awake during the day and asleep at night, through the gradual reduction of daytime sleep and introduction of normal night-time sleep routines. It is important to identify secondary gains of a disturbed routine, which may include opportunities for a close relationship with a parent or avoidance of school attendance or academic work. Medication such as melatonin may occasionally be used briefly as an adjunct to behavioural techniques.

Family therapy

We have already emphasised the importance of a systemic perspective in somatising disorders. The family's concerns should be addressed at the outset, but also regularly reviewed. The family can play a key part in helping the child to learn new coping strategies and in reducing family behaviours that may be reinforcing the symptoms. Family work can be used to address parental psychopathology or stress that may be contributing to the child's presentation. Family work is also used for psychoeducational purposes to introduce a carefully paced rehabilitation and explain the nature of the illness and its treatment (Chalder, 1999). This might include: exploration of the family's illness beliefs and alternatives; helping parents to manage physical symptoms and other kinds of behaviour; and enabling recovering children to negotiate differently and more directly with their parents.

A systemic approach is useful in helping the family and professional systems to work together successfully for the benefit of the young person. Systemic work may be undertaken on a day or in-patient basis in paediatric or CAMHS settings. In illnesses with unexplained physical symptoms, there is great potential for conflicting views and beliefs – for example, whether the young person should be attempting normal activities, or whether this would be physically harmful to them. Using a systemic approach to clarify the beliefs and attitudes of all those involved in the care and rehabilitation (family and professionals) facilitates a more consistent management strategy between professionals, which in turn helps family engagement with the treatment. This is also useful when the young person's presentation has conflicting aspects, for example fearing activity *v.* wanting to recover, as the different professionals contributing to the treatment plan may get caught up with one side of these views. Skills in this area are particularly useful when different family members have polarised views on the young person's illness and management.

Psychopharmacology

The use of medication can be considered but no psychotropics are licensed specifically for somatising disorders in children and adolescents and there is limited available evidence. However, medication may be helpful if comorbid disorders such as depression or anxiety have been identified, and it may also enable the rehabilitation process to proceed more easily in children without diagnosed comorbidity. For example, an open-label trial of citalopram for paediatric recurrent abdominal pain showed improvement in both the pain and symptoms of anxiety and depression (Campo *et al*, 2004). Occasionally, benzodiazepines may be helpful for short-term use in treating associated anxiety, for example, while waiting for selective serotonin reuptake inhibitors to take effect (Campo, 2008).

Education and school liaison

Addressing school attendance, learning and problems with peer groups is particularly important. Establishing the extent of the problem and helping the young person and family recognise its relevance is crucial in aiding recovery from the symptomatic presentation. Addressing excessive academic and emotional demands (which are frequently self-imposed by the child) is also worthwhile. The approach to peer group interaction problems will depend on the young person and their pre-existing skills, and may require interventions such as cognitive–behavioural, didactic social skills or problem-solving techniques. Liaison with education professionals is essential, and undertaking a cognitive assessment may also provide useful information.

Rehabilitation

Rehabilitation is necessary to minimise the impact of persisting symptoms. It encourages a focus on improving functioning, not just curing symptoms. Rehabilitation involving graded activity programmes with family cognitive–behavioural treatment has been shown to be effective for chronic fatigue (Stulemeijer et al, 2005). In severe cases, 'restrained rehabilitation', a coordinated multidisciplinary package that takes seriously the importance of a correct pace and identification of unacknowledged reluctances, is recommended (Calvert & Jureidini, 2003). This is because the planning of a return to a more appropriate lifestyle requires great care and attention to timing. It may be important to discourage hasty overactivity and (apparently paradoxically) to encourage regular rest. This enforces an appropriate pace and prevents relapses with severe physical symptoms. It also gives a clear message to the family that the professional takes seriously their own statements about the severity of the illness and the time required to recover. This approach may be used skilfully to remove any inappropriate secondary gains that are reinforcing the young person's behaviour. Another aspect of rehabilitation involves gradually shifting the burden of responsibility from clinician to parent and patient.

Other management

Monitoring daily variations in specific symptoms and associated impairments is useful. Dietary habits should also be addressed, as these may have altered. Muscle relaxation may be useful for headaches, and graded physical exercise may be useful for muscular problems and fatigue. Rest periods, distraction techniques and relaxation techniques (e.g. guided imagery) may also be useful in fatigue and recurrent pains. Work carried out in school settings and out-patient clinics for children and adolescents has shown that tension headaches can be substantially improved by relaxation training (Garralda, 2005). Practical management strategies should be introduced for paroxysmal non-epileptic events. Integrating the work of mental health clinicians with that of physiotherapists and any other specialists, such as rheumatologists, is essential to ensure a shared formulation and management plan, for example where there are physical problems secondary to immobility. Patient support groups may be helpful, although in some circumstances they may take a different viewpoint

211

from the professionals and may undermine the therapeutic work being done. Progress in terms of symptoms and functioning at home and in the community needs to be regularly monitored and reassurance provided that if objective signs of organic disease are present they will be investigated appropriately. Psychiatric admission may be required if progress is not made with out-patient treatment or the child is very incapacitated and there is associated psychopathology.

Treatment for factitious disorders

Management of factitious disorders follows the same principles as for any other somatising presentation, but special care should be taken to engage the parents, with the aim of preventing them from being punitive when the factitious nature of the symptom becomes apparent. Unfortunately, young people whose factitious presentations are severe and intractable are more likely to come from families in which problems with open and trusting relationships are evident, making work with all the family difficult.

Treatment in severely disturbed, disrupted or broken families

Sometimes, management in the organised way described for most families is simply not possible. Complicating factors include physical, sexual or emotional abuse or attachment disorder in the aetiology, numerous coexisting psychological symptoms, including conduct problems and self-harm, somatising disorders in the parents, and other major social dysfunction in the child or family. The child may be living in a family with significant ongoing relationship difficulties or may have been placed in a substitute family. In either case, professionals may have major difficulties in engaging the parents. If possible, the principles and practice of management described above should be used. But in some cases, damage limitation may have to be the main objective: responding to crises and periods of emotional distress with an intervention relevant to the mood disorder or self-harming phase, or helping to find an appropriate educational or substitute home environment. Preventing unnecessary medical interventions is important for young people with severe disruption of social circumstances and relationships, but even this may be difficult if the young person is moved to a different part of the country.

When CAMHS referral is not taken up by the family

Unfortunately, despite the best efforts of paediatric and child mental health professionals, a proportion of families with a child who has a severe somatising disorder refuse any treatment associated with a mental health service. This can be frustrating for CAMHS professionals, especially when a young person with severe symptoms and impairments is living a very restricted life. It is important to remember that CAMHS professionals can still make a useful contribution in these circumstances, working

---

Box 13.4 Liaison roles of child and adolescent mental health services in the management of problem families

Support: Advise and enable professionals to make optimum interventions and keep the biopsychosocial formulation in mind

Containment: Help professionals avoid unnecessary investigations and treatment

Prevention of avoidable impairment: Keep an overview of the effect on the patient of the disorder and the family's response to it

---

with the health, education and other professionals to whom the family does allow access (Box 13.4). Supporting these professionals in keeping a perspective on the illness is a useful role, and enables them to provide some basic mental health interventions, such as information on sleep hygiene, basic cognitive–behavioural techniques and, possibly, prescription of antidepressants. They might also advise a paediatric play worker or practice counsellor who is able to spend time with the young person. The purpose is not to encourage delivery of interventions by those without appropriate training, but to work with them on principles of management in key areas, to give young people and their families an opportunity to develop trust in an accepting, emotionally congruent and sympathetic professional. The person (e.g. paediatrician, play worker, practice counsellor) who has been able to develop a relationship with the family can also encourage the family to consider engagement with CAMHS for more intensive and appropriate treatment in the future. Another aspect of the CAMHS liaison role is to help the paediatrician (and others) to retain the biopsychosocial formulation in mind, rather than seeing a puzzling physical problem.

Naturally, someone with a chronic, severe and untreated problem is unlikely to make a quick recovery, but without such indirect CAMHS support, the paediatrician's or GP's urge to reinvestigate without good reason may become overwhelming. Thus, CAMHS can help to contain the situation, preventing harm from unnecessary investigations and treatments. Some families repeatedly seek new specialists and interventions, and professionals, including the GP, may need help to resist pressure to make referrals for yet more opinions. It is important that children and families are not prevented from receiving necessary advice from experts but, in principle, such experts should be approached by the first specialist for second opinions, rather than by the family, who may involve professionals not fully informed about the background and previous investigations and formulation.

Another consideration is to keep under review the extent to which the somatising disorder and the family's management may be causing avoidable impairment to the young person's development. Rarely, despite parents' good intentions, the intensity of their wish to undertake major pharmacological and surgical interventions, and/or their insistence on a disabled lifestyle for their child, leaves the professional uneasy about whether the young person's welfare is being safeguarded. Such concerns are always uncomfortable to face and will of course require careful discussion with paediatric colleagues before local safeguarding professionals are contacted. Occasionally it is indeed necessary to involve Social Services and child protection legislation to ensure the well-being of the patient.

Outcomes and continuities

The range of disorders described in this chapter is wide and the interventions and outcomes equally broad. It is difficult to make robust predictions of outcome of the somatising disorders at different ages, and the literature appears to give inconsistent results. This problem is compounded by the existence of a group of sufferers and families who find it difficult to engage with active treatments. Outcomes will vary depending on severity of symptoms, resulting impairment and possible risk factors (e.g. personality difficulty and family support). However, reassuringly the majority of children with somatising disorders seen in specialist services recover, although symptoms can persist in some and others will experience a relapsing illness.

Outcomes may be considered in relation to the future risk of (a) psychiatric disorders or symptoms, (b) continuing unexplained physical symptoms and (c) more widespread somatising problems. It has become increasingly clear that the experience of excess or chronic physical symptoms in childhood and adolescence is associated with psychiatric disorders, especially depression and anxiety. It has also been shown that individuals with somatic symptoms in childhood are more likely to have psychiatric disorders in adulthood (Zwaigenbaum et al, 1999; Campo et al, 2001; Fearon & Hotopf, 2001), even if comorbid psychiatric symptoms were not apparently present in childhood. We do not yet know which young people will, as they develop, acquire the ability to express emotional distress verbally and whether they differ from those who continue to present somatising disorders, either with or without other psychological symptoms.

Concerning specific disorders, adjustment disorders characterised by physical and emotional symptoms are by definition short-lived, as are transient dissociative (conversion) reactions. In general, these disorders show poor continuity with adult presentations. One study of conversion disorder showed that, even though 85% recovered, 35% had a mood or anxiety disorder at 4-year follow-up (Pehlivantürk & Unal, 2002). Factitious disorders often have a similar clinical course: the index episode usually resolves completely, but the underlying difficulties remain and are associated with other psychiatric presentations later. Those who had childhood recurrent abdominal pain have been found to have high levels of anxiety, poor social outcomes, perceived susceptibility to physical impairments and hypochondriacal beliefs in adulthood (Campo *et al*, 2001).

The long-term outcomes of well-defined somatoform disorders in childhood and adolescence are rarely reported, although symptom-specific groups (e.g. complex regional pain syndrome, usually seen as a form of somatoform pain disorder) have been described. A study by Murray *et al* (2000) describes recovery times following diagnosis (itself sometimes more than 2 years after symptom onset) of between 0 and 140 weeks (median 7 weeks), but 27.5% of patients relapsed. Clinically, any of the long-lasting severe somatoform disorders may show continuities into adulthood. This is consistent with the results of studies of adults with somatoform disorders that suggest that many began in adolescence or even earlier.

Chronic fatigue is a better-researched area for both treatment and outcome, with studies of adults, adolescents and children providing information about positive factors for recovery. These include engagement with psychiatric services (Vereker, 1992); clear physical precipitants of the illness; onset at the start of a new school year; ongoing immunological abnormalities; and better maternal health and socioeconomic status (Rangel *et al*, 1999). It is suggested that these children are at greater risk of developing further psychiatric disorders post-recovery (Garralda & Chalder, 2005). Two-thirds of children do recover, but their recovery can be slow, taking years. In a relatively small study of adolescents, persistent symptoms were predicted by personality difficulties and personality disorder (Rangel *et al*, 2000*b*).

Conclusion

This chapter has provided an overview of the management and outcomes of somatising disorders, using the evidence base as far as possible. However, with the exception of the relatively larger literature on chronic fatigue and recurrent abdominal pain, somatising conditions remain one of the most neglected areas of research in child and adolescent psychiatry. Recognition of these disorders and their responsiveness to vigorous treatment is a continuing major problem. The challenges continue once recognition has occurred: a non-pejorative terminology is needed, to be shared with paediatricians; and treatment research using rigorous definitions must approach the strength level of randomised controlled trials. The new classification systems introduced into DSM-5 (American Psychiatric Association, 2013) and anticipated in ICD-11 will influence research efforts into these disorders. Despite the research limitations, there is a wealth of clinical material in the literature, and the development of collaborations between centres and between disciplines to achieve a better evidence base forms an exciting prospect for future research and treatment of these impairing disorders.

References

American Psychiatric Association (2013) *Diagnostic and Statistical Manual of Mental Disorders (5th edn) (DSM-5)*. APA.

Ani C, Reading R, Lynn R, *et al* (2013) Incidence and 12-month outcome of non-transient childhood conversion disorder in the UK and Ireland. *British Journal of Psychiatry*, **202**, 413–418.

Calvert P, Jureidini J (2003) Restrained rehabilitation: an approach to children and adolescents with unexplained signs and symptoms. *Archives of Disease in Childhood*, **88**, 399–402.

Campo JV (2008) Disorders primarily seen in medical settings. In *Clinical Manual of Child and Adolescent Psychopharmacology* (ed RL Findling), pp. 375–423. American Psychiatric Publishing.

Campo JV (2012) Annual Research Review: Functional somatic symptoms and associated anxiety and depression – developmental psychology in paediatric practice. *Journal of Child Psychology and Psychiatry*, **53**, 575–592.

Campo JV, Di Lorenzo C, Chiappetta L, *et al* (2001) Adult outcomes of pediatric recurrent abdominal pain: do they just grow out of it? *Pediatrics*, **108**, E1.

Campo JV, Perel JM, Lucas A, *et al* (2004) Citalopram treatment of pediatric recurrent abdominal pain and comorbid internalizing disorders: an exploratory study. *Journal of the American Academy of Child & Adolescent Psychiatry*, **43**, 1234–1242.

Chalder T (1999) Family oriented cognitive behavioural treatment for adolescents with chronic fatigue syndrome. In *Chronic Fatigue Syndrome: Helping Children and Adolescents* (Association for Child Psychology and Psychiatry Occasional Paper OP16) (ed E Garralda), pp. 19–23.

Chalder T, Berelowitz G, Pawlikowska T, *et al* (1993) Development of a fatigue scale. *Journal of Psychosomatic Research*, **37**, 147–153.

Chalder T, Goodman R, Hotopf M, *et al* (2003) Epidemiology of chronic fatigue syndrome and self reported myalgic encephalomyelitis in 5–15 year olds: cross sectional study. *BMJ*, **327**, 654–655.

Dell ML, Campo JV (2011) Somatoform disorders in children and adolescents. *Psychiatric Clinics of North America*, **34**, 643–660.

Eminson M, Benjamin S, Shortall A, *et al* (1996) Physical symptoms and illness attitudes in adolescents: an epidemiological study. *Journal of Child Psychology and Psychiatry*, **37**, 519–528.

Fearon P, Hotopf M (2001) Relation between headache in childhood and physical and psychiatric symptoms in adulthood: national birth cohort study. *BMJ*, **322**, 1145–1148.

Fiertag O, Taylor S, Tareen A, *et al* (2012) Somatoform disorders. In *IACAPAP e-Textbook of Child and Adolescent Mental Health* (ed JM Rey), sect. I, ch. 1. International Association for Child and Adolescent Psychiatry and Allied Professions.

Garber J, Walker SL, Zeman J (1991) Somatization symptoms in a community sample of children and adolescents: further validation of the Children's Somatization Inventory. *Psychological Assessment*, **3**, 588–595.

Garralda ME (2005) Functional somatic symptoms and somatoform disorders in children. In *A Clinician's Handbook of Child and Adolescent Psychiatry* (eds C Gillberg, R Harrington, HC Steinshausen), pp. 246–268. Cambridge University Press.

Garralda ME (2008) Somatization and somatoform disorders. *Psychiatry*, **7**, 353–356.

Garralda ME (2010) Unexplained physical complaints. *Child Adolescent Psychiatric Clinics of North America*, **19**, 199–209.

Garralda ME, Chalder T (2005) Chronic fatigue syndrome in childhood. *Journal of Child Psychology and Psychiatry*, **46**, 1143–1151.

Gowers SG, Harrington RC, Whitton A, *et al* (1999) Brief scale for measuring the outcomes of emotional and behavioural disorders in children: Health of the Nation

Outcome Scales for Children and Adolescents (HoNOSCA). *British Journal of Psychiatry*, **174**, 413–416.

Kozlowska K (2001) Good children presenting with conversion disorder. *Clinical Child Psychology and Psychiatry*, **6**, 575–591.

Kozlowska K, Nunn KP, Rose D, *et al* (2007) Conversion disorder in Australian pediatric practice. *Journal of the American Academy of Child & Adolescent Psychiatry*, **46**, 68–75.

Larsson B (1992) Behavioural treatment of somatic disorders in children and adolescents. *European Child and Adolescent Psychiatry*, **1**, 82–88.

Lask B (1986) The high-achieving child. *Postgraduate Medical Journal*, **62**, 143–145.

Lask B, Fosson A (1989) *Childhood Illness: The Psychosomatic Approach*. John Wiley & Sons.

Lieb R, Pfister H, Mastaler M, *et al* (2000) Somatoform syndromes and disorders in a representative population sample of adolescents and young adults: prevalence, comorbidity and impairments. *Acta Psychiatrica Scandinavica*, **101**, 194–208.

McGrath PJ, Reid GJ (1995) Behavioral treatment of pediatric headache. *Pediatric Annals*, **24**, 486–491.

Murray CS, Cohen A, Perkins T, *et al* (2000) Morbidity in reflex sympathetic dystrophy. *Archives of Disease in Childhood*, **82**, 231–233.

Pehlivantürk B, Unal F (2002) Conversion disorder in children and adolescents: a 4-year follow-up study. *Journal of Psychosomatic Research*, **52**, 187–191.

Rangel L, Garralda E, Levin M, *et al* (1999) Psychiatric adjustment in adolescents with a history of chronic fatigue syndrome. *Journal of the American Academy of Child & Adolescent Psychiatry*, **38**, 1515–1521.

Rangel L, Garralda E, Levin M, *et al* (2000a) The course of severe chronic fatigue syndrome. *Journal of the Royal Society of Medicine*, **93**, 129–134.

Rangel L, Garralda E, Levin M, *et al* (2000b) Personality in adolescents with chronic fatigue syndrome. *European Child and Adolescent Psychiatry*, **9**, 39–45.

Robins PM, Smith SM, Glutting JJ, *et al* (2005) A randomized controlled trial of a cognitive-behavioral family intervention for pediatric recurrent abdominal pain. *Journal of Pediatric Psychology*, **30**, 397–408.

Sanders MR, Shepherd RW, Cleghorn G, *et al* (1994) The treatment of recurrent abdominal pain in children: a controlled comparison of cognitive-behavioral family intervention and standard pediatric care. *Journal of Consulting and Clinical Psychology*, **62**, 306–314.

Stulemeijer M, de Jong LW, Fiselier TJ, *et al* (2005) Cognitive behaviour therapy for adolescents with chronic fatigue syndrome: randomised controlled trial. *BMJ*, **330**, 14.

Vereker MI (1992) Chronic fatigue syndrome: a joint paediatric-psychiatric approach. *Archives of Disease in Childhood*, **67**, 550–555.

Walker LS, Greene JW (1991) The functional disability inventory: measuring a neglected dimension of child health status. *Journal of Pediatric Psychology*, **1**, 39–58.

Walker LS, Williams SE, Smith CA, *et al* (2006) Parent attention versus distraction: impact on symptom complaints by children with and without chronic functional abdominal pain. *Pain*, **122**, 43–52.

Whiting P, Bagnall AM, Sowden AJ, *et al* (2001) Interventions for the treatment and management of chronic fatigue syndrome: a systematic review. *Journal of the American Medical Association*, **286**, 1360–1368.

World Health Organization (1992) *The ICD-10 Classification of Mental and Behavioural Disorders: Clinical Descriptions and Diagnostic Guidelines*. WHO.

Wright B, Partridge I, Williams C (2000) Management of chronic fatigue syndrome in children. *Advances in Psychiatric Treatment*, **6**, 145–152.

Zwaigenbaum L, Szatmari P, Boyle MH, *et al* (1999) Highly somatizing young adolescents and the risk of depression. *Pediatrics*, **103**, 1203–1209.

CHAPTER 14

Evaluating psychological treatments for children with autism

Patricia Howlin

Once considered to be a very rare condition, diagnosed mainly in children with severe intellectual impairments and no or very limited language, it is now known that autism can occur in individuals of all cognitive and linguistic levels and that its effects are lifelong. Awareness of this wider spectrum has resulted in a steady decrease in age at first diagnosis (Fountain *et al*, 2011) and an increase in prevalence estimates from approximately 4 per 10 000 in the 1970s to around 1 per 100 (Baird *et al*, 2006). These changes have resulted in much greater research into the effectiveness of different interventions and there has been a particular focus on developing programmes for newly diagnosed preschool children. The present chapter focuses on current evidence for the effectiveness of psychosocial interventions, but further information on a wide range of other interventions can be found at the Research Autism website (www. researchautism.net). The aim of this website, which is associated with the UK National Autistic Society, is to review the published evidence on interventions in popular use. Over 100 interventions are currently listed, and the quality of evidence (both favourable and unfavourable) is rated by independent experts. The website covers developmental, educational, psychological, pharmacological and 'alternative' or 'complimentary' therapies (e.g. pet therapies, special diets and vitamin supplements, and some potentially hazardous interventions such as chelation, testosterone regulation and hyperbaric oxygen).

Interventions for children with autism

There are a number of psychologically based interventions for which the evidence base is improving. These include interventions designed to enhance cognitive and behavioural functioning, and those that focus on the specific deficits associated with autism, particularly in the areas of communication and social skills.

Behavioural interventions

The effectiveness of behaviourally based strategies for children with autism was initially demonstrated in the 1960s, although the focus then was predominantly on the elimination of 'undesirable' behaviours, notably tantrums, aggression and self-injury, with frequent use of aversive procedures, including electric shock.

Throughout the 1970s, treatment was largely conducted on an in-patient hospital basis, often with very little involvement of the child's family. The procedures used to improve skills such as social interaction and communication were frequently highly prescriptive and inflexible, and took little account of individual factors such as the child's developmental level or the family situation. Over time, however, behavioural approaches have become more individually based, with parents now playing an integral role.

Applied behavioural analysis is a particular way of analysing the possible cause(s) of behavioural deficits or excesses and developing specific, behaviour-based strategies to treat them. Behavioural programmes typically involve a range of different strategies, with an emphasis on the reinforcement of desired behaviour. Two major components of these programmes, which have been extensively researched, are discrete trial training and pivotal response training. Discrete trial training focuses specifically on developing skills in a step-by-step manner (using chaining, shaping and fading techniques), systematic identification of reinforcers, continuous monitoring of progress, and generalisation to progressively less structured and more natural environments. Pivotal response training also aims to foster generalisation to the child's everyday environment and, as the name suggests, focuses on pivotal aspects of behaviour such as motivation and responsivity to multiple stimuli. It includes components such as child choice, turn-taking and other maintenance strategies, and makes use of naturalistic settings and teaching procedures to enhance language, play and social behaviour.

Early intensive behavioural intervention

The home-based preschool behavioural programme Early Intensive Behavioural Intervention (EIBI), also known as the UCLA Young Autism Project), exemplifies the most intensive use of behavioural techniques. It was developed by Lovaas (1987) for 2- to 6-year-old children with autism. Intervention involves at least 2 years of 40 hours per week therapy and necessitates the input of professional consultants and behavioural therapists as well as family members. Systematic reviews of interventions following the Lovaas model (Magiati *et al*, 2012) suggest that these programmes are generally more effective in improving cognitive and language skills than standard care or 'eclectic' interventions. However, the impact on adaptive behaviours or core symptoms of autism is limited, and in all EIBI studies there are some children who fail to improve. This has led to attempts to identify the characteristics of the children who do and do not respond to early intensive intervention. Although initial IQ and language ability (especially receptive language) show some relationship with outcome, the effect of other variables (e.g. age at onset of treatment and severity of autism) is much less consistent. Critics of these highly structured EIBI programmes – which in the UK can cost around £35 000–£40 000 per child – note the enormous amount of time, money and energy required by the families involved, the restricted curriculum and the limited range of outcome measures used. The fact that the children are taught mainly in a one-to-one setting at home, rather than learning with and from their peers, is a further issue of concern.

The Early Start Denver Model (ESDM)

Concerns about the limited scope of the Lovaas EIBI programmes have resulted in the emergence of treatment models that are broader and more developmental in scope. The Early Start Denver Model (ESDM), for example, although behaviourally based, focuses specifically on the interaction between the child and their social environment and its developers report significant gains on tests of IQ, language and adaptive behaviour (Dawson et al, 2010). There is even a suggestion, from very preliminary electroencephalogram (EEG) data, that the programme may 'normalise' brain activity (Dawson et al, 2012). However, not all children respond equally well to the programme, and research into the factors that appear to be related to progress indicates that pretreatment variables such as functional use of objects, imitation and goal-understanding appear to be better predictors than age, IQ, social attention or intensity of treatment (Vivanti et al, 2013).

Parent training in behavioural techniques

Although research on the ESDM programme suggests that the results are more limited when treatment is short-term and delivered by parents rather than expert therapists (Rogers et al, 2012), some other randomised controlled trials (RCTs) have reported positive effects of teaching parents how to apply behavioural techniques in the home setting. Thus, Jocelyn et al (1998) and Tonge et al (2006) recorded significant improvements in parents' mental health, knowledge of autism and perception of control, together with language gains in the children involved, after relatively short, low-intensity parent-training programmes. Roberts et al (2011) also found that improvements in children's language and adaptive behaviours and in parents' quality of life were greater in a group receiving parent training plus a centre-based programme for the children, than for families in an individualised home-based programme.

Communication-based programmes

Functional communication training

Despite the general effectiveness of behavioural approaches for children with autism, it has become increasingly evident that programmes with a specific emphasis on teaching speech have little impact, particularly for children with more severe receptive and expressive impairments (Howlin, 2006). Recent approaches therefore have focused on enhancing broader communicative abilities, rather than emphasising spoken language.

For example, techniques derived from applied behavioural analysis have been used to increase functional communication skills. Analysis of the underlying function of many so-called challenging behaviours indicates that these are frequently a reflection of children's very limited communication skills. Failure to understand what is going on around them and the inability to express their needs and feelings verbally leave many children with no effective means of communicating other than by actions, which may be aggressive or disruptive in nature. Systematic analysis of the communicative function of such behaviours and teaching the child to communicate the same needs but in a different and more acceptable way (e.g. using signs, gestures or electronic aids) has been shown in many single-case and case-series studies to reduce disruptive behaviours, while at the same time establishing more effective communication skills (Mancil, 2006).

Signing and picture systems

Although various signing and picture systems (e.g. Makaton language; Walker, 1976) have been developed over the years to improve the communication skills of non-verbal children with autism, the evidence base for these is generally weak. The one exception, which has been systematically evaluated in RCTs, is the Picture Exchange Communication System (PECS; Bondy & Frost, 1998), a picture-based approach to enhance communication and understanding. The programme follows a set sequence of stages, beginning with prompting the child to make requests and culminating in the child learning to comment spontaneously by verbal or non-verbal means.

Single-case and case-series studies have reported significant increases in spontaneous communication (verbal and non-verbal), improvements in social interaction and joint attention, and reductions in behavioural problems. Randomised controlled trials indicate rather more limited effects. For example, Howlin et al (2007) found that in classes where teachers had training and ongoing consultation in PECS, pupils with autism showed significant increases in their use of PECS in the classroom. However, there were no improvements in spoken language or scores on formal language tests and no changes in autism symptoms. Furthermore, treatment effects were not maintained when intervention ceased and consultancy visits were no longer provided. Yoder & Stone (2006) also reported some positive effects of PECS on spontaneous communication but again not all children responded equally well (individual responses to interventions are discussed below).

Improving social reciprocity and parent–child interactions

Several recent programmes designed to foster development in young children with autism have focused on facilitating parent–child communication. For example, in a large-scale multicentre RCT, the Preschool Autism Communication Trial (PACT), Green et al (2010) investigated the efficacy of a programme that focuses on parent–child synchrony. They found significant improvements in parental synchrony with their child, child initiations and parent–child shared attention. However, there were no significant changes in severity of autism symptoms or the child's behaviour in school.

The Hanen More Than Words programme also focuses on parent–child interaction, turn-taking and reciprocity (Hanen Centre, 2011). An initial study suggested that parents in the programme showed improved communication and coping skills, and a reduction in stress; children showed increased vocabulary and communication skills, and a reduction in behavioural problems (McConachie et al, 2005). However, a more recent trial (Carter et al, 2011) found no effects of the programme on parental responsivity or children's communication. Moreover, certain children, notably those with higher levels of object interest, made less progress in the programme than children in the non-treatment group.

The EarlyBird programme (National Autistic Society, 2013) is based on a format similar to More Than Words and is designed specifically to support parents in the period between diagnosis of autism and the child's transition to nursery or school. The focus is on helping parents to improve children's social communication skills, as well as providing guidance on how to develop effective management strategies. Although there are no independent evaluations of the effect of EarlyBird on children's development, parents report less stress and more positive perceptions of their child after participation in the programme.

Another intervention, again based on principles similar to those of More Than Words, is the Responsive Education and Prelinguistic Milieu Teaching (RPMT) technique (Yoder & Stone, 2006). This focuses on three main strategies for increasing language: helping parents to learn to follow the child's lead (because children learn best with things that interest them); increasing motivation to communicate (e.g. by placing desired objects just beyond reach); and using social games to provide natural reinforcement. The technique has been shown to have positive effects on joint attention, turn-taking and child initiations.

Programmes focusing on social and emotional competence and understanding

Several interventions have been developed to improve some of the more fundamental deficits associated with autism, notably those related to imagination, and social and emotional understanding. Most of these rely on case–control or case-series designs, although more RCTs are beginning to appear.

Joint attention and symbolic play

Deficits in these areas are among the earliest signs of developmental abnormality shown by young children with autism. In a series of RCTs, Kasari and colleagues (2006, 2008, 2010) evaluated the efficacy of short-term programmes to enhance joint attention or symbolic play in children as young as 21 months, many of whom were already receiving EIBI. Both approaches resulted in improvements in expressive language, but other changes were specific to the intervention received. Thus, children in the joint attention groups made most improvement in joint attention and initiation; those in the symbolic play groups made more gains in symbolic and interactive play.

Theory of mind

There are many different programmes designed to address the impairments in 'theory of mind' (ToM) that are characteristic of autism, and a number of RCTs (e.g. Begeer *et al*, 2011) have been carried out. However, although training appears to improve competence on tasks related to the specific aspects of ToM that are taught, generalisation to other domains is very limited. There is no evidence of improvements in day-to-day social functioning and no studies have examined the long-term effect of intervention (the longest follow-up studies are around 2 months). Furthermore, even when participants do demonstrate improvements on trained tasks, there is the question of whether success is achieved by routes very different from those involved in typical development. In other words, have the children truly improved their ability to 'mind read', or have they simply developed alternative strategies to solve the tasks presented to them?

Social skills

Strategies designed to help children with autism improve social competence and social understanding include social skills groups, peer training, social scripts, structured joint play activities and manualised programmes. Despite the widespread use of these strategies in clinical and educational settings, recent reviews (Begeer *et al*, 2011; Cappadocia & Weiss, 2011; Kasari & Patterson, 2012) highlight the methodological problems associated with research in this area. These include the lack of a universal definition of social skills, failure to specify primary outcome measures, the very wide range of procedures and participants involved, divergent theoretical backgrounds and the variety of settings. There is now a growing number of successful RCTs of social skills interventions, but the impact on functioning in real-life settings has still to be demonstrated.

Social stories

'Social stories' (Gray, 1995) are frequently used by teachers and clinicians to improve social performance and understanding. Social stories can involve various formats, but typically utilise simple, cartoon-type drawings to help even very young children with autism understand why they experience specific social problems, why other people react as they do and how behaviour might be modified in future. Although there are several positive accounts of efficacy, group sizes tend to be small, experimental controls are generally absent and, as with social skills training more generally, the evidence base remains limited. Two recent systematic reviews of social stories (Karkhaneh et al, 2010; Kokina & Kern, 2010) note the limitations of much research in this area and conclude that the effects, although often moderately positive, are variable. Issues such as generalisation and maintenance of treatment effects also need to be addressed. On the whole, social stories seem to be more effective when used to reduce inappropriate behaviours than to increase social skills and when used in general education settings.

General educational programmes

Although there are positive reports of the effects of many different specialist educational programmes, evidence from randomised or other well-controlled trials is very sparse and, as yet, there is no evidence that any one particular programme is superior to others. Comparisons of highly specialised behavioural programmes with non-specialist 'eclectic' educational provision generally indicate that the former are significantly more likely to result in greater progress in preschool children, but the findings are not consistent (Magiati et al, 2012).

Teaching and Education of Autistic and Related Communication-Handicapped Children (TEACCH)

This widely used programme combines developmental, educational and behavioural strategies to enhance communication and minimise behavioural problems (Schopler, 1997). There is a specific focus on environmental structure and predictability, minimal dependence on verbal instruction and maximum use of visual cues.

Although significant gains have been reported in child behaviour, adaptive skills, cognitive ability and parent satisfaction, with some generalisation to non-treatment settings, comparative studies are few, sample sizes small, and the results tend to be inconsistent. For example, Tsang *et al* (2007) compared the progress of 18 preschool children receiving TEACCH with that of a control group of 16 children in eclectic nursery education. After 6 months, the TEACCH group showed greater improvement in perception and motor skills, but no significant changes in IQ or communication; the control group showed greater improvement in daily living skills.

Learning Experiences and Alternative Program for Preschoolers and their Parents (LEAP)

This inclusive intervention model uses peer-mediated interventions, errorless learning, incidental teaching, pivotal response training and positive behaviour support. In a comparison of the full LEAP programme with its manual-only version, Strain & Bovey (2011) found that after 2 years, children in the full programme showed significantly greater improvements on measures of cognitive, language and social skills, problem behaviours and autism symptoms than controls. However, many teachers required almost the full 2-year training period to reach an adequate level of fidelity to the programme.

School-based EIBI

In a study in mainstream preschool and kindergarten settings, Eikeseth *et al* (2012) found that, after 2 years, children receiving EIBI had higher IQ and adaptive behaviour scores than children in eclectic programmes. Nevertheless, improvement in IQ was less than in some other EIBI studies, and it often proved difficult for teaching staff to achieve the recommended number of weekly intervention hours. Moreover, some staff required several months of training and in some schools there was opposition to the use of EIBI, leading to drop out from the programme.

Interventions for mental health problems

Cognitive–behavioural therapy

Young people with autism have a greatly increased risk of mental health difficulties, particularly anxiety and depression (Simonoff *et al*, 2008) and there is growing use of cognitive–behavioural strategies with this group. However, there is little information to indicate for which individuals CBT is likely to be most effective, or which CBT-based procedures are potentially most successful for young people with autism. To date, positive results are reported for difficulties related to anxiety, anger management and social problems (for a review see Moree & Davis, 2010) and there is also some evidence supporting mindfulness therapy for young people with autism and mental health problems (Singh *et al*, 2011). Nevertheless, there remains the question of how far techniques focusing on cognitions can be successfully adapted for use with individuals for whom abstraction, imagination and social/emotional understanding are fundamentally impaired. The question of whether cognitive–behavioural approaches can offer more than behavioural approaches requires far more research.

How to determine what works for whom

As is clear from the above, there is no evidence that any one type of intervention is consistently more effective than another for children with autism. The findings also indicate that the effects of an intervention are often relatively circumscribed. Thus, for example, programmes to improve non-verbal communication do just that – they do not tend to have a significant impact on verbal skills or broader cognitive functioning. Similarly, programmes with a focus on parent–child interactions tend to result in changes in the child at home with their parents, but there is little evidence of improvement in the child's functioning in other areas. It is important to note, too, that until relatively recently, almost all intervention studies have presented their findings in terms of group or average improvements and this frequently obscures individual differences in response to treatment.

The focus of recent research, therefore, has shifted from attempts to demonstrate that one programme is better than another – an unduly simplistic aim given the heterogeneity of autism – to attempts to identify factors that may predict which subgroups of children are most likely to respond to particular interventions. For example, within behavioural programmes, there is some indication that pivotal response training may be more successful for children who are making more social initiations pre-intervention (Koegel *et al*, 1999), whereas functional use of objects, imitation and goal understanding appear to be the best predictors of outcome among children receiving the ESDM programme (Vivanti *et al*, 2013). A study of the effects of an inclusive group educational programme for toddlers with autism revealed that those with low social avoidance at baseline made more gains than those with high social avoidance initially (Ingersoll *et al*, 2001). Another study explored the differential effects of training to enhance either joint attention or symbolic play (Kasari *et al*, 2008). Overall, joint attention training had a greater impact on expressive language than symbolic play training, and the effect was most significant for children with the lowest levels of language pre-treatment.

In a study comparing PECS with RPMT, although RPMT significantly enhanced turn-taking, joint attention and initiation, initiations only increased in children who already had some joint attention skills (Yoder & Stone, 2006). The RPMT technique also seemed to have greater effect when used by mothers who were more responsive to their children. Children exposed to PECS, on the other hand, showed an increase in requesting behaviour, although this effect was found only in children with initially low levels of initiation/joint interaction and higher levels of object exploration. In another RCT of PECS, children with poorer language and greater severity of autistic symptoms showed less response to training and little improvement in spontaneous communication compared with children with initially higher levels of expressive language (Gordon *et al*, 2011).

There are many unexplored factors (child, family and environmental) that may also have a major effect on outcome. For example, in the LEAP study (Strain & Bovey, 2011) neither child behaviour nor family socioeconomic status predicted outcome – what was most important was the fidelity with which teachers implemented the programme. There has been little systematic exploration of optimal methods for identifying variables that are most likely to moderate or mediate the effects of treatment. Furthermore, certain factors, such as functional use of objects, that seem to predict a positive outcome for some interventions (e.g. ESDM: Vivanti *et al*, 2013; RPMT: Yoder & Stone, 2006) appear to be associated with a negative outcome in others (e.g. More Than Words: Carter *et al*, 2011).

Evaluating treatment outcomes

Finally, there is the issue of how best to assess the success of an intervention. Many instruments commonly used to assess treatment outcomes were never designed to measure change, and recent studies (e.g. Dawson *et al*, 2010; Green *et al*, 2010) have failed to demonstrate significant improvements in core symptoms of autism measured by standard diagnostic instruments such as the Autism Diagnostic Observation Schedule (ADOS) and Autism Diagnostic Interview (ADI). Other research, particularly that involving EIBI, has focused on IQ, but even a statistically significant increase in IQ scores does not necessarily result in improvements in behaviour or practical day-to-day skills. Future outcome studies need to place greater emphasis on developing ecologically valid measures that more accurately reflect a child's ability to function successfully in the social environment.

Future directions

Autism is a complex and heterogeneous condition that has a pervasive effect on functioning from infancy through to adult life. The search for effective treatments has been ongoing for many decades, but recent reviews highlight the poor quality of much intervention research and the failure of any one treatment to demonstrate superiority over all others. There are concerns, too, that interventions proven to work in highly controlled experimental settings (efficacy trials) may prove less effective in real-life settings. It is also important to note that those interventions with a strong evidence base have been evaluated primarily with children and families from White, often middle-class, backgrounds; their effectiveness for ethnically diverse groups remains untested (Kasari & Patterson, 2012).

Nevertheless, it is clear that a variety of approaches, although not 'cures' for autism, can result in improvements in many areas, including communication, social functioning and behaviour. It is also evident that the effects of treatment are highly variable. Much larger intervention trials are now needed to explore the moderating and mediating variables that can help to predict individual, not just group, outcomes in response to any intervention and to avoid exposing children and families to treatments that, for them, are inappropriate or even deleterious.

Finally, it is important to recognise that autism persists throughout life. The types of intervention needed in early childhood (which focus mainly on behaviour and communication) may be very different from those required in adolescence or adulthood (when social, emotional and mental health problems may be of more concern). Thus, there is a need for provision that can both monitor and meet individuals' changing needs over the years, and that does not come to an abrupt end when they reach school-leaving age. There is currently little support to facilitate the transition from childhood to adulthood and the provision of specialised adult services for individuals with autism remains woefully inadequate. This is a major challenge for the future (Howlin *et al*, 2013).

References

Baird G, Simonoff E, Pickles A, *et al* (2006) Prevalence of disorders of the autism spectrum in a population cohort of children in South Thames: the Special Needs and Autism Project (SNAP). *Lancet*, **368**, 210–215.

Begeer S, Gevers C, Clifford P, *et al* (2011) Theory of Mind training in children with autism: a randomized controlled trial. *Journal of Autism and Developmental Disorders*, **41**, 997–1006.

Bondy AS, Frost LA (1998) The Picture Exchange Communication System. *Seminars in Speech and Language*, **19**, 373–389.

Cappadocia M, Weiss J (2011) Review of social skills training groups for youth with Asperger Syndrome and High Functioning Autism. *Research in Autism Spectrum Disorders*, **5**, 70–78.

Carter AS, Messinger DS, Stone WL, *et al* (2011) A randomized controlled trial of Hanen's 'More Than Words' in toddlers with early autism symptoms. *Journal of Child Psychology and Psychiatry*, **52**, 729–816.

Dawson G, Rogers S, Munson J, *et al* (2010) Randomized, controlled trial of an intervention for toddlers with autism: the Early Start Denver Model. *Pediatrics*, **125**, 17–23.

Dawson G, Jones EGH, Merkle K, *et al* (2012) Early behavioral intervention is associated with normalized brain activity in young children with autism. *Journal of the American Academy of Child & Adolescent Psychiatry*, **51**, 1150–1159.

Eikeseth S, Klintwall L, Jahr E, *et al* (2012) Outcome for children with autism receiving early and intensive behavioral intervention in mainstream preschool and kindergarten settings. *Research in Autism Spectrum Disorders*, **6**, 829–835.

Fountain C, King M, Bearman P (2011) Age of diagnosis for autism. *Journal of Epidemiology and Community Health*, **65**, 503–510.

Gordon K, Pasco G, McElduff F, *et al* (2011) A communication-based intervention for nonverbal children with autism: What changes? Who benefits? *Journal of Consulting and Clinical Psychology*, **79**, 447–457.

Gray C (1995) *My Social Stories Book*. Jessica Kingsley.

Green J, Charman T, McConachie H, *et al* (2010) Parent-mediated communication-focused treatment in children with autism (PACT): a randomised controlled trial. *Lancet*, **375**, 2152–2160.

Hanen Centre (2011) More Than Words® – The Hanen Program® for Parents of Children With Autism Spectrum Disorder. Hanen Centre (http://www.hanen.org/Programs/For-Parents/More-Than-Words.aspx). Accessed 15 August 2013.

Howlin P (2006) Augmentative and alternative communication systems for children with autism. In *Social and Communication Development in Autism Spectrum Disorders* (eds T Charman, W Stone), pp. 236–66. Guilford Press.

Howlin P, Gordon K, Pasco G, *et al* (2007) The effectiveness of Picture Exchange Communication System (PECS) training for teachers of children with autism: a pragmatic, group randomised controlled trial. *Journal of Child Psychology and Psychiatry*, **48**, 473–481.

Howlin P, Moss P, Savage S, *et al* (2013) Social outcomes in mid- to later adulthood among individuals diagnosed with autism and average nonverbal IQ as children. *Journal of the American Academy of Child & Adolescent Psychiatry*, **52**, 572–581.

Ingersoll B, Schreibman L, Stahmer A (2001) Brief report: differential treatment outcomes for children with autistic spectrum disorder based on level of peer social avoidance. *Journal of Autism and Developmental Disorders*, **31**, 343–349.

Jocelyn LJ, Casiro OG, Beattie D, *et al* (1998) Treatment of children with autism: a randomized controlled trial to evaluate a caregiver-based intervention program in community day-care centers. *Journal of Developmental Behavior and Pediatrics*, **19**, 26–34.

Karkhaneh M, Clark B, Ospina MB, *et al* (2010) Social stories to improve social skills with autism spectrum disorder: a systematic review. *Autism*, **14**, 641–662.

Kasari C, Patterson S (2012) Interventions addressing social impairment in autism. *Current Psychology Reports*, **14**, 713–725.

Kasari C, Freeman S, Paparella T (2006) Joint attention and symbolic play in young children with autism: a randomized controlled intervention study. *Journal of Child Psychology and Psychiatry*, **47**, 611–620.

Kasari C, Paparella T, Freeman S, *et al* (2008) Language outcome and autism: randomized comparison of joint attention and play interventions. *Journal of Consulting and Clinical Psychology*, **76**, 125–137.

Kasari C, Gulsrud C, Wong C, *et al* (2010) Randomized controlled caregiver mediated joint engagement intervention for toddlers with autism. *Journal of Autism and Developmental Disorders*, **10**, 1045–1056.

Koegel LK, Koegel RL, Shoshan Y, *et al* (1999) Pivotal response intervention. II: Preliminary long-term outcome data. *Journal of the Association for Persons with Severe Handicaps*, **24**, 186–198.

Kokina A, Kern L (2010) Social Story interventions for students with autism spectrum disorders: a meta-analysis. *Journal of Autism and Developmental Disorders*, **40**, 812–826.

Lovaas OI (1987) Behavioral treatment and normal educational and intellectual functioning in young autistic children. *Journal of Consulting and Clinical Psychology*, **55**, 3–9.

Magiati I, Tay XW, Howlin P (2012) Early comprehensive interventions for children with autism spectrum disorders: a critical synthesis of recent review findings. *Neuropsychiatry*, **2**, 543–570.

Mancil GR (2006) Functional communication training: a review of the literature related to children with autism. *Education and Training in Developmental Disabilities*, **41**, 213–224.

McConachie H, Randle V, Hammal D, *et al* (2005) A controlled trial of a training course for parents of children with suspected autism spectrum disorder. *Journal of Paediatrics*, **147**, 335–340.

Moree BN, Davis TE (2010) Cognitive-behavioral therapy for anxiety in children diagnosed with autism spectrum disorders: modification trends. *Research in Autism Spectrum Disorders*, **4**, 346–354.

National Autistic Society (2013) EarlyBird. NAS (http://www.autism.org.uk/earlybird). Accessed 15 Aug 2013.

Roberts J, Williams K, Carter M, *et al* (2011) Randomised controlled trial of two early intervention programs for young children with autism: centre-based with parent program and home-based. *Research in Autism Spectrum Disorders*, **5**, 1553–1566.

Rogers SJ, Estes A, Lord C, *et al* (2012) Effects of a brief Early Start Denver model (ESDM)-based parent intervention on toddlers at risk for autism spectrum disorders: a randomized controlled trial. *Journal of the American Academy of Child & Adolescent Psychiatry*, **51**, 1052–1065.

Schopler E (1997) Implementation of TEACCH philosophy. In *Handbook of Autism and Pervasive Developmental Disorders* (2nd edn) (eds DJ Cohen, FR Volkmar), pp. 767–798. John Wiley & Sons.

Simonoff E, Pickles A, Charman T, *et al* (2008) Psychiatric disorders in children with autism spectrum disorders: prevalence, comorbidity, and associated factors in a population-derived sample. *Journal of the American Academy of Child & Adolescent Psychiatry*, **47**, 921–929.

Singh NN, Lancioni GE, Singh AD, *et al* (2011) Adolescents with Asperger syndrome can use a mindfulness-based strategy to control their aggressive behavior. *Research in Autism Spectrum Disorders*, **5**, 1103–1109.

Strain, P. S & Bovey, E. H (2011) Randomized, controlled trial of the LEAP model of early intervention for young children with Autism Spectrum Disorders. *Topics in Early Childhood Special Education*, **31**, 133–154.

Tonge B, Brereton A, Kiomall M, *et al* (2006) Effects on parental mental health of an education and skills training program for parents of young children with autism: a randomized controlled trial. *Journal of the American Academy of Child & Adolescent Psychiatry*, **45**, 561–569.

Tsang SKM, Shek DTL, Lam LI, *et al* (2007) Brief report: application of the TEACCH program on Chinese pre-school children: does culture make a difference? *Journal of Autism and Developmental Disorders*, **37**, 390–396.

Vivanti G, Dissanayake C, Zierhut C, *et al* (2013) Brief report: predictors of outcomes in the Early Start Denver Model delivered in a group setting. *Journal of Autism and Developmental Disorders*, **43**, 1717–1724.

Walker M (1976) *Manual of Language Programmes for Use with the Revised Makaton Vocabulary*. Makaton Charity.

Yoder PJ, Stone WL (2006) A randomized comparison of the effect of two pre-linguistic communication interventions on the acquisition of spoken communication in preschoolers with autism spectrum disorders. *Journal of Speech and Language Hearing Research*, **49**, 698–711.

CHAPTER 15

Attention-deficit hyperactivity disorder: assessment and treatment[†]

Peter Hill

Attention-deficit hyperactivity disorder (ADHD) is a heterogeneous neurobehavioural syndrome with a multifactorial aetiology, present since early childhood and commonly having other conditions comorbid with it. The essential components are extreme and impairing inattention, hyperactivity and impulsivity. It is four times more common in boys, so the male pronoun is used in this chapter.

In the UK, the syndrome is recognised as equivalent to the combined presentation type of ADHD in the American DSM-5 (American Psychiatric Association, 2013). This comprises both hyperactive/impulsive and inattentive symptoms. In the USA, additional DSM-5 subtypes of predominantly inattentive presentation and predominantly hyperactive/impulsive presentation are recognised, but this practice is less prevalent in the UK, although the unofficial term 'attention-deficit disorder' (equivalent to ADHD – predominantly inattentive presentation) is used in some educational documents. The standards for UK diagnostic practice are often more stringently applied than in the USA, and generally correspond to the ICD-10 criteria for hyperkinetic disorder, which is essentially a severe form of combined ADHD (World Health Organization, 1992). The UK prevalence rate for combined ADHD is just under 5%, at 3–4% in boys and just under 1% in girls (Ford *et al*, 2003). The overall UK rate for hyperkinetic disorder is about 1.5%, with a similar male excess (Meltzer *et al*, 2000). There is widespread underdiagnosis.

Inattention is a broad concept that refers not just to difficulties in focusing and sustaining attention but includes vulnerability to distraction and poor self-organisation. This results in careless mistakes and a failure to follow through satisfactorily on set tasks, particularly if these contain cognitive demands. Typically, tasks are left unfinished, and the affected individual is likely to be demonstrably distractible.

[†]This is a revision of a 1996 article by Mary Cameron and Peter Hill. Mary Cameron died at a young age and this revision is dedicated to her memory.

Hyperactivity refers to a general increase in the tempo and amount of apparently purposeful but ineffectual activity, as well as an increase in the number of purposeless, minor movements (fidgeting) or whole-body movements (restlessness). It includes excessive talkativeness and noisiness.

Impulsiveness is characterised by sudden unconsidered actions: repeatedly interrupting others, blurting out answers prematurely in class, failure to wait for one's turn and butting into other people's activities. It commonly has a quality of impatient social disinhibition. In some individuals it is mainly evident in reckless behaviour; things are done suddenly without heed for danger or adverse consequences.

Current UK practice does not usually recognise hyperactive/impulsive presentation subtypes, thus conforming more to ICD-10 criteria, and takes the threshold for clinical diagnosis of ADHD to be at least six items on each of the two axes of inattention and hyperactivity/impulsivity (Box 15.1).

Box 15.1   Attention-deficit hyperactivity disorder items in DSM-5

Inattention

- Careless with detail
- Fails to sustain attention
- Appears not to listen
- Does not finish instructed tasks
- Has poor self-organisation
- Avoids tasks requiring sustained mental effort
- Loses things
- Is easily distracted
- Seems forgetful

Hyperactivity/impulsivity

- Fidgets
- Leaves seat when should be seated
- Runs/climbs excessively and inappropriately
- Noisy in play
- Shows persistent motor overactivity unmodified by social context
- Blurts out answers before question completed
- Fails to wait turn or in queue
- Interrupts others' conversation or games
- Talks excessively for social context

For combined-type ADHD, at least six items from each of the above lists must:

- all occur 'often'
- be pervasive (present in more than one type of situation)
- be present from an early age (below 6 years)
- impair the child's normal functioning
- not be better explained by another condition.

(After American Psychiatric Association, 2013)

These must be:

(a) excessive compared with what is normal for a child of that age or developmental ability

(b) present from an early age (less than 7 years)

(c) pervasive, i.e. present in more than one type of social situation; they will be most obvious when self-control is required or when cognitively demanding tasks are set

(d) associated with impaired personal function.

It is apparent that elements of inattention, hyperactivity and impulsivity exist in the general population, so that the clinical syndrome of ADHD represents an extreme the end of a spectrum of normal variation. It can be conceptualised as a categorical condition by the application of diagnostic rules, but it is not qualitatively distinct from such variation.

It is difficult to diagnose ADHD with confidence in preschool children as preschool hyperactivity does not necessarily persist into the school years. Furthermore, it may not be easy for first-time parents to distinguish normal childhood exuberance and brief but developmentally appropriate attention spans from clinically significant variation. Preschool children may not spend enough time in social situations outside the home for pervasiveness of symptoms and impairment to be established.

Neurobiology

A large number of imaging studies have shown abnormalities in brain structure and functioning in children with ADHD (Rubia, 2012). These include reduced volumes of:

- frontal and parietotemporal cortex
- basal ganglia
- splenium of the corpus callosum
- cerebellum.

This is almost certainly due to delayed maturation, estimated as a 2-year delay. Some recent longitudinal studies noted by Rubia show that these volume deficits can be corrected over time by stimulant medication. Diffusion tensor imaging work indicates an additional widespread deficit in white matter interconnectivity. In parallel with this, functional magnetic resonance imaging (fMRI) studies have shown repeatedly that there is underfunctioning of frontostriatal pathways and underactivation of several prefrontal cortical areas, consistent with the reduced cognitive executive functioning found in neuropsychological research. In other words, a wider deficit in motivational and inhibitory networks has been identified. The emerging picture is of a generally underconnected and underfunctioning immature brain as far as higher attentional, social and affective functioning are concerned.

None of these findings, although replicated, are yet useful in clinical diagnostic practice and there is no place for routine imaging. Nevertheless, illustrations from the studies are of great interest to parents and children.

Assessment

The aims of assessment are:

- confirmation of clinical features of ADHD and establishing their level of severity across more than one setting (e.g. home and school)
- evaluating impairment: social, educational and emotional
- exclusion of differential diagnoses (anxiety, intellectual disability)
- detection of comorbid disorders and problems
- elucidation of aetiological risk factors thought to maintain the clinical picture
- physical appraisal of cardiovascular fitness and growth status
- evaluation of parental attitudes to the child and to treatment.

Before clinical contact: children and school-age teenagers

Parent- or teacher-completed rating scales can be used to identify individuals for a specialist clinic and to focus questioning at an initial appointment. It is possible to screen using the parent-scored Strengths and Difficulties Questionnaire (SDQ) (Goodman, 1997). Although a score of 7 from the sum of items 2, 10, 15, 21 and 25 has been used to identify probable cases of ADHD in epidemiological studies, there may be advantages in using a lower score (5 or 6), since a false-positive rate will matter less when selecting individuals for clinical assessment.

Questionnaires specifically focused on ADHD, such as the Conners 3 (Conners, 2008) or the CADDRA ADHD Checklist (Canadian ADHD Resource Alliance, 2011), can mislead because wording such as 'often' (derived from DSM-IV-TR: American Psychiatric Association, 2000) can be interpreted variously. It may be better to use them in clinic (for pretreatment baseline measures), when such wording can be clarified at interview. Rating scale scores alone are insufficient for diagnosis.

Although a school report or questionnaire collected before a first appointment can save time with primary school children, with secondary school children it is wise to wait until the child is seen to clarify which teacher is best placed to be approached.

Assessment process at a first appointment

Assessment is a clinical procedure. There is no need for routine investigations such as brain scans, electroencephalograms (EEGs) or electrocardiograms (ECGs). A few centres use computerised tools such as the QbTest (Vogt & Williams, 2011) or a qualitative EEG, but as things stand these cannot substitute for clinical judgement.

Interview with parent(s)

It is inadequate merely to check key items for a diagnosis of ADHD, since comorbidity and differential diagnoses will be missed. A preferable approach is to take a history of presenting problems and check through other behavioural systems and emotions in the standard way. Follow with a developmental history and a family history (especially for ADHD and cardiac morbidity in early adult life). While facts are being elicited, consider family atmosphere and attitudes to the child, ADHD and medication.

Specific questioning on the following may reveal aetiological, intensifying or perpetuating risk factors, each of which will only apply to some children:

- features of ADHD in relatives (including parents)
- mother's alcohol, nicotine or illicit drug intake during pregnancy
- early birth or low birth weight
- failure to regain birth weight in the first 2 weeks of life
- adoption after 6 months
- early exposure to environmental lead
- early closed head injury with sustained loss of consciousness
- persistent lack of sleep
- dietary problems
- ongoing family discord.

It makes sense to take an educational history: schools attended, levels of attainment, disciplinary problems and friendships.

Parents should be asked to complete a rating scale such as the Conners 3-P (Conners, 2008) or SNAP-IV-C (Swanson, 2007). Adolescents can complete the self-report Conners 3-SR (Conners, 2008).

Box 15.2 Dyspraxia screen

- Static tremor (outstretched arms and fingers)
- Static balance (standing on one leg for 20 seconds)
- Normal walking and running
- Heel–toe (tight-rope) walk
- Modified Fog's test (walking on the medial sides of the feet with knees apart, then on the lateral sides with knees together): check for dystonic wrist and arm movements
- Finger–nose test
- Thumb to each fingertip in rapid sequence
- Rapid alternating rotation at wrists ('polish a round doorknob') with outstretched arm
- Joint mobility in fingers, thumbs, elbows and knees, and check for flat feet
- Writing their own name and address
- Drawing a man

Observation and physical examination of the child

A child with ADHD may be attentive and self-contained during a very brief individual interview. Observing the child during an interview with the parents as well as seeing the child alone provides a total of at least an hour's worth of sustained observation and much can be learnt from this.

Constructional toys are useful: give an instruction to build something and then look for completion and persistence, as well as coordination. Any clues from the parental account that might indicate dyspraxia should lead to a brief physical examination (Box 15.2).

Check hearing by speaking a number softly but with just a little resonance at 1 metre distance on each side. Listening to speech and assessing compliance with instructions screens for speech and language problems. A husky voice can indicate vocal abuse from excessive talkativeness.

It is wise to check for weak auditory short-term and working memory, since this is a common associated impairment and may be the only factor in purely inattentive ADHD. This can be done quickly using a digit span test (a random sequence of numbers spoken at a rate of one per second). Norms are given in Table 15.1.

Because stimulants can (rarely) slow growth, it is important to record and chart baseline height and weight. Stimulants, and occasionally atomoxetine, can produce an elevation of blood pressure and tachycardia. It is therefore necessary to carry out a clinical examination of the cardiovascular system.

A detailed neurological examination is not likely to yield much of significance, but it can reassure parents, particularly if they raise the topic of brain damage. Watch the child as he leaves the room, since this is the time when tics are likely to be most evident, having been voluntarily suppressed during the assessment.

Interview with an older child or teenager

Even a brief interview with the young person provides an opportunity to learn further about family, peer group and school life. There may be antisocial activities and risky behaviours such as unprotected sex or substance misuse that are unknown to parents.

Table 15.1 Norms for digit span recall

Age, years	Number of digits successfully recalled	
	Forwards	Backwards
6	5	3
10	6	4
14	7	5

Further information

It is crucial to obtain a school report and rating scale to confirm pervasiveness of symptoms. The Conners 3 (Conners, 2008) offers broad scope for an initial assessment and includes the 10-item Conners ADHD Index (Conners 3AI), which is convenient for follow-up by teachers or parents. Some clinicians like to use the SKAMP (items 81–90 of the 90-item SNAP-IV-C; Swanson 2007) for teacher follow-up because of its face validity. Some estimation of academic achievement is needed to evaluate impairment, detect possible comorbid dyslexia, and provide a baseline for assessing treatment impact.

Differential diagnosis

Simple misbehaviour

Marked, but age- (or mental age-) appropriate boisterousness, disobedience or cheekiness is the most common differential. The central issue is whether this is excessive for the child's age or developmental level. Teachers are in an excellent position to make this comparison through daily experience of observing the child in a group of children his own age. Explosive temper or excitability are often referred to by parents or peers as 'being a bit hyper'. Rating scales will help clarification.

Disruptive behaviour disorders

Oppositional-defiant disorder and conduct disorder may be differential diagnoses as well as comorbid conditions, since restlessness and inattention are common among disruptive children generally. Furthermore, there has been a long history of professionals placing more emphasis on diagnosing these conditions, which has led to a view of ADHD as essentially an antisocial, angry condition. The diagnosis of conduct disorder requires repetitive, persistent and serious antisocial, aggressive or defiant behaviour. In practice, the distinction between ADHD and disruptive behaviour disorders can be difficult to make because of comorbidity.

Disinhibited attachment disorder

Disinhibited attachment disorder can develop in children who have not had the opportunity to form selected secure emotional attachments because of the lack of sensitive or consistent parental care. Such children may present as distractible or restless, with attentional problems and social disinhibition. In some clinics, heated discussions arise as to whether inattentive restlessness is fundamentally ADHD or represents an attachment disorder. This is usually futile, as NICE recommends treating ADHD symptoms when these are present, irrespective of putative aetiology

(National Institute for Health and Clinical Excellence, 2008), and in any case both conditions may well be comorbid.

Generalised anxiety disorder

Generalised anxiety disorder can yield inattentiveness and restlessness, but social disinhibition and impulsiveness are less likely to be present.

Autism spectrum conditions

Mild autism spectrum conditions can present with inattentiveness and it can be difficult to separate inattention arising from a lack of interest in complying with another person's instructions from inattention as a component of ADHD.

Bipolar disorder

Juvenile bipolar disorder has historically been invoked as a differential diagnosis, but there should be no confusion if the requirement for a sustained period of elevated mood with associated grandiosity in bipolar disorder is maintained.

Comorbidity

All the disorders that need to be differentiated from ADHD can also be comorbid conditions. In addition to the above, the other conditions that are frequently encountered are listed in Box 15.3 and need to be considered in any clinical assessment.

Box 15.3 Conditions commonly comorbid with attention-deficit hyperactivity disorder

- Autism spectrum conditions
- Depression
- Disinhibited attachment disorder
- Dyscalculia
- Dyslexia
- Dyspraxia (developmental coordination disorder) and dysgraphia
- Generalised anxiety disorder
- Juvenile bipolar disorder
- Oppositional-defiant disorder/conduct disorder
- Sleep disorders
- Specific language impairment
- Substance misuse
- Tic disorders/Tourette syndrome

Impairment

For a diagnosis of ADHD it is necessary to go further than establishing the presence of characteristic symptoms; there must be documentation that impairment exists. This is not a single measure but should involve checking several domains of the individual's life. NICE recommends a helpful list (National Institute for Health and Clinical Excellence, 2008). The Weiss Impairment Scales, WFIRS-P for parents (Weiss *et al*, 2004) and the corresponding self-completed WFIRS-S for teenagers (Weiss, 2007), are useful instruments.

Tests

It is not necessary to carry out a full psychological assessment on each child unless there are major educational problems that need exploration. Blood tests (e.g. for iron, lead or thyroid function), brain imaging, EEGs and ECGs are similarly not routine, but should be considered on their merits in each case.

Formulation

Using parental information, school information, considering impairment and its impact, and one's own observations, it should now be possible to:

- establish a diagnosis of ADHD
- exclude alternative diagnoses
- identify comorbid problems and diagnoses.

Completing an ADHD-RS-IV at interview with the parents enables a measure of severity. The scale lists the diagnostic items shown in Box 15.1, worded to correspond to the text of DSM-5, and these are each rated 0–3 for frequency (rarely, sometimes, often, very often) by the interviewer so that the maximum possible score is 54. A readily available equivalent, the CADDRA ADHD Checklist (Canadian ADHD Resource Alliance, 2011) uses severity (not at all, somewhat, pretty much, very much) rather than frequency, with comparable scoring. Most children with ADHD seen in clinics will score higher than the mid-thirties.

In addition, it is particularly useful to ask for a short list of key problems that can be stated in language understandable by all family members and entered onto a simple linear or five-point scale. This may be the best way of identifying operationalised goals of treatment against which progress can be measured.

Treatment: general principles

As things stand in 2013, optimal treatment approaches in the UK follow the principles derived from the NICE guidelines (National Institute for

Health and Clinical Excellence, 2008) and include three components: psychoeducation, parental handling and medication. Although dietary treatments, neurofeedback and cognitive therapy may yield worthwhile advances in the future, their evidence base is small and they remain essentially experimental.

School-based measures include both those addressing behaviour and those promoting learning. There is a potential role for schools in promoting social competence through social skills groups of peers (which are hard to set up in clinics). Active liaison between clinic and school, usually through the special educational needs coordinator (SENCO), is crucial once parental permission is granted.

Psychoeducation

It is apparent from the VOICES study (Singh *et al*, 2012) that many children with diagnosed ADHD do not understand what it is. It also seems likely that parents, some teachers and some primary healthcare professionals are less well informed than would be desirable. Newspaper journalism and the internet are not always helpful. Discussion with both parents and child, and letters to or discussions with schools and primary healthcare, can make the following points.

- ADHD is at the extreme end of a spectrum of difficulties with attention, activity and impulse control in the general population.
- ADHD rarely exists on its own. Most children with ADHD will have other problems, such as difficulties with anger, socialisation, physical coordination, short-term memory or learning. What is seen as ADHD is often actually an associated oppositional-defiant or conduct disorder.
- ADHD is based on known neurological dysfunction that can be demonstrated in research even if this is not yet defined sufficiently to be useful in clinical practice. Pictures from fMRI studies are helpful in making this point.
- The brains of children with ADHD show about 2 years' delay in growth and development of the frontoparietal cortex.
- Research shows that a child with ADHD has particular problems with motivation ('allocating mental effort') and learning from experience.
- Medication can partially compensate for these shortcomings in brain development and motivational learning.
- It is helpful to see the ADHD as something that gets in the way of success ('His ADHD stops you being the sort of parent you want to be', 'The ADHD gets in the way of learning at school and he can't just turn it off').

Parental handling

Clinics may simply refer parents to parenting classes. This is broadly in line with NICE recommendations (National Institute for Health and Clinical

Excellence, 2008) but needs some thought. Parents who have brought up their child's older siblings successfully may feel (and be) patronised. It may be better to discuss two simple points with parents:

- a child with ADHD requires more than standard parenting if he is to learn and prosper
- it is particularly hard to be an effective parent of a child with ADHD, as the ADHD works against the child's ability to learn and the parent's sense of competence.

And recommend that they:

- set a small number of household rules, couched in language that is specific and understandable by all ('Schoolbag always packed before going to bed')
- get beyond simply trying to control disobedience, overexcitement or hyperactivity and set out to have opportunities for a good time with their child, showing him love and appreciation
- keep verbal instructions short and clear
- include positive comments, praise and encouragement, linked with a points incentive system where appropriate
- consider deals ('Get your homework done and OK'd by me, then you can go out'), but ensure that the child's action precedes the reward or the parent's half of the deal
- use a simple disciplinary system such as '1-2-3 Magic' (www.123magic.com)
- avoid harsh punishment, harsh judgements and condemnations
- keep the child's social life alive, but arrange brief play dates with structured activities to avoid overexcited mayhem or fights
- keep as calm as possible
- plan ahead to avoid trouble.

Families containing a child with ADHD need support from a local network if available or from the National Attention Deficit Disorder Information and Support Service (ADDISS). The strain on families is extensive, with parental depression, strained marital relationships and family break-up all common. Bear in mind that a child with ADHD is likely to have siblings and one or both parents who also have ADHD.

Medication

Stimulants (methylphenidate or dexamfetamine) are the mainstay of medication in ADHD, particularly following the initial findings of the Multimodal Treatment of Attention Deficit Hyperactivity Disorder (MTA) study (MTA Cooperative Group, 1999). They are highly effective (effect size 0.8–1.2) against all three symptom areas of ADHD, long-established (>50 years) and relatively safe. Methylphenidate is recommended by NICE as an initial agent (National Institute for Health and Clinical Excellence, 2008), although some individuals will respond better to dexamfetamine. Both competitively block the dopamine transporter which provides presynaptic reuptake of dopamine from the synapse.

A physical examination must be carried out before prescribing. Potential adverse effects on cardiovascular functioning (very mildly raised blood pressure and pulse rate) mean it is also necessary to check that there are no significant cardiac symptoms and no family history of sudden cardiac death in early adulthood.

Two single-dose trials of 5 and 10 mg of standard (immediate release) methylphenidate on separate days, each given 1 hour before an assigned task that involves simulated or actual schoolwork, with the effect observed by a parent, form a powerful and sensitive predictor of likely effect. Such trials can also identify the few children who become excited or irritable after taking the drug. The trial approach can subsequently be extended to school days, comparing morning and afternoon effects following a morning dose. The clinical duration of a single dose of methylphenidate is 3–4 hours.

There is no standard dose of methylphenidate or dexamfetamine, so it is necessary to titrate dose against effect. Simply obtaining a positive result is not good enough; one aims for an optimal result in terms of either general symptom relief or achievement against a specific goal.

An excessive dose produces a vacant expression and diminished social responsiveness. To avoid this it is important to obtain reports from school, since blood levels will be maximal there and have declined by return home.

Most children will move from immediate-release methylphenidate to extended-release preparations such as Equasym XL®, Medikinet XL® or Concerta XL®. These each have differing pharmacokinetic properties with differing release patterns across the day. It is important to track symptoms or deficits across the school day and choose the appropriate preparation accordingly.

Although it has been conventional for drug marketing authorisations ('licences') to cite a 60 mg maximum daily dose of methylphenidate, this has no scientific backing and in practice it is often necessary to exceed this. NICE makes the same point (National Institute for Health and Clinical Excellence, 2008).

Dexamfetamine can be tried in a similar fashion, using doses approximately half those required for methylphenidate. There are no extended-release preparations of dexamfetamine available in the UK, but the prodrug lisdexamfetamine provides extended effect for 12–13 hours following a single dose. It is inert when taken, but is converted into dexamfetamine by red blood cells.

Stimulant medication commonly suppresses appetite during the day. This is occasionally associated with slowing of weight growth and, less commonly, with slowing of height growth. Existing follow-up studies are weak, but do not show an effect on ultimate adult height. Nevertheless, height and weight should be monitored 6 monthly and the dose adjusted accordingly.

If stimulants are given too late in the day, there is the risk that sleep onset will be delayed. This can be dealt with by simple sleep hygiene advice or, if necessary, melatonin. Other side-effects include abdominal pain, headache and very rarely a skin rash or Raynaud's phenomenon. Some children feel socially constrained or suffer lowering of mood and, occasionally, irritability. Auditory hallucinations are rare and alarming but they do not endure once the medication is discontinued.

Children for whom school behaviour and achievement are the key problems do not necessarily need medication at weekends or holidays. In similar vein, the optimal dose regimen may differ from day to day. One treats for the day in question. There is no need to offer a 'course' of treatment or allow for accumulation, since stimulants are eliminated or metabolised on the day of administration. Occasionally it is necessary to increase the dose after a few months in order to maintain the effect, probably because of reactive upgrading of the dopamine transporter.

Stimulants are controlled drugs and not all general practitioners will prescribe them, in spite of NICE recommendations for shared care protocols between specialist clinics and primary care (National Institute for Health and Clinical Excellence, 2008). The introduction of specialist ADHD nurses, especially those who can prescribe, has been a major service development.

Children who are anxious, have tics or pre-existing sleep problems, or who need treatment that covers early mornings and evenings will probably need atomoxetine. This is a noradrenaline reuptake inhibitor with similar effects to stimulants, but it does not affect sleep onset, so can be given at night or twice daily. Its side-effect profile includes occasional nausea, irritability and low mood that reverse promptly on discontinuation. Side-effects can be minimised by gradually increasing the dose (starting with 10 mg daily for 7 days and increasing the daily dose by capsule size (18 mg, 25 mg, 40 mg, 60 mg, 80 mg, ...) each week when initiating. Dose is conventionally 1.2–1.8 mg/kg/day. Atomoxetine is not a controlled drug.

Treatment of hyperactive, disorganised or aggressive behaviour in the early morning or evening is hard to achieve with stimulants alone, and either a switch to atomoxetine or supplementation with clonidine should be considered if behavioural management techniques fail.

Treatment: assessing progress

If the symptom count (e.g. score on the ADHD-RS-IV) is very high and it is apparent that ADHD pervades most aspects of the child's life, then the impact of treatment can be titrated against an overall measure (e.g. the ADHD-RS-IV or Conners 3).

Yet there are instances when one or two specific issues caused by ADHD are key problems to be tackled, and in such cases a goal-setting approach makes sense. An individualised simple linear analogue or five-point scale can be constructed. For instance, a child may be repeatedly disciplined at school for calling out impulsively in class. A baseline frequency can be obtained and a simple scale constructed (e.g. called out more than once a lesson, once a lesson, twice a day, once a day, not at all) for an identified day in each week. Progress can be assessed against this in a way that is visible to child, parent and clinician.

Adherence to prescribed treatment is low, especially among teenagers.

Prognosis

A proportion of children will improve with maturation, but it is important to note that although hyperactivity wanes with age, impulsivity and inattention do so at a slower rate. Generally speaking, about 15% of children who show a full ADHD picture in late childhood will have a full diagnosis in early adult life, but 50% will show an attenuated picture characterised by troublesome inattentiveness, impulsiveness and personal disorganisation. Yet generally speaking, the impact of educational and social failure and the persistence of comorbid antisocial behaviours, alcohol and drug misuse, and high rates of mood disorders may be more of a problem in adult life than persisting symptoms or diagnosis of ADHD.

The NICE guideline recommends transition arrangements for teenagers with ADHD who are graduating to adult psychiatric services, specifically the use of the care programme approach and a full assessment following transition to determine comorbidity and impairment (National Institute for Health and Clinical Excellence, 2008). It is evident that local arrangements vary, from special adult ADHD clinics to absorption into generic mental health teams.

References

American Psychiatric Association (2000) *Diagnostic and Statistical Manual of Mental Disorders (4th Edn Text Revision) (DSM-IV-TR)*. American Psychiatric Association.

American Psychiatric Association (2013) *Diagnostic and Statistical Manual of Mental Disorders (5th edn) (DSM-5)*. APA.

Canadian ADHD Resource Alliance (2011) *ADHD Checklist*. CADDRA (http://caddra.ca/cms4/pdfs/caddraGuidelines2011ADHDChecklist.pdf). Accessed 22 Jan 2014.

Conners CK (2008) *Conners 3rd Edition (Conners 3)*. Multi-Health Systems.

Ford T, Goodman R, Meltzer H (2003) The British Child and Adolescent Mental Health Survey 1999: the prevalence of DSM-IV disorders. *Journal of the American Academy of Child & Adolescent Psychiatry*, **42**, 1203–1211.

Goodman R (1997) The Strengths and Difficulties Questionnaire: a research note. *Journal of Child Psychology and Psychiatry*, **38**, 581–586.

Meltzer H, Gatward R, Goodman R, *et al* (2000) *The Mental Health of Children and Adolescents in Great Britain*. TSO (The Stationery Office).

MTA Cooperative Group (1999) A 14-month randomized clinical trial of treatment strategies for attention-deficit/hyperactivity disorder. *Archives of General Psychiatry*, **56**, 1073–1086.

National Institute for Health and Clinical Excellence (2008) *Attention Deficit Hyperactivity Disorder: Diagnosis and Management of ADHD in Children, Young People and Adults* (NICE Clinical Guideline 72). NICE.

Rubia K (2012) ADHD: what have we learned from neuroimaging? *Cutting Edge Psychiatry in Practice*, **2**, 16–21.

Singh I, Baker L, Thomas K (2012) *Voices On Identity, Childhood, Ethics and Stimulants: Children Join the Debate (VOICES Final Report)*. ADHD VOICES.

Swanson J (2007) *The SNAP-IV Teacher and Parent Rating Scale*. University of California, Irvine.

Vogt C, Williams T (2011) Early identification of stimulant treatment responders, partial responders and non-responders using objective measures in children and adolescents with hyperkinetic disorder. *Child and Adolescent Mental Health*, **16**, 144–149.

Weiss M (2007) *Weiss Functional Impairment Rating Scale – Self Report (WFIRS-S)*. Canadian ADHD Resource Alliance.

Weiss M, Wasdell M, Bomben M (2004) *Weiss Functional Impairment Rating Scale – Parent Report (WFIRS-P)*. Canadian ADHD Resource Alliance.

World Health Organization (1992) *The ICD-10 Classification of Mental and Behavioural Disorders: Clinical Descriptions and Diagnostic Guidelines*. WHO.

CHAPTER 16

Schizophrenia

Chris Hollis

Schizophrenia is one of the most devastating psychiatric disorders to affect children and adolescents. Although extremely rare before the age of 10, the incidence of schizophrenia rises steadily through adolescence to reach its peak in early adult life. The clinical severity, impact on development and poor prognosis of child- and adolescent-onset schizophrenia reinforce the need for early detection, prompt diagnosis and effective treatment.

The current concept of schizophrenia in children and adolescents evolved from a different perspective held during much of the 20th century. Until the early 1970s, the term childhood schizophrenia was applied to children who would now be diagnosed with autism. Kolvin's landmark studies distinguished children with early-onset (autistic) symptoms beginning in the first 2 years of life from children with a relatively 'late-onset' psychosis with onset of symptoms after age 6 or 7, which closely resembled adult schizophrenia (Hollis, 2008). Importantly, in ICD-9 (1978) and DSM-III (1980) the separate category of childhood schizophrenia was removed, and the same diagnostic criteria for schizophrenia were applied across the age range. The validity of the diagnosis of schizophrenia in childhood and adolescence is supported by follow-up studies into adulthood that show a high level of diagnostic stability (Hollis, 2000).

This chapter focuses on children and young people who meet ICD-10 (World Health Organization, 1992) or DSM-5 (American Psychiatric Association, 2013) diagnostic criteria for schizophrenia. I use the term 'adolescent schizophrenia' as short-hand to refer to child and adolescent cases with onset up to 17 years of age. I examine evidence for continuities and discontinuities between adolescent schizophrenia and adult-onset schizophrenia in terms of aetiology, premorbid features, clinical presentation, course and outcome, and treatment response. My goal is to summarise what is currently known about adolescent schizophrenia and to indicate the extent and limitations of the evidence base for clinical diagnosis, management and treatment.

Epidemiology

Incidence and prevalence

Gillberg *et al* (1986) calculated age-specific prevalences for all psychoses (including schizophrenia, schizophreniform disorder, affective psychosis, atypical psychosis and drug psychoses) using Swedish case-register data on 13- to 18-year-olds with psychotic illnesses. In 41% of cases the diagnosis was schizophrenia. At 13 years of age, the prevalence for all psychoses in the general population was 0.9 per 10 000, showing a steady increase during adolescence, reaching a prevalence of 17.6 per 10 000 at age 18 years.

Gender ratio

Males are over-represented in many clinical studies of childhood-onset schizophrenia (Russell et al, 1989; Spencer & Campbell, 1994). However, other studies of predominantly adolescent-onset schizophrenia have described an equal gender ratio (Hollis, 2000).

Aetiology and risk factors

Genetics

Twin studies have suggested the heritability of schizophrenia to be as high as 83% (Cannon et al, 1998). However, one of the most significant implications of twin, adoption and family studies in schizophrenia is that they challenge the idea that what is inherited is a categorical psychiatric disorder. Similar to autism, genetic studies in schizophrenia have shown that the genetic liability to schizophrenia extends to schizotypal personality disorders and other conditions viewed as lying on the broader schizophrenia spectrum (Erlenmeyer-Kimling et al, 1995). These results suggest that what is inherited in schizophrenia is likely to be underlying neurodevelopmental and psychological traits that interact with environmental factors to determine liability to the disorder.

Candidate genes in childhood-onset schizophrenia

The National Institute of Mental Health (NIMH) study of childhood-onset schizophrenia has contributed much to the literature. It reported an association between two overlapping genes G70 and G32 on chromosome 13 (13q33.2) and childhood-onset schizophrenia (Addington et al, 2004). Another intriguing finding of the study is an association between the dysbindin-1 gene on chromosome 6 (DTNBP1 6p22.3) and poor premorbid social and academic adjustment (Rapoport et al, 2005). In addition, polymorphisms of the GAD1 (glutamic acid decarboxylase) gene have been associated with both childhood-onset schizophrenia and abnormal frontal grey matter loss (Addington et al, 2005). Finally, neuregulin 1 susceptibility haplotypes have been associated with abnormal developmental trajectories for both grey and white matter in this population (Addington et al, 2007).

Cytogenetic abnormalities

The NIMH study also revealed a high rate of previously undetected cytogenetic abnormalities, including velocardiofacial syndrome (VCFS) in

4 of the 80 young people (5%) involved (Sporn *et al*, 2004a). Velocardio-facial syndrome is associated with progressive cortical grey matter loss in children and adolescents who are not yet showing psychotic symptoms, suggesting that one or more genes mapping to chromosome region *22q11* is responsible for a high-risk phenotype (Sporn *et al*, 2004a). The overall high rate of various cytogenetic abnormalities (seen in 10% of the NIMH sample) suggests the possibility of more subtle genomic instability similar to that seen in autism (Rapoport *et al*, 2005). This idea is supported by the high rate of small structural deletions/duplications that disrupt genes seen in early-onset schizophrenia (Walsh *et al*, 2008).

Cannabis and schizophrenia

Acute intoxication with cannabis and other illicit substances, such as stimulants and hallucinogens, can precipitate psychotic symptoms or exacerbate existing psychotic illness. Cannabis confers an overall two-fold increased risk of later schizophrenia (Arseneault *et al*, 2004). In the Dunedin cohort, Arseneault *et al* (2002) showed that the association was strongest for the youngest cannabis users, with 10.3% of those who were using cannabis at 15 years of age developing schizophreniform disorder by the age of 26. So far, cannabis use has not been directly implicated in adolescent schizophrenia – possibly because of the relatively lower prevalence of cannabis use in younger adolescents and a short duration between exposure and psychotic outcome. However, cannabis use is associated with earlier age at onset of schizophrenia in adults (Arendt *et al*, 2005). Studies of gene–environment interaction (Caspi *et al*, 2005), taken together with human (Dean *et al*, 2003) and animal (Pistis *et al*, 2004) neuropharmacological studies, suggest that cannabis may enhance the risk of schizophrenia in vulnerable individuals during a critical period of adolescent brain development.

Neurobiology of schizophrenia

Structural brain abnormalities

The brain changes reported in childhood-onset schizophrenia appear to be very similar to those described in adult schizophrenia, supporting the idea of an underlying neurobiological continuity. Children with childhood-onset schizophrenia (onset at less than 13 years of age) in the NIMH study had smaller brains, with larger lateral ventricles and reduced prefrontal lobe volume, than healthy young people (Jacobsen & Rapoport, 1998). As in adult studies, reduced total cerebral volume is associated with negative symptoms of schizophrenia (Alaghband-Rad *et al*, 1997). Childhood-onset patients have a higher rate of developmental brain abnormalities than controls, including an increased frequency of cavum septum pellucidum (Nopoulos *et al*, 1998). In patients with adolescent schizophrenia there is evidence of ventricular enlargement and reduced volume of the prefrontal cortex and thalamus (James *et al*, 2004).

Progressive brain changes

Longitudinal imaging studies in adolescent schizophrenia show a fourfold greater reduction in cortical volume than in healthy adolescents (Rapoport *et al*, 1999). Most strikingly, the pattern of the exaggerated grey matter loss is identical to the pattern of normal development, suggesting amplification of a normal developmental process (Rapoport & Gogtay, 2007). Progressive changes appear to be time-limited to adolescence, and the rate of volume reduction in frontal and temporal structures is associated with premorbid developmental impairment and baseline symptom severity, declining as individuals reach adult life (Giedd *et al*, 1999).

The clinical phases of schizophrenia

Premorbid social and developmental impairments

Adolescent schizophrenia is associated with poor premorbid functioning and early developmental delays (Alaghband-Rad *et al*, 1995; Hollis, 1995, 2003). Similar types of developmental and social impairments in childhood have been reported in adult-onset schizophrenia, but premorbid impairments appear to be more common and severe in adolescent schizophrenia. In the Maudsley study of adolescent schizophrenia (Hollis, 2003) significant early delays were particularly common in the areas of language (20%), reading (30%) and bladder control (36%). A consistent characteristic in the premorbid phenotype is impaired sociability, with about a third of individuals with adolescent schizophrenia having significant premorbid difficulties in social development affecting the ability to make and keep friends.

Premorbid IQ in adolescent schizophrenia is reduced and lower than in adult schizophrenia (Alaghband-Rad *et al*, 1995; Hollis, 2000). In about a third of child- and adolescent-onset cases, the young person has an IQ below 70, with the whole distribution of IQ shifted down compared with both adolescent affective psychoses and adult schizophrenia.

Premorbid psychopathology

A diverse range of clinical diagnoses, including attention-deficit hyperactivity disorder (ADHD), conduct disorder, anxiety, depression and autism spectrum disorders, may precede the diagnosis of schizophrenia in children and adolescents (Schaeffer & Ross, 2002). However, there is a lack of any specific premorbid diagnosis that could practically aid early clinical identification of those at high risk of schizophrenia. A more promising line of research has demonstrated a strong link between self-reported psychotic symptoms in childhood and later schizophrenia (Poulton *et al*, 2000). In the Dunedin cohort study, psychotic symptoms at age 11 increased the risk of schizophreniform disorder at age 26 but not of other psychiatric diagnoses. Relative to the rest of the cohort, those identified at age 11 with 'strong' psychotic symptoms also had significant impairments in motor development, receptive language and IQ (Cannon *et al*, 2002). Although none of these individuals met criteria for a diagnosis of schizophrenia during adolescence, it appears that isolated or attenuated psychotic symptoms, in combination with pan-developmental impairment, constitute a significant high-risk premorbid phenotype.

Is it possible to identify young people 'at risk' of psychosis and schizophrenia?

Research has examined the feasibility of detecting and treating young people in the 'at-risk' stage, prior to the development of psychosis. This approach rests on three assumptions:

1 it is possible to detect such people
2 these people will be at markedly increased risk of later psychosis
3 an effective intervention will reduce this risk.

There is evidence to support assumptions 1 and 2 in people with a strong family history of psychosis, who are therefore at high genetic risk (Miller *et al*, 2001), and in those reporting particular perceptual abnormalities (Klosterkotter *et al*, 2001).

Various criteria have been developed in an attempt to identify a 'high-risk' phenotype. Features typically include: transient or attenuated psychotic symptoms; a decline in psychosocial functioning; and enhanced familial risk of psychosis. Early studies conducted in specialist centres suggested that up to 50% of 'high-risk' individuals made the transition to a firm diagnosis of a psychotic disorder within 12 months (Yung *et al*, 2003). However, more recent studies suggest that transition rates are considerably lower, at 10–15% (Fusar-Poli *et al*, 2012), and that the 'high-risk' phenotype is clinically heterogeneous and unstable over time (van Os & Murray, 2013). Mood disorder and substance misuse are particularly prevalent in these samples. Given the low rate of transition to frank psychosis in these help-seeking and functionally impaired individuals, treating the presenting problems (e.g. depression, substance misuse and paranoia) may be a more sensible strategy than intervening with the primary purpose of preventing the onset of psychosis.

Prodromal symptoms and onset of psychosis

Before the onset of psychosis, young people typically enter a prodromal phase characterised by a gradual but marked decline in social and academic functioning that precedes active psychotic symptoms. An insidious deterioration prior to the onset of psychosis is typical of the presentation of adolescent schizophrenia, and is more common in schizophrenia than in affective psychoses (Hollis, 2008). Non-specific behavioural changes such as social withdrawal, declining school performance, and uncharacteristic and odd behaviour begin, on average, over a year before the onset of positive psychotic symptoms. In retrospect, it can be seen that these behavioural changes were often early negative symptoms, which had their onset well before positive symptoms such as hallucinations and delusions.

Early recognition of the disorder is difficult, as premorbid cognitive and social impairments gradually shade into prodromal symptoms before the onset of active psychotic symptoms. Prodromal symptoms can include odd ideas, eccentric interests, change in affect, and unusual or bizarre perceptual experiences. Although these features can also occur in schizotypal personality disorder and autism spectrum disorder, in a schizophrenic prodrome there is usually progression to more severe dysfunction.

Diagnosis of schizophrenia in children and adolescents

Clinical characteristics

Even if strict adult definitions of schizophrenia (DSM-5 or ICD-10) are applied, there are age-dependent variations in phenomenology. Adolescent schizophrenia is characterised by a more insidious onset, negative symptoms, greater disorganisation (incoherence of thought and disordered sense of self), hallucinations in different modalities and, for relatively fewer patients, systematised or persecutory delusions (Green *et al*, 1992).

A wide variety of anomalous perceptual experiences may occur at the onset of an episode of schizophrenia, leading to a sense of fear or puzzlement which may constitute a delusional mood and herald a full psychotic episode. These anomalous experiences may include the sense that familiar places and people and their reactions have changed in some subtle way. These experiences may result from a breakdown between perception and memory (of familiar places and people) and associated affective responses (salience given to these perceptions). For example, a young person at the onset of illness may study their reflection in the mirror for hours because it looks strangely unfamiliar, or misattribute threatening intent to an innocuous comment, or experience family members or friends as being unfamiliar, leading to a secondary delusional belief that they have been replaced by a double or alien. In summary, some clinical phenomena in schizophrenia can be understood in terms of a loss of normal contextualisation and coordination of cognitive and emotional processing.

Clinical assessment

The assessment of a child or adolescent with possible schizophrenia should include a detailed history, mental state and physical examinations and laboratory tests. A baseline psychometric assessment is also desirable. A detailed understanding of specific cognitive deficits in individual cases of adolescent schizophrenia can be particularly helpful in guiding education and rehabilitation. The neurological examination should focus on abnormal involuntary movements and other signs of extrapyramidal dysfunction.

Physical investigations

Physical investigations and laboratory tests in suspected cases of child- and adolescent-onset schizophrenia are listed in Table 16.1. It is usual to obtain a full blood count, liver and thyroid function tests and a drug screen (urine or hair analysis). The high yield of cytogenetic abnormalities reported in childhood-onset schizophrenia (Nicholson *et al*, 1999) suggests the value of cytogenetic testing, including karyotypying for sex chromosome aneuploidies and fluorescent *in situ* hybridisation (FISH) for 22q11.2 deletion syndrome (22q11DS or velocardiofacial syndrome).

Developmental issues in assessment

The child's cognitive level will influence their ability to understand and express complex psychotic symptoms such as passivity phenomena, thought alienation and hallucinations. In younger children, careful distinctions have to be made between developmental immaturity and psychopathology. For example, distinguishing true hallucinations from normal subjective phenomena like dreams and communication with imaginary friends may be difficult for younger children. Developmental maturation can also affect the spatial localisation of hallucinations. Internal localisation of hallucinations

Table 16.1 Physical investigations in child- and adolescent-onset psychoses

Investigation	Target disorder
Urine drug screen	Drug-related psychosis (amphetamines, ecstasy, cocaine, LSD and other psychoactive compounds)
Electroencephalogram (EEG)	Complex partial seizures/temporal lobe epilepsy
Magnetic resonance imaging (MRI) brain scan	Ventricular enlargement, structural brain anomalies (e.g. cavum septum pellucidum)
	Enlarged caudate (typical antipsychotics)
	Demyelination (metachromatic leukodystrophy)
	Hypodense basal ganglia (Wilson's disease)
Serum copper and ceruloplasmin	Wilson's disease
Urinary copper	
Arylsulphatase A (white blood cell)	Metachromatic leukodystrophy
Karyotyping/cytogentics (fluorescent *in situ* hybridisation (FISH))	Sex chromosome aneuploidies, velocardiofacial syndrome (22q11 microdeletion)

LSD, lysergic acid diethylamide.

is more common in younger children and makes these experiences more difficult to subjectively differentiate from inner speech or thoughts. Formal thought disorder may also appear very similar to the pattern of illogical thinking and loose associations seen in children with immature language development. Negative symptoms can appear very similar to non-psychotic language and social impairments, and can also be easily confused with anhedonia and depression.

Differential diagnosis

Psychotic symptoms in children and adolescents are diagnostically non-specific, occurring in a wide range of functional psychiatric and organic brain disorders. The differential diagnosis of children and adolescents with suspected schizophrenia is summarised in Box 16.1. Referral for a neurological opinion is recommended if neurodegenerative disorder is suspected (see below).

Affective, schizoaffective and 'atypical' psychoses

The high rate of positive psychotic symptoms found in adolescent-onset major depression and mania can lead to diagnostic confusion. Affective psychoses are most likely to be misdiagnosed as schizophrenia if a

---

Box 16.1 Differential diagnosis of schizophrenia in childhood and adolescence

Psychoses

Affective psychoses (bipolar/major depressive disorder)

Schizoaffective disorder

Atypical psychosis

Developmental disorders

Autism spectrum disorders (Asperger syndrome)

Developmental language disorder

Schizotypal personality disorder

Organic conditions

Drug-related psychosis (amphetamines, ecstasy, lysergic acid diethylamide (LSD), phencyclidine (PCP))

Complex partial seizures (temporal lobe epilepsy)

Wilson's disease

Metachromatic leukodystrophy

Schneiderian concept of schizophrenia is applied, with its emphasis on first-rank symptoms. Because significant affective symptoms also occur in about one-third of patients with first-episode schizophrenia, it may be impossible to make a definitive diagnosis on the basis of a single cross-sectional assessment. In DSM-5 the distinction between schizophrenia, schizoaffective disorder and affective psychoses is determined by the relative predominance and temporal overlap of psychotic symptoms (hallucinations and delusions) and affective symptoms (elevated or depressed mood). Given the difficulty in applying these rules with any precision, there is a need to identify other features to distinguish between schizophrenia and affective psychoses. Irrespective of the presence of affective symptoms, the most discriminating symptoms of schizophrenia are an insidious onset and the presence of negative symptoms (Hollis, 2008). Similarly, complete remission from a first psychotic episode within 6 months of onset is the best predictor of a diagnosis of affective psychosis (Hollis, 2008). Schizoaffective and atypical psychoses are diagnostic categories with low predictive validity and little longitudinal stability (Hollis, 2000).

Autism spectrum disorders

Some children with autism or Asperger syndrome have social and cognitive impairments that overlap closely with the premorbid phenotype described in schizophrenia. Furthermore, children on the autism spectrum can also develop psychotic symptoms in adolescence. In the NIMH childhood-onset schizophrenia sample, 19 individuals (25%) had a lifetime diagnosis of autism spectrum disorder; of these, 1 was diagnosed with autism, 2 with Asperger syndrome and 16 with pervasive developmental disorder not otherwise specified (PDD-NOS) (Sporn *et al*, 2004*b*). Although some children with autism spectrum disorders show a clear progression into classic schizophrenia, others show a more episodic pattern of psychotic symptoms without the progressive decline in social functioning and negative symptoms characteristic of adolescent schizophrenia.

Often it is only possible to distinguish between schizophrenia and an autism spectrum disorder by taking a careful developmental history that details the age at onset and pattern of autistic impairments in communication, social reciprocity and interests/behaviours.

Neurodegenerative disorders

Rare neurodegenerative disorders with onset in late childhood and adolescence can mimic schizophrenia. The most important examples are Wilson's disease (hepatolenticular degeneration) and metachromatic leukodystrophy. These disorders usually involve significant extrapyramidal symptoms (e.g. tremor, dystonia and bradykinesia) or other motor abnormalities (e.g. unsteady gait) and a progressive loss of skills (dementia) that can aid the distinction from schizophrenia. Suspicion of a neurodegenerative disorder is one of the clearest indications for brain magnetic resonance imaging (MRI) in adolescent psychoses. Adolescents with schizophrenia show relative reduction in grey matter and sparing of white matter. In contrast, metachromatic leukodystrophy is characterised by frontal and occipital white matter destruction and demyelination. In Wilson's disease, hypodense areas are seen in the basal ganglia, together with cortical atrophy and ventricular dilatation. The pathognomonic Kayser–Fleisher ring in Wilson's disease begins as a greenish-brown crescent-shaped deposit in the cornea above the pupil (this is most easily seen during slit lamp examination). In Wilson's disease there is increased urinary copper excretion, and reduced serum copper and serum ceruloplasmin levels. The biochemical marker for metachromatic leukodystrophy is reduced arylsulfatase-A (ASA) activity in white blood cells. This enzyme deficiency results in a deposition of excess sulfatides in many tissues, including the central nervous system.

Treatments

Pharmacological treatments

Because of the very small number of trials of antipsychotics conducted with child and adolescent patients, it is necessary to extrapolate most evidence on drug efficacy from studies in adults. However, it should be noted that children and adolescents show a greater sensitivity to a range of antipsychotic-related adverse events, including extrapyramidal side-effects (EPSE) and treatment resistance with traditional antipsychotics (Kumra et al, 1998), and weight gain, obesity and metabolic syndrome with atypical antipsychotics (de Hert et al, 2011).

Head-to-head comparisons of atypical and typical antipsychotics (e.g. risperidone v. olanzapine v. haloperidol) in adolescents with schizophrenia have reported similar efficacy against psychotic symptoms, but a differing profile of adverse effects (Sikich et al, 2008). These findings broadly replicate results from the NIMH-funded Clinical Antipsychotic Trials of Intervention Effectiveness (CATIE) pragmatic study that found no overall difference in effectiveness between typical and atypical antipsychotics in adults, whereas there were differences in tolerability and side-effect profiles (Lieberman et al, 2005). In younger patients (children and adolescents), EPSE are more common with haloperidol and high-dose risperidone than with olanzapine. Weight gain and obesity are most common with olanzapine, less common with risperidone and least common with haloperidol. Sedation is greater with olanzapine and haloperidol than with risperidone (Toren et al, 2004). Further evidence is emerging that children and adolescents experience more rapid and serious weight gain on olanzapine and risperidone than do adults (de Hert et al, 2011). Morbid obesity (body mass index BMI >90th percentile) is found in up to 50% of adolescents and young people chronically treated with atypical antipsychotics (Theisen et al, 2001). Complications of obesity include hyperglycaemia (type 2 diabetes), hyperlipidemia and hypercholesterolemia. It is recommended that dietary advice (reducing carbohydrate intake) combined with regular exercise should be prescribed before initiating antipsychotics in children and adolescents.

Baseline investigations and monitoring

Before starting treatment with antipsychotic medication a physical examination should include height, weight (BMI), cardiovascular examination, including pulse and blood pressure, and a neurological examination for evidence of abnormal movements. Baseline laboratory investigations include prolactin, fasting blood glucose and plasma lipids. Weight should be recorded weekly for the first 6 weeks on antipsychotic medication, repeated at 12 weeks and then every 6 months. Physical examination, laboratory investigations and review of adverse effects should be repeated 6 monthly while a young person is receiving antipsychotic medication (National Institute for Health and Clinical Excellence, 2013).

Summary

Choice of antipsychotic is determined largely by the profile of adverse effects, as most drugs, with the possible exception of clozapine, show similar efficacy. The growing awareness of the adverse effect profiles of different drugs and greater sensitivity to these effects in children and adolescents means that drug choice should be a collaborative exercise, tailored to the needs and preferences of the young person and their family.

Psychosocial interventions

Family interventions

Psychosocial family interventions have a number of principles in common. First, it is useful for families to understand schizophrenia as an illness, as patients are then less likely to be seen as responsible for their symptoms and behaviour. Second, the family is not implicated in the aetiology of the illness. Instead, the burden borne by the family in caring for a disturbed or severely impaired young person is acknowledged. Third, the intervention is offered as part of a broader multimodal package that includes drug treatment.

An important issue when working with parents of children and adolescents with schizophrenia is to recognise that the illness typically results in a bereavement process for the loss of their 'normal' child. Parents will often value a clear diagnosis of schizophrenia, as it can provide an explanation for previously unexplained perplexing and disturbed behaviour. Understanding schizophrenia as a disorder of the developing brain can also relieve feelings of guilt commonly expressed by parents and carers.

Cognitive–behavioural therapy

Cognitive–behavioural therapy (CBT) has been shown to improve the short-term (6-month) outcome of adults with schizophrenia who have antipsychotic-resistant positive symptoms (Turkington & Kingdon, 2000). The National Institute for Health and Care Excellence (NICE) clinical guideline recommends that children and young people with psychosis and schizophrenia should be offered family interventions and individual CBT in conjunction with antipsychotic medication (National Institute for Health and Clinical Excellence, 2013). This recommendation reflects extrapolation of evidence and guidance in adult schizophrenia, as direct evidence is currently lacking for the benefit of family interventions or CBT in adolescent schizophrenia.

Course and outcome

Short-term course

Adolescent schizophrenia characteristically runs a chronic course, with only a minority of cases making a full symptomatic recovery from the first psychotic episode. The Maudsley follow-up study (Hollis, 2008) found that only 12% of young people with schizophrenia admitted to hospital were in full remission on discharge, compared with 50% of those with affective psychoses. The short-term outcome of schizophrenia presenting in early life appears to be worse than that of a first episode in adulthood. If full recovery does occur, then it is most likely within the first 3 months of onset of psychosis. In the Maudsley study, adolescent-onset patients who were still psychotic after 6 months had only a 15% chance of achieving full remission, whereas over half of those who had active psychotic symptoms for less than 3 months made a full recovery (Hollis, 2008). The clinical implication is that the course over the first 6 months of illness is the best predictor of remission.

Long-term outcome

A number of long-term follow-up studies of child- and adolescent-onset schizophrenia all describe a typically chronic, unremitting long-term course, with severely impaired functioning in adult life (Hollis, 2008). However, the generally poor outcome of early-onset schizophrenia conceals considerable heterogeneity. In most studies, about one-fifth of young patients have a good outcome with only mild impairment, whereas at the other extreme about one-third are severely impaired, requiring intensive social and psychiatric support.

Prognostic factors

The predictors of poor outcome in adolescent-onset schizophrenia include premorbid social and cognitive impairments, a prolonged first psychotic episode, extended duration of untreated psychosis and the presence of negative symptoms (Hollis, 2008).

Organisation of treatment services

It is a paradox that patients with child- or adolescent-onset schizophrenia have the most severe form of the disorder, yet they often receive inadequate and poorly coordinated services. Possibly this is because the responsibility for schizophrenia is seen to lie with adult psychiatric services, which have a remit that typically does not extend to patients under 18 years of age. In the UK, services for adolescents with psychosis and schizophrenia are provided by community-based child and adolescent mental health services (CAMHS) or, in some areas, by early intervention in psychosis (EIP) teams, which provide services for young people from age 14 upwards. The NICE clinical guideline for psychosis and schizophrenia in children and young people recommends that the assessment of young people with psychosis in EIP services should include access to a psychiatrist with training in child and adolescent mental health (National Institute for Health and Clinical Excellence, 2013). However, there remain significant gaps in the provision of comprehensive services for adolescents with schizophrenia, including access to crisis and assertive outreach services and psychosocial interventions.

Conclusion

The past decade has seen a dramatic growth in our understanding of the clinical course and neurobiological underpinnings of adolescent schizophrenia. It is now clear that adult-based diagnostic criteria have validity in this age group and the disorder has clinical and neurobiological continuity with schizophrenia in adults. Adolescent schizophrenia is a severe variant of the adult disorder associated with greater premorbid impairment, a higher familial risk, and more severe clinical course and poorer outcome. The poor outcome of children and adolescents with schizophrenia has highlighted the need to target early and effective treatments and develop specialist services for this group.

References

Addington AM, Gornick M, Sporn AL, et al (2004) Polymorphisms in the 13q33.2 gene G72/G30 are associated with childhood-onset schizophrenia and psychosis not otherwise specified. Biological Psychiatry, 55, 976–980.

Addington AM, Gornick M, Duckworth J, et al (2005) GAD1 (2q31.1), which encodes glutamic acid decarboxylase (GAD67), is associated with childhood-onset schizophrenia and cortical gray matter loss. Molecular Psychiatry, 10, 581–588.

Addington AM, Gornick MC, Shaw P, et al (2007) Neuregulin 1 (8p12) and childhood-onset schizophrenia: susceptibility haplotypes for diagnosis and brain development trajectories. Molecular Psychiatry, 12, 195–205.

Alaghband-Rad J, McKenna K, Gordon CT, et al (1995) Childhood-onset schizophrenia: the severity of premorbid course. Journal of the American Academy of Child & Adolescent Psychiatry, 34, 1273–1283.

Alaghband-Rad J, Hamburger SD, Giedd J, *et al* (1997) Childhood-onset schizophrenia: biological markers in relation to clinical characteristics. *American Journal of Psychiatry*, **154**, 64–68.

American Psychiatric Association (2013) *Diagnostic and Statistical Manual of Mental Disorders (5th edn) (DSM-5)*. APA.

Arendt M, Rosenberg R, Foldager L, *et al* (2005) Cannabis-induced psychosis and subsequent schizophrenia-spectrum disorders: follow-up study of 535 incident cases. *British Journal of Psychiatry*, **187**, 510–515.

Arseneault L, Cannon M, Poulton R, *et al* (2002) Cannabis use in adolescence and risk for adult psychosis: longitudinal prospective study. *BMJ*, **325**, 1212–1213.

Arseneault L, Cannon M, Witton J, *et al* (2004) Causal association between cannabis and psychosis: examination of the evidence. *British Journal of Psychiatry*, **184**, 110–117.

Cannon M, Caspi A, Moffitt TE, *et al* (2002) Evidence for early childhood, pandevelopmental impairment specific to schizophreniform disorder: results from a longitudinal birth cohort. *Archives of General Psychiatry*, **59**, 449–456.

Cannon TD, Kaprio J, Lonnqvist J, *et al* (1998) The genetic epidemiology of schizophrenia in a Finnish twin cohort: a population-based modeling study. *Archives of General Psychiatry*, **55**, 67–74.

Caspi A, Moffitt TE, Cannon M, *et al* (2005) Moderation of the effect of adolescent-onset cannabis use on adult psychosis by a functional polymorphism in the catechol-O-methyltransferase gene: longitudinal evidence of a gene × environment interaction. *Biological Psychiatry*, **57**, 117–1127.

de Hert M, Dobbelaere M, Sheridan EM, *et al* (2011) Metabolic and endocrine adverse effects of second-generation antipsychotics in children and adolescents: a systematic review of randomized, placebo controlled trials and guidelines for clinical practice. *European Psychiatry*, **26**, 144–158.

Dean B, Bradbury R, Copolov DL (2003) Cannabis-sensitive dopaminergic markers in post mortem central nervous system: changes in schizophrenia. *Biological Psychiatry*, **53**, 585–592.

Erlenmeyer-Kimling L, Squires-Wheeler E, Adamo UH, *et al* (1995) The New York High Risk Project: psychoses and Cluster A personality disorders in offspring of schizophrenic parents at 23 years of follow-up. *Archives of General Psychiatry*, **52**, 857–865.

Fusar-Poli P, Bonoldi I, Yung AR, *et al* (2012) Predicting psychosis: meta-analysis of transition outcomes in individuals at high clinical risk. *Archives of General Psychiatry*, **69**, 220–229.

Giedd JN, Jefferies NO, Blumenthal J, *et al* (1999) Childhood-onset schizophrenia: progressive brain changes during adolescence. *Biological Psychiatry*, **46**, 892–898.

Gillberg C, Wahlstrom J, Forsman A, *et al* (1986) Teenage psychoses – epidemiology, classification and reduced optimality in the pre-, peri- and neonatal periods. *Journal of Child Psychology and Psychiatry*, **27**, 87–98.

Green W, Padron-Gayol M, Hardesty A, *et al* (1992) Schizophrenia with childhood onset: a phenomenological study of 38 cases. *Journal of the American Academy of Child & Adolescent Psychiatry*, **31**, 968–976.

Hollis C (1995) Child and adolescent (juvenile onset) schizophrenia: a case control study of premorbid developmental impairments. *British Journal of Psychiatry*, **166**, 489–495.

Hollis C (2000) The adult outcomes of child and adolescent-onset schizophrenia: diagnostic stability and predictive validity. *American Journal of Psychiatry*, **157**, 1652–1659.

Hollis C (2003) Developmental precursors of child- and adolescent-onset schizophrenia and affective psychoses: diagnostic specificity and continuity with symptom dimensions. *British Journal of Psychiatry*, **182**, 37–44.

Hollis C (2008) Schizophrenia and allied disorders. In *Rutter's Child and Adolescent Psychiatry* (5th edn) (eds M Rutter, D Bishop, D Pine, *et al*), pp. 737–758. Blackwell Publishing.

Jacobsen LK, Rapoport JL (1998) Research update. *Childhood-onset schizophrenia: implications for clinical and neurobiological research. Journal of Child Psychology and Psychiatry*, **39**, 101–113.

James ACD, Smith DM, Jayaloes JS (2004) Cerebellar, prefrontal cortex, and thalamic volumes over two time points in adolescent-onset schizophrenia. *American Journal of Psychiatry*, **161**, 1023–1029.

Klosterkotter J, Hellmich M, Steinmeyer EM, *et al* (2001) Diagnosing schizophrenia in the initial prodromal phase. *Archives of General Psychiatry*, **58**, 158–164.

Kumra S, Jacobsen LK, Lenane M, *et al* (1998) Case series: spectrum of neuroleptic-induced movement disorders and extrapyramidal side-effects in childhood-onset schizophrenia. *Journal of the American Academy of Child & Adolescent Psychiatry*, **37**, 221–227.

Lieberman JA, Stroup TS, McEvoy JP, *et al* (2005) Effectiveness of antipsychotic drugs in patients with chronic schizophrenia. *New England Journal of Medicine*, **353**, 1209–1223.

Miller P, Lawrie SM, Hodges A, *et al* (2001) Genetic liability, illicit drug use, life stress and psychotic symptoms: preliminary findings from the Edinburgh study of people at high risk for schizophrenia. *Social Psychiatry and Psychiatric Epidemiology*, **36**, 338–342.

National Institute for Health and Clinical Excellence (2013) *Psychosis and Schizophrenia in Children and Young People: Recognition and Management* (NICE Clinical Guideline 155). NICE.

Nicholson RM, Giedd JN, Lenane M, *et al* (1999) Clinical and neurobiological correlates of cytogenetic abnormalities in childhood-onset schizophrenia. *American Journal of Psychiatry*, **156**, 1575–1579.

Nopoulos PC, Giedd JN, Andreasen NC, *et al* (1998) Frequency and severity of enlarged septi pellucidi in childhood-onset schizophrenia. *American Journal of Psychiatry*, **155**, 1074–1079.

Pistis M, Perra S, Pillolla G, *et al* (2004) Adolescent exposure to cannabinoids induces long-lasting changes in the response to drugs of abuse of rat midbrain dopamine neurons. *Biological Psychiatry*, **56**, 86–94.

Poulton R, Caspi A, Moffitt TE, *et al* (2000) Children's self-reported psychotic symptoms and adult schizophreniform disorder: a 15-year longitudinal study. *Archives of General Psychiatry*, **57**, 1053–1058.

Rapoport JL, Gogtay N (2007) Brain neuroplasticity in healthy, hyperactive and psychotic children: insights from neuroimaging. *Neuropsychopharmacology Reviews*, **33**, 181–197.

Rapoport JL, Giedd J, Blumenthal J, *et al* (1999) Progressive cortical change during adolescence in childhood-onset schizophrenia: a longitudinal magnetic resonance imaging study. *Archives of General Psychiatry*, **56**, 649–654.

Rapoport JL, Addington AM, Frangou S (2005) The neurodevelopmental model of schizophrenia: update 2005. *Molecular Psychiatry*, **10**, 434–449.

Russell AT, Bott L, Sammons C (1989) The phenomena of schizophrenia occurring in childhood. *Journal of the American Academy of Child & Adolescent Psychiatry*, **28**, 399–407.

Schaeffer JL, Ross RG (2002) Childhood-onset schizophrenia: premorbid and prodromal diagnostic and treatment histories. *Journal of the American Academy of Child & Adolescent Psychiatry*, **41**, 538–545.

Sikich L, Frazier JA, McLellen J, *et al* (2008) Antipsychotics in early-onset schizophrenia and schizoaffective disorder: findings from The Early-Onset Schizophrenia Spectrum Disorders (TEOSS) study. *American Journal of Psychiatry*, **165**, 1420–1431.

Spencer EK, Campbell M (1994) Children with schizophrenia: diagnosis, phenomenology and pharmacotherapy. *Schizophrenia Bulletin*, **20**, 713–725.

Sporn AL, Addington AM, Reiss AL, *et al* (2004a) 22q11 deletion syndrome in childhood-onset schizophrenia: an update. *Molecular Psychiatry*, **9**, 225–226.

Sporn AL, Addington AM, Gogtay N, *et al* (2004b) Pervasive developmental disorder and childhood-onset schizophrenia: co-morbid disorder or phenotypic variant of a very early onset illness? *Biological Psychiatry*, **55**, 989–994.

Theisen FM, Linden A, Geller F, *et al* (2001) Prevalence of obesity in adolescent and young adult patients with and without schizophrenia and in relationship to antipsychotic medication. *Journal of Psychiatric Research*, **35**, 339–345.

Toren P, Ratner S, Laor N, *et al* (2004) Benefit–risk assessment of atypical antipsychotics in the treatment of schizophrenia and comorbid disorders in children and adolescents. *Drug Safety*, **27**, 1135–1156.

Turkington D, Kingdon D (2000) Cognitive–behavioural techniques for general psychiatrists in the management of patients with psychoses. *British Journal of Psychiatry*, **177**, 101–106.

van Os J, Murray R (2013) Can we identify and treat 'schizophrenia light" to prevent true psychotic illness? *BMJ*, **346**, f304, doi: 10.1136/bmj.f304.

Walsh T, McClellan JM, McCarthy SE, *et al* (2008) Rare structural variants disrupt multiple genes in neurodevelopmental pathways in schizophrenia. *Science*, **320**, 539–43.

World Health Organization (1992) *The ICD-10 Classification of Mental and Behavioural Disorders: Clinical Descriptions and Diagnostic Guidelines*. WHO.

Yung AR, Philips LJ, Yuen HP, *et al* (2003) Psychosis prediction: 12–month follow up of a high risk ('prodromal') group. *Schizophrenia Research*, **60**, 21–32.

CHAPTER 17

Tourette syndrome

Mary Robertson

Tourette syndrome is named after the French physician Georges Gilles de la Tourette. A complex neuropsychiatric disorder with onset in childhood, it is characterised by multiple motor tics and one or more vocal/phonic tics, lasting longer than a year (World Health Organization, 1992; American Psychiatric Association, 2013).

The impact of this disorder is significant and a plethora of studies by several groups have examined the quality of life (QoL) of young people who are affected by Tourette syndrome (Table 17.1). Despite different schedules, the results have been remarkably consistent, and also concordant with adult data, showing that people with Tourette syndrome have a reduced QoL compared with healthy individuals. Employment status, tic severity, as well as greater emotional and behavioural difficulties, obsessive–compulsive behaviours, obsessive–compulsive disorder (OCD), attention-deficit hyperactivity disorder (ADHD), anxiety and depression all adversely affect the QoL (Robertson, 2012); in addition, functional impairment is increased. Only two out of the eleven QoL studies (Bernard *et al*, 2009; Eddy *et al*, 2011*a*) did not find that tic severity affected QoL.

A Tourette-specific quality of life scale has now been validated (the Gilles de la Tourette Syndrome–Quality of Life scale (GTS-QOL; Cavanna *et al*, 2008) and a version for children and adolescents has been published in Italian (C&A-GTS-QOL; Cavanna *et al*, 2013*a*). Cavanna *et al* (1212) examined 46 young people with Tourette syndrome aged 6–16 years and reassessed them again 13 years later using the GTS-QOL. Tic severity, premonitory sensations and family history of Tourette syndrome were identified as childhood predictors of a poorer QoL in adulthood, and tic severity adversely affected the physical, psychological and cognitive domains of QoL. Cavanna *et al* (2013*b*) compared child- and parent-reported QoL and everyday functioning in a group of 75 youngsters with Tourette syndrome. Although, somewhat surprisingly, no differences were found between young people who had Tourette syndrome only and young people who had Tourette syndrome and comorbid psychiatric disorders, there were differences in scores for total, school and home activities impairment. Furthermore, the parents and youngsters did not necessarily share similar views about the impact of Tourette syndrome on functioning.

Several studies have demonstrated that the parents of youngsters with Tourette syndrome have more difficulties than other parents. In

Table 17.1 The effect of Tourette syndrome on the young person's quality of life (QoL)

Reference	Country	Sample size, n	Schedule/ questionnaire	Results	Factors associated with reduced QoL
Storch et al, 2007	USA	59	Self-report Parent report	QoL lower in Tourette's than in healthy controls; QoL higher in Tourette's than in psychiatric controls	Tic severity; probably also OCB/ OCD and ADHD
Bernard et al, 2009	USA	56	TACQOL	QoL relates primarily to comorbid ADHD and OCD; in ADHD inattentive symptoms associated with lower QoL	ADHD (inattention) Not tics
Cutler et al, 2009	UK	57	Self-report	QoL significantly lower in Tourette's than in healthy controls	Tic severity; ADHD; OCB
Pringsheim et al, 2009a	Canada	71	Child Health Questionnaire	Tourette's significantly affected only family activities domain Comorbid ADHD & OCD reduced QoL in all domains	ADHD symptom severity was most important predictor of reduced QoL
Hao et al, 2010	China	1335	PedsQL 4.0	Tourette's scored lower than controls on all	Not stated
Conelea et al, 2011	USA	232	HRQoL	Functional impairment in Tourette's	Tic severity; comorbid psychiatric conditions
Eddy et al, 2011a	UK & Italy	50	YQOL-R	Reduced QoL in Tourette's	Depression; OCD; ADHD Not tic severity
Eddy et al, 2011b	UK & Italy	50	YQOL-R	Reduced QoL in Tourette's	Tic severity; OCD; ADHD

(continued)

Table 17.1 *(Continued)*

Reference	Country	Sample size, *n*	Schedule/questionnaire	Results	Factors associated with reduced QoL
Yi *et al*, 2011	China	174	Subjective self-report	QoL lower in Tourette's than in healthy controls	QoL negatively related to age, course, symptom severity, total child behavioural problems; positively related to family active-cultural orientation
Cavanna *et al*, 2013*b*	Italy	75	C&A-GTS-QOL (self-report) IRS-P (parents)	Tourette's only v. Tourette's+OCD: no group differences; differences for Total & School impairment & Home activities scores	QoL in youngsters with Tourette syndrome is more complex than in adults
Eddy *et al*, 2012	Italy	50	YQOL-R	QoL higher in Tourette's only than in Tourette's+OCD and/or ADHD	OCD and/or ADHD: lower scores on Total and Relationship domains; ADHD: lower scores on Self and Relationship domains; OCD: more widespread QoL problems

ADHD, attention-deficit hyperactivity disorder; C&A-GTS-QOL, Gilles de la Tourette Syndrome – Quality of Life Scale for Children and Adolescents; HRQoL, health-related quality of life assessment; IRS-P, Impairment Rating Scale – Parent; OCB, obsessive–compulsive behaviour; OCD, obsessive–compulsive disorder; PedsQL 4.0, Pediatric Quality of Life Inventory, version 4; TACQOL, TNO-AZL (Netherlands Organisation for Applied Scientific Research Academic Medical Centre) Questionnaires for Children's Health-Related Quality of Life; YQOL-R, Youth Quality of Life Instrument – Research Version.

Source: modified and updated from Robertson, 2011, 2012.

both uncontrolled studies (using standardised schedules) and normative data, more 'stress' (e.g. parental burden, parental psychopathology) was reported, with one of the main stressors being child-care difficulties. Parenting stress was related to the child's gender, age, school situation and Tourette severity, the parents' age and family income, with a significant negative correlation found between lack of social support and parenting stress. Multiple linear regression analysis found disease severity and family income to be the variables with the greatest predictive power for parenting stress, accounting for 42% of the variance (Lee *et al*, 2007). In the only controlled study, using the General Health Questionnaire (GHQ-28) to assess parents' mental health and the Child and Adolescent Impact Assessment to assess caregiver burden, parents of children with Tourette syndrome were more psychiatrically impaired than parents of children with asthma (Cooper *et al*, 2003). In summary, studies have shown considerable parenting stress, caregiver burden and psychopathology in the parents of youngsters with Tourette syndrome. As only one study was controlled, this is a fruitful area for further research.

Epidemiology and prevalence

Tourette syndrome has now been described almost worldwide. Males are more commonly affected, with the male/female ratio being 3 or 4 to 1. Clinical characteristics are similar irrespective of the country of origin, highlighting the biological nature of Tourette syndrome. In some instances it seems that within families, the affected males have tics whereas the females have obsessive–compulsive behaviours.

Tourette syndrome was once considered to be rare, but a comprehensive review shows that at least eight studies with similar multistaged methods documented remarkably consistent findings and suggests a global prevalence of between 0.4 and 3.8% for youngsters between the ages of 5 and 18 years, with a calculated prevalence (from raw data) of 1% worldwide, apart from Sub Saharan Africa (Robertson, 2008*a*,*b*). In the UK, two definitive prevalence studies have been undertaken. Hornsey *et al* (2001) reported a prevalence of 0.76–1.85%. Scharf *et al* (2012) subsequently examined prevalence using a general practitioner database (the population-based Avon Longitudinal Study of Parents and Children, known as the ALSPAC study). They reported a prevalence of Tourette syndrome in 13-year-olds of 0.3% (as narrowly defined) and 0.7% (as defined more broadly). Several other recent studies are all roughly in accord with the figure of 1% worldwide. The prevalence of Tourette syndrome in special educational populations, such as individuals with intellectual disabilities and emotional and behavioural disorders, is much higher, and in the case of autism spectrum disorders (ASD) the rate of Tourette syndrome is as high as 6–11% (for individual references see Robertson, 2008*a*,*b*).

Aetiological theories

Aetiological suggestions for Tourette syndrome include genetic factors and environmental influences. The latter might be infections and neuro-immunological effects, pre- and/or perinatal difficulties, psychosocial stressors and/or androgen influences. The idea that the aetiology of Tourette syndrome is psychological has now been discredited.

No single gene has been identified to date, and although the scientific community has been enthused by the 'discovery' of various genes (e.g. *SLITRK1*), it is likely that more than one gene is responsible. For full reviews of the genetics of Tourette syndrome see O'Rourke *et al* (2009) and Deng *et al* (2012). Recent genetic data implicate a genetic variant of HTR2C, a rare functional mutation in the *HDC* gene encoding L-histidine decarboxylase, and the *DLGAP3* gene. Another study conducted a genome-wide linkage analysis in a large high-risk Utah pedigree examining a qualitative trait (a diagnosis of Tourette syndrome) and a quantitative phenotype based on tic severity. Two regions of interest were found: chromosome 3p for the Tourette syndrome phenotype and chromosome 1p for tic severity (Knight *et al*, 2010). These results are all exciting, but emphasise the need for studies on large numbers of individuals using rare variants, sib-pair analysis, extended pedigrees or large cohorts. At least two international collaborative efforts are in place. Of importance is the fact that in the vast majority of individuals with Tourette syndrome the chromosomes are normal (Robertson & Trimble, 1993).

Perhaps stimulated by the fact that no gene(s) have been positively implicated in Tourette syndrome, neuroimmunological theories have been a focus of interest. These include hypotheses of (i) autoimmunity and (ii) lowered immunity. These neuroimmunological theories, possibly operating via the process of molecular mimicry, began when Swedo *et al* (1998) described a group of 50 children with OCD and tic disorders, designated as paediatric autoimmune neuropsychiatric disorders associated with streptococcal infections (PANDAS). The diagnostic criteria included: presence of OCD and/or a tic disorder, prepubertal symptom onset (usually acute and dramatic), association with group A beta-haemolytic streptococcal (GABHS) infections, episodic course of symptom severity and association with neurological abnormalities. The relapsing, remitting course was associated with significant psychopathology, including emotional lability, separation anxiety, night-time fears, bedtime rituals, cognitive deficits, oppositional behaviours and hyperactivity. It must be emphasised that PANDAS and Tourette syndrome are not the same entity.

Recently, researchers have found laboratory evidence of GABHS infections in some patients with Tourette syndrome, and/or documented in several controlled studies that some individuals with Tourette syndrome have increased anti-basal ganglia antibodies (ABGAs). One suggestion in this context is that people with Tourette syndrome have a predisposition to autoimmune responses, as indicated by the reduced frequency of regulatory T-cells which induce tolerance towards self-antigens. Another is that there may be a general lowered immunity, as evidenced by an immunoglobulin A (IgA) dysgammaglobulinaemia. Low levels of IgA may then lead to increased risk of upper respiratory tract infections (see Robertson, 2012).

It has been suggested by Leckman (2003) that the mothers of children with tics are 1.5 times as likely to have experienced a complication during pregnancy than the mothers of children who did not have tics. Among monozygotic twins discordant for Tourette syndrome, the index twins with Tourette syndrome have had lower birth weights than their unaffected twins. It has also been demonstrated that the severity of maternal life stress during pregnancy, and severe nausea and/or vomiting during the first trimester are risk factors for tic disorders in offspring. Other studies have shown that prematurity, low birth-weight, low Apgar scores and more frequent maternal prenatal visits were associated with Tourette syndrome (e.g. Leckman, 2003). One controlled study (Burd *et al*, 1999) demonstrated that people who developed Tourette syndrome had had more pre- and perinatal difficulties than a control group. Maternal smoking during pregnancy has been associated with: (a) a diagnosis of Tourette syndrome (Motlagh *et al*, 2010; Zhang *et al*, 2012); (b) increased tic severity (Matthews *et al*, 2006); and (c) an increased likelihood of comorbid ADHD in Tourette syndrome (Prinsgsheim *et al*, 2009b; Cui & Zheng, 2010; Motlagh *et al*, 2010). Finally, Leckman and his group have suggested that androgen exposure ('prenatal masculinisation of the brain') may also be important in the aetiopathogenesis of Tourette syndrome and tic-related disorders. Thus, the aetiopathology of Tourette syndrome is much more complex than previously recognised, with complicated genetic mechanisms, some infections, pre- and perinatal difficulties, maternal smoking, life stressors and androgens affecting the phenotype (Leckman, 2003; Robertson, 2012).

Clinical features

The age at onset of Tourette syndrome ranges from 2 to 21 years, with a mean of 7 years commonly reported. The onset of vocal tics is usually some months to years later, many studies reporting a delay of around 11 years. Tics usually begin in the head and face, and eye blinking is often the first (and one of the most common) tics. Tics can be simple (e.g. blinking, eye rolling) or complex (e.g. touching, hopping). Simple vocal tics include sniffing, throat clearing, gulping, snorting and coughing. Complex vocal tics include barking, making animal noises and uttering strings of words. Tics characteristically wax and wane, are usually preceded by premonitory sensations, diminish during goal-directed behaviour and increase with emotional excitement and fatigue. Other important and characteristic features include echolalia (copying what others say), echopraxia (copying what others do), palipraxia (repeating one's action) and palilalia (repeating the last word or part of one's sentences). Non-obscene socially inappropriate behaviour and self-injurious behaviour are both common and difficult to treat.

Echo phenomena have long been understood to be part of Tourette syndrome, described by Gilles de la Tourette himself in 1885. In one study, echo phenomena were significantly associated with the longer duration and severity of Tourette syndrome, as well as measures of obsessionality, depression and anxiety (Robertson *et al*, 1988). Echo phenomena are healthy in children up to 36 months of age, but in older children clinicians should investigate for neuropsychiatric pathology. Echo phenomena are a feature of Tourette syndrome, with patients echoing both healthy movements and tics, although, as expected, echoes were predominantly part of the tic repertoire (Ganos *et al*, 2012*a*).

Coprolalia has been widely misunderstood as a pathognomonic feature. It denotes inappropriate, involuntary, out-of-context swearing, often disguised by the patient and without offensive intent. Instead of the whole swear word, many individuals say only part of the word (e.g. 'fu fi') and disguise it, for example, by coughing. It occurs in about 20–30% of patients of Tourette syndrome clinics and begins within 5 years of tic onset. It seldom occurs in community samples. The Tourette Syndrome Association in the USA suggests that as few as 10–15% of all people with Tourette syndrome have this feature. Many physicians are still under the misapprehension that coprolalia must be present in order to make the diagnosis. Coprolalia is often used in the media as a symptom of Tourette syndrome, probably because its sensational effect increases viewing numbers. It has been suggested that copropraxia (the inappropriate making of obscene gestures) occurs in about 6–18% of clinic patients (Robertson *et al*, 1988; Freeman *et al*, 2009). The latter authors have also documented that coprophenomena are associated with tic severity, repetitive behaviours, the amount of comorbid psychiatric disorders and the number of anti-tic medications taken.

The peak of tic severity is around 10–12 years of age. Symptoms usually begin with transient bouts of tics, but by 10 years, most children notice nearly irresistible urges that precede the tics. These premonitory sensations appear to be in the child's conscious awareness and are likely to reflect a defect in sensorimotor gating because they intrude and become a source of distraction. Premonitory sensations are common, occur with the majority of tics and may be either localised (around the area of the tic) or generalised (covering a wide area of the body). They have been likened to the 'urge' or 'tight' sensation before a sneeze and, as with the sneeze in healthy people, they are usually relieved by the tics (Kwak *et al*, 2003). It has been understood that most people can suppress tics, and that this is in part due to the premonitory sensations. In a recent study, however, it was demonstrated that there was no correlation between the perceived strength of premonitory sensations and the ability to suppress tics: in other words, the urges and tic inhibition are not directly related (Ganos *et al*, 2012*b*).

Over the course of hours, tics occur in bouts, with a regular inter-tic interval (Leckman *et al*, 2006). It has been suggested that there may be a fractal, deterministic and possibly chaotic process in the tic time series (short-term bouts, and longer-term waxing and waning) (Peterson & Leckman, 1998).

Comorbidity with Tourette syndrome

The comorbid psychiatric disorders most commonly seen in Tourette syndrome include ADHD, obsessive–compulsive behaviours, OCD and ASD. The relationships between these and Tourette syndrome are complex and are summarised in Table 17.2.

An investigation embracing 3500 clinic patients with Tourette syndrome worldwide demonstrated that at all ages, 88% of individuals had reported comorbidity/psychopathology. The most common was ADHD, followed by obsessive–compulsive behaviours and OCD. Anger control problems, sleep difficulties, coprolalia and self-injurious behaviours reached high levels only in patients with comorbid disorders. Males were more likely than females to have comorbid disorders (Freeman *et al*, 2000). This has also been shown to be true in community studies, with around 90% of people with Tourette syndrome having attracted other diagnoses (for studies, see Robertson, 2012). Thus, both in clinic populations and in the community, only about 10% of people with just Tourette syndrome ('Tourette syndrome only') have tics and 90% have comorbid psychiatric diagnoses.

Relatively recently, research groups have separated individuals with Tourette syndrome into subgroups on the basis of clinical symptoms, specifically separating those with and without ADHD. Thus, they have examined children with Tourette syndrome only, and compared them with groups such as Tourette syndrome plus ADHD, ADHD only, and unaffected controls. Youngsters with Tourette syndrome only did not differ from unaffected controls on many ratings, including aggression, delinquency or conduct difficulties. By contrast, children with Tourette syndrome plus ADHD were significantly above unaffected controls, and similar to those with ADHD only, on the indices of disruptive behaviours. Studies further showed that youngsters with Tourette syndrome plus ADHD demonstrated more internalising and behaviour problems and poorer social adaptation than children with Tourette syndrome only or controls. Of importance is that youngsters with Tourette syndrome only were not significantly different from unaffected controls on most measures of externalising behaviours and social adaptation, but had more internalising symptoms. In summary, individuals with Tourette syndrome only appear to be similar to healthy controls and, except for the internalising problems, significantly different from those with Tourette syndrome plus ADHD, and this clearly has major management and prognostic implications (Robertson, 2006*a*).

Table 17.2 Comorbid disorders and coexistent psychopathology in young people with Tourette syndrome

	Incidence	Aetiology/possible associations	Comments	Further information
Comorbid disorders				
Attention-deficit hyperactivity disorder	Most common: 21–90%; Mean: 60%	Genetic in a subgroup	Also common in clinic, community and epidemiological studies	Robertson & Eapen, 1992; Walkup et al, 1999; Freeman et al, 2000; Robertson, 2006a
Obsessive–compulsive behaviours/disorder	Common: 27–32% in clinics	Integral part of Tourette's; share genetic influences	OCB is egosyntonic; OCD is egodystonic	Freeman et al, 2000; Robertson, 2000
Autism spectrum disorders	6–11%	Genetic in a subgroup; also probably non-specific & there may be general neurodevelopmental problems		Robertson, 2011
Self-injurious behaviour	30%	Difficult to treat	Mild SIB related to OCB, severe related to impulsivity; mild & severe related to tic severity	Robertson et al, 1989; Mathews et al, 2004
Non-obscene socially inappropriate behaviour	Common (30–60%)	Possibly related to impulsivity, ADHD or conduct disorder; not related to OCB/OCD	One-third have social difficulties as a result of NOSI	Kurlan et al, 1996
Coexistent psychopathology				
Depression	13–76%	Multifactorial; not genetic	Depression more common in Tourette's than in healthy controls	Robertson, 2006b
Anxiety	Common (range 19–80%)	Secondary to having Tourette's; some suggest anxiety pre-dates tics		Robertson, 2003
Personality disorders	Common (64%)	Probably related to childhood ADHD, ODD, conduct disorder	Whole spectrum of personality disorders: not restricted to OCPD	Robertson et al, 1997

(continued)

Feature	Frequency	Description	Reference
Dysphoria	Fairly common with almost all antipsychotics	Side-effect of anti-Tourette's medication	Robertson, 2000, 2003
School phobia/separation anxiety	Not common, but noted	May be side-effect of anti-Tourette's medication	Robertson, 2000, 2003
Rage or explosive outbursts	20%	Associated with ADHD, tic severity, lower age at tic onset, prenatal exposure to tobacco	Chen et al, 2013
Sleep problems	Very common: 75%	Night terrors, insomnia, nightmares, sleep-walking, sleep-talking/walking, nocturnal enuresis, bruxism	Robertson et al, 1988
Cognitive dulling/drowsiness	32% (some studies)	Side-effect of anti-Tourette's medication	Robertson et al, 1988, Robertson, 2000
Dyslexia, dyspraxia, reading difficulties	6%		Lees et al, 1984
Schizophrenia	Very rare	Co-occurs by chance	Few isolated case reports
Examinations: IQ (WAIS/WISC) MSE Neurological EEG CT scans		Average IQ: 100 None psychotic Normal in 67% n.a.d. in 63–74% n.a.d. in 97%	Lees et al, 1984; Robertson et al, 1988
		Focal dystonia, chorea, mild dysdiadochokinesia, tonic torticollis, spasmodic dysphonia, cavum septum pellucidum cavities (in headbangers)	
Total comorbidity and/or psychopathology	88–90%	Mixed Figures same in clinical and epidemiological studies	Freeman et al, 2000; Khalifa & von Knorring, 2003, 2005

ADHD, attention-deficit hyperactivity disorder; CT, computed tomography; EEG, electroencephalogram; MSE, mental state examination; n.a.d., nothing abnormal detected; NOSI, non-obscene socially inappropriate behaviour; OCB, obsessive–compulsive behaviour; OCD, obsessive–compulsive disorder; OCPD, obsessive–compulsive personality disorder; ODD, oppositional defiant disorder; SIB, self-injurious behaviour; WAIS, Wechsler Adult Intelligence Scale; WISC, Wechsler Intelligence Scale for Children. Source: modified and updated from Robertson, 2011, 2012.

In other controlled studies, young people with Tourette syndrome have been shown to have more obsessional symptoms than control participants. Importantly, the obsessive–compulsive behaviours encountered in Tourette syndrome are statistically and clinically different from those behaviours in OCD (for a review, see Robertson, 2000, 2003). The obsessive–compulsive behaviours in people with Tourette syndrome include thoughts (obsessions) of violence, sex and aggression and actions (compulsions) concerning touching of self and/or others, symmetry and ordering. This differs from many people with OCD, who are often more preoccupied with dirt, germs and contamination. It is also clear that there is a genetic link between Tourette syndrome and obsessive–compulsive behaviours (Eapen *et al*, 1993).

It has long been documented that Tourette syndrome and ASD have clinical similarities and share many symptoms. Recently, evidence has been emerging from phenomenological, epidemiological and pathogenetic perspectives (State, 2010) that Tourette syndrome and ASD overlap. It has been suggested that shared molecular pathways affect the development of both disorders: examples include disruption of the *NRXN1*, *NLGN4X* and *CNTNAP2* genes (Clarke *et al*, 2012; Eapen, 2012).

It seems likely that the disorders discussed in this section are comorbid with Tourette syndrome because they have neurodevelopmental similarities, clinical similarities and in some cases are probably genetically related.

Coexistent psychopathology

The most common coexistent psychopathologies found in Tourette syndrome include depressive illness, depressive symptoms, anxiety, phobias, intellectual disabilities and, in adolescents and adults, personality disorder. These appear to be coexisting rather than comorbid, as they are unlikely to share a genetic underpinning. The psychoses, such as bipolar affective disorder, are probably related to other disorders such as OCD and ADHD, whereas schizophrenia is rare and the two disorders co-occur only by chance (Robertson, 2003, 2012). The relationships between Tourette syndrome, comorbid disorders and coexistent psychopathology are summarised in Table 17.2.

There is some exciting evidence emerging that specific aspects of the aetiology, phenotype and indeed endophenotype (e.g. specific brain changes related to a particular clinical type) may be found in Tourette syndrome and this is a worthwhile direction for future research (Robertson & Eapen, 2013).

Aggression and behavioural difficulties

The genetic predisposition to aggression in humans appears to be greatly affected by the relationship between polymorphic genetic variants (particularly functional polymorphisms in the monoamine oxidase A

(MAOA) and serotonin transporter (5-HTT) genes) and anatomical changes in the limbic system of aggressive people (Pavlov *et al*, 2012). The MAOA genotype is associated with aggressive behaviour, especially in interaction with childhood trauma or other early adverse events, and particularly so in males. Among individuals who have experienced childhood trauma or other early adverse events, the low-expressing variant (MAOA-L) seems to be related to greater aggression in males, whereas the high-expressing variant (MAOA-H) may be associated with more aggression in females (Verhoeven *et al*, 2012).

McGrath *et al* (2012) used structural equation modelling to examine genotype–phenotype interaction in young adult women, focusing on the MAOA gene and problem behaviours. Results showed that a main effect of the MAOA genotype (genetic material) and an MAOA–physical maltreatment interaction was an association with conduct problems (behavioural difficulties). Marquez *et al* (2013), using rat models, showed changes in some brain areas due to excess expression of the MAOA gene in peripubertally stressed animals. In adulthood, these rats showed increased aggression, which was reversed by treatment with an MAOA-inhibiting drug.

Early stress might lead to an upset of social hierarchy status, with resultant social consequences (aggression/fighting), although this is not fully understood (Cordero & Sandi, 2007; Timmer *et al*, 2011). It has been suggested that aggressive behaviours are probably influenced by both genetic (e.g. the MAOA gene) and epigenetic (e.g. risk to the fetus, pre- and perinatal difficulties) factors (Liu, 2011). For example, violence or aggression to women during pregnancy can result in obstetric problems and altered personality in offspring if the child has an individual vulnerability. There are, of course, also cultural theories of aggression, for example that it is related to the male dominance in society or that children learn it from their early role models such as parents.

As already mentioned, one of the most common comorbidities in youngsters with Tourette syndrome is ADHD (Robertson, 2012). Compared with unaffected peers, adults with Tourette syndrome are more likely to have personality disorders (e.g. Robertson *et al*, 1997). In youngsters with both Tourette syndrome and ADHD (compared with Tourette syndrome alone) there are significantly more disruptive behaviours (Robertson, 2006*a*), and adults with Tourette syndrome have additional problems with substance misuse, aggression and forensic encounters (Haddad *et al*, 2009). Some of the explanations may be integral to Tourette syndrome, whereas others may well be generic, as outlined above.

In conclusion, it appears that as far as psychopathology and in particular aggressive behaviours are concerned, there are genetic influences (e.g. MAOA genotype), epigenetic factors (e.g. risk to fetus, perinatal difficulties) and also environmental effects (e.g. early-life stressors). It is likely that these factors also apply to the aggressive and behavioural difficulties found in people with Tourette syndrome, which in many cases have been associated with comorbid ADHD.

Types of Tourette syndrome

There have been many studies indicating that Tourette syndrome is not a unitary condition as suggested, indeed stipulated, by both American Psychiatric Association (DSM-5) and World Health Organization (ICD-10) diagnostic criteria. In an early study of 90 people with Tourette syndrome, Robertson et al (1988) reported a high incidence of obsessionality, depression and hostility. Importantly, depression was not related to medication. Aggression, hostility and obsessionality were significantly associated with some core features of Tourette syndrome, including copro- and echo-phenomena and a family history of the syndrome. The first study to formally investigate the phenotype was that of Alsobrook & Pauls (2002), who used hierarchical cluster analysis (HCA) and principal component factor analysis (PCFA) and reported four significant factors, which accounted for 61% of the variance. These were: aggressive phenomena (e.g. kicking, temper fits and argumentativeness); motor and vocal/phonic tics only; compulsive phenomena; and tapping and absence of grunting. Since then there have been many other analytical studies conducted on clinical cohorts (e.g. Storch et al, 2007; Grados & Mathews, 2008; Robertson et al, 2008; Cavanna et al, 2011; McGuire et al, 2013), and all have reported more than one type or phenotype. In addition, a large multiply affected pedigree living in the community which had originally been assessed by Robertson & Gourdie (1990) was also submitted to HCA and PCFA by Robertson & Cavanna (2007) and again four types (phenotypes) were found. Moreover, in all studies that examined for it, one type was 'pure Tourette syndrome', i'e. motor and vocal tics only. This is in agreement with the clinical data of Freeman et al (2000) and community data of Khalifa & von Knorring (2003, 2005), who found that only about 10% of all individuals with Tourette syndrome have only motor and vocal tics. Although not directly comparable, all studies using HCA, PCA or latent class analysis (LCA) have shown two or more factors, in terms of both tics and psychopathology.

All these studies add to the growing body of evidence that Tourette syndrome is not a unitary condition. Thus, one is able to conclude that the Tourette syndrome phenotype is heterogeneous and not unitary as previously suggested and shown in DSM and ICD. In conclusion, whether using complex statistical methods (e.g. HCA, PCA, LCA) or material derived from clinical or community settings, one type (phenotype) or clinical presentation of Tourette syndrome consists of 'pure simple motor and vocal tics only', whereas other phenotypes include complex tics and the comorbid disorders, various coexistent psychopathologies and complex behaviours.

Assessment

The assessment of patients with Tourette syndrome requires a thorough personal and family history, as well as full mental state and neurological examinations. Several standardised schedules may be useful for accurately diagnosing Tourette syndrome, assessing the response to medication and in research. These include: the National Hospital Interview Schedule (Robertson & Eapen, 1996); the Yale Global Tic Severity Scale (Leckman *et al*, 1989); the self-rated Premonitory Urge for Tics Scale (Woods *et al*, 2005); the Motor Tic, Obsession and Compulsion, and Vocal Tic Evaluation Survey (MOVES; Gaffney *et al*, 1994); the Hopkins Motor and Vocal Tic Severity Scale (Walkup *et al*, 1992); the Rush Video-Based Tic Rating Scale (Goetz *et al*, 1987); and the Diagnostic Confidence Index (Robertson *et al*, 1999). For reviews of these scales see Robertson (2011) and Robertson & Cavanna (2008). The physician-rated Diagnostic Confidence Index and the self-rated MOVES are useful for the practising clinician, as they will ensure that the main symptoms for diagnosis (Diagnostic Confidence Index) and severity (MOVES) are assessed. The Diagnostic Confidence Index highlights the phenomenological characteristics of tics, including the presence of coprolalia, echolalia and palilalia, complex tics, premonitory urges/sensations, relief after tics, suppressibility, rebound, suggestibility, variability of tics, and the waxing and waning course (Robertson *et al*, 1999).

Familiarity with Tourette syndrome, as well as training by an expert, are important for implementing the majority of these scales. However, a good clinician, given time, will be able to elicit symptoms, make a diagnosis and give correct treatment and management.

Many clinicians would suggest blood sampling for copper and ceruloplasmin (to exclude Wilson's disease) and acanthocytes (to exclude neuroacanthosis) as good practice, but genetic testing for Huntingdon's disease would only be undertaken exceptionally. Neuroimaging in research studies shows differences between patients with Tourette syndrome and controls, and endophenotypes (brain changes specific to Tourette syndrome) have been suggested (Robertson & Eapen, 2013): in routine practice, however, computed tomography, electroencephalograms (EEGs) and electrocardiograms (ECGs) are usually non-contributory. These investigations are usually only warranted to exclude any other diagnosis such as myoclonic (jerking) or petit mal (blinking) epilepsy or chorea with rheumatic fever.

Management and treatment

The treatment for all individuals with Tourette syndrome includes psychoeducation, reassurance and explanation. In many mild cases and young people this may in fact suffice. Medication is the mainstay for the majority of symptoms of Tourette syndrome and many of the comorbid conditions and coexistent psychopathologies. New strategies include the successful and side-effect-free habit reversal training and comprehensive behavioural intervention for tics. Injection of botulinum toxin into the periorbital tissues and vocal cords has yet to be fully evaluated, and deep brain stimulation for severe and refractory tics in adults also needs further study (see Robertson 2011, 2012).

Table 17.3 includes the main managements and medications for Tourette syndrome currently available and used by many clinicians. Empirical evidence of efficacy, ranked A to D ('good' to 'minimal'), has been collated from double-blind trials (best evidence), large series (some evidence) and case reports (minimal or anecdotal evidence) and also personal experience, which, although anecdotal, covers many patients and is representative of clinic populations.

Behavioural methods for adult and child patients may be useful alone or in combination with medications for many aspects of Tourette syndrome. Relatively recently, habit reversal training has been shown to be significantly better than or equal to supportive psychotherapy and better than the waiting list for adults with Tourette syndrome. Comprehensive behavioural intervention for tics was found to be helpful for young people (Piacentini et al, 2010). Exposure and response prevention has also proved very successful in the treatment of tics, and a novel non-pharmacological treatment using self-hypnosis was successful in 26 (almost 80%) of 33 children (see Robertson, 2012). In recent European guidelines, behavioural therapies are recommended as a first-line treatment of Tourette syndrome, albeit on the basis of evidence less strong than for habit reversal training (Verdellen et al, 2011).

Medication is often required for the treatment of moderate to severe tics and psychopathologies in patients with Tourette syndrome. Double-blind trials have demonstrated that many medications (Table 17.3) are superior to placebo. Importantly, the dose given for Tourette syndrome is small compared with the dose for schizophrenia or mania. Thus, a daily dose of 0.5–3 mg of haloperidol may be sufficient in Tourette syndrome, whereas 30 mg may be required in severe mania or schizophrenia in adults. Tetrabenazine can also be effective and is prescribed mainly by neurologists: a side-effect can be depression. Clonidine (or guanfacine in the USA) can be given for tics, impulse control and ADHD (and it may also help with insomnia). A baseline ECG is advisable, as is regular monitoring of pulse and blood pressure. One can commence at a dose of 25 µg, increasing gradually to 150 µg daily. It is advisable to take blood for a baseline prolactin, as many antipsychotic medications result in hyperprolactinaemia, which can have endocrinal repercussions (Robertson, 2000, 2012).

Antidepressants, especially the selective serotonin reuptake inhibitors (SSRIs), are useful for depression (e.g. fluoxetine at a standard dose of 20 mg/day) and obsessive–compulsive behaviours or OCD (e.g. fluoxetine at 40–60 mg/day). Clomipramine (a tricyclic antidepressant) may also be useful in obsessive–compulsive behaviours or OCD, but it usually has more side-effects than the SSRIs and is dangerous in overdose. In the obsessive–compulsive behaviours and OCD associated with Tourette syndrome, a small dose of an antipsychotic is useful as an augmentation agent. A less used but successful treatment is botulinum toxin injected

Table 17.3 Main strategies of the management of the motor and vocal/phonic tics of Tourette syndrome in young people, showing the current evidence

Treatment	Empirical evidence[a]	Comments	Reference/further information
Haloperidol (antipsychotic)	A: good	Three DBTs show haloperidol better than placebo Has many adverse side-effects; used worldwide: in many countries is the only drug licensed for Tourette syndrome	Scahill et al, 2006; Robertson, 2011
Risperidone (antipsychotic)	A: good	Four RCTs in both adults and children Subsequent reports of serious adverse effects: increase in weight and glucose abnormalities (diabetes); in common use worldwide	Scahill et al, 2006; Robertson, 2011
Pimozide (antipsychotic)	A: good	Four DBTs show that pimozide and haloperidol have equal efficacy, and pimozide fewer adverse side-effects than haloperidol Some reports of prolonged QTc interval with pimozide; widely used	Scahill et al, 2006; Robertson, 2011
Sulpiride (antipsychotic)	B: adequate = 1DBT + other evidence > 150 patients	One DBT showed that sulpiride was superior to placebo; one small case series and two large case series (249 patients) showed that sulpiride improved motor and vocal tics and had few side-effects Widely used in UK; unavailable in USA and Canada	Robertson, 2011
Tiapride (antipsychotic)	B: adequate = 2 small DBTs only or open label or larger case reports (> 100 patients)	One DBT v. placebo (number of patients not given) and one DBT (10 patients) showed tiapride superior to placebo Widely used in Europe (most common in Russia and Germany); unavailable in UK, USA, Canada	Chouza et al, 1982; Eggers et al, 1988
Aripiprazole (antipsychotic)	B: adequate = 1 DBT, other open trials & numerous series & case reports - now totalling well over 350 patients	Positive successful reports in 222 patients; pilot study in China showed aripiprazole to be effective and safe, with transient minimal side-effects; treated 20 adults for 56 months successfully; series of 100 patients treated successfully; multicentre controlled study in China showed it as effective as tiapride Becoming first-line treatment in many dedicated Tourette's clinics in UK and Europe	Robertson, 2011; Cui et al, 2010; Neuner et al, 2012; Wenzel et al, 2012; Liu et al, 2011

(continued)

277

Table 17.3 *(continued)*

Treatment	Empirical evidence[a]	Comments	Reference/further information
Clonidine	A: good	Six DBTs showed clonidine (tablets and transdermal patches) superior to placebo	Robertson, 2011
Botulinum toxin	B: adequate	One DBT showed decreased tics, decreased urges; one series of 30 in open label study showed decreased tics, decreased urges, improved QoL hypophonia in 80% of the 30: other case series and reports showed positive results	Robertson, 2011
Atomoxetine	B: adequate	Two DBTs showed reduced tics and ADHD	Robertson, 2011
Tetrabenazine	D: minimal	Two studies (86 patients) report success; no DBTs; depression is common side-effect; used mainly by neurologists	Robertson, 2011
Habit reversal training	A: good	RCTs show it to be better than psychotherapy, and waiting list to be as effective as other behavioural methods	Robertson, 2011
Exposure and response prevention	A: good	More evidence for habit reversal training than for exposure and response prevention	Verdellen *et al*, 2011
Comprehensive behavioural intervention for tics	A: good	Good improvement	Piacentini *et al*, 2010
Deep brain stimulation	Not indicated for young people	Just over 100 patients with Tourette syndrome have had DBS for severe refractory symptoms with good effect; at present only recommended in research centres with strict protocols	Hariz & Robertson, 2010

DBT, double-blind trial; QoL, quality of life; RCT, randomised controlled trial.
a. A, good, 2–3 DBTs; B, adequate, 1 DBT, >150 patients; C, fair, 1 double-blind trial only, or open label trial or case series/case reports, <150 patients; D, minimal, only case reports, small series.
Modified from Robertson (2011) & Scahill *et al* (2006).

into affected areas (e.g. the vocal cords for loud distressing vocal tics and coprolalia); treatment is usually done by a neurologist with special expertise, in expert clinics. It is important to know that the response to individual antipsychotics is idiosyncratic; a patient may respond to one but not another and, unfortunately, not to a second trial of an original medication, if discontinued.

Recently, the newer atypical (second-generation) antipsychotics have been shown to be useful in treating Tourette syndrome. The main side-effects are weight increase and, in some individuals, precipitation of diabetes or metabolic syndrome. It is therefore advisable to check fasting glucose levels in patients receiving the atypicals, especially if they have put on weight. Atypical antipsychotics used successfully in treating Tourette syndrome include risperidone, olanzapine, quetiapine, ziprasidone and aripiprazole. In both the literature and my clinical experience, patients treated with antipsychotics can have raised prolactin levels, which in some cases requires discontinuation of the drugs (Robertson, 2012). Rickards *et al* (2012) have reported findings from a survey of European prescribing practices in Tourette syndrome which showed that, in the management of various symptom clusters, risperidone was most frequently prescribed for tics, sertraline for obsessive–compulsive behaviours and methylphenidate for ADHD. The use of aripiprazole has gained momentum in Europe, the UK and USA, and one controlled trial in China showed it to be as effective as tiapride (Liu *et al*, 2011). Aripiprazole is therefore rated B in Table 17.3.

As stated earlier, clonidine has been used in the treatment of Tourette syndrome and of ADHD, and thus it may well be a useful treatment for individuals with both disorders. Good evidence for the safety and efficacy of the combination of stimulants and clonidine comes from a large randomised double-blind trial including over 130 children who had ADHD and a tic disorder and were treated with clonidine alone, methylphenidate alone, clonidine and methylphenidate, or placebo (Tourette's Syndrome Study Group, 2002). Compared with placebo, the greatest benefit was with the combination of clonidine and methylphenidate. Of importance was that the proportion of participants reporting a worsening of tics was no higher in those treated with methylphenidate than in those receiving clonidine or placebo.

Thus, it does appear from evidence-based studies that stimulants, if used judiciously in patients with Tourette syndrome or tics and comorbid ADHD, do not necessarily increase tics. In addition, the combination of stimulants and clonidine appears to be safe. Atomoxetine is a relatively new agent for the treatment of ADHD and it may prove useful in the treatment of Tourette syndrome plus ADHD – further research is needed.

Deep brain stimulation is used worldwide for Parkinson's disease, tremor and dystonia, and even for depression, OCD and Tourette syndrome (e.g. Hariz & Robertson, 2010). It has been used in over 100 people with Tourette syndrome, but only those with severe refractory illness. It is unlikely that it would be used in youngsters under the age of 20.

Continuity into adult life

It was initially thought that Tourette syndrome was lifelong. Several studies have now reported that tic severity reduces during adolescence and it seems that by the age of 18, tics decrease in many patients. Only greater tic severity in childhood has been associated with increased tic severity at follow-up. Although the prognosis of Tourette syndrome is better than originally thought concerning tic symptomatology (for a review, see Robertson, 2008a,b), the comorbidity often changes with age (Rizzo et al, 2012) and the psychopathology (e.g. depression) worsens with age (e.g. Robertson, 2006b).

In an elegant study, Pappert et al (2003) followed up a group of 56 individuals with Tourette syndrome who had been videotaped according to a strict protocol between 1978 and 1991, when they were 8- to 14-year-olds. Thirty-one of the original cohort, now aged over 20, were contacted and included in a follow-up video study. A rater assessed the 62 tapes and rated 5 tic domains: the two videotapes for each participant were compared for each tic domain, as well as a composite tic disability score. Results showed that 90% of the adults still had tics. Many patients who had suggested that they were tic free were not, as no less than 50% had objective evidence of tics. The mean tic disability score reduced significantly with age. All tic domains improved with age and there were significant improvements for motor tics. The improvements in tic disability were not related to medication, as only 13% of the adults were receiving medication for tics, compared with 81% of the children. The authors concluded that although tics improve with time, most adults have persistent tics.

Rizzo et al (2012) investigated 100 people with Tourette syndrome who were assessed at onset and at follow-up 10 years later to evaluate the severity of the tics and the presence of comorbid disorders and coexistent psychopathologies. Impairment was also evaluated. At 10-year follow-up, 58% of the 38 individuals with 'pure' Tourette syndrome (i.e. no comorbidity) persisted with the same 'pure' clinical phenotype, whereas 42% had changed to a 'Tourette plus OCD' phenotype. In the Tourette plus OCD subgroup, 55% required medication and fared better than those with initial comorbidities, who also had a significantly reduced quality of life.

Conclusion

Tourette syndrome is now recognised to be common, affecting 1% of the population almost worldwide. The aetiology is more complex than was once thought, and is widely accepted to be genetic in most individuals, although no single gene has been identified. Other behaviours, however, such as obsessive–compulsive behaviours and OCD, are widely recognised phenotypes of the putative gene(s). Newer evidence is that some cases of ADHD and ASD also share some genetic underpinning. Other aetiopathological suggestions include environmental influences, such as infections, neuroimmunological effects, pre- and/or perinatal difficulties, psychosocial stressors and/or androgen influences. The old idea that Tourette syndrome is psychological and to be treated with psychoanalysis has now been discredited.

Exciting evidence is emerging that specific aspects of the aetiology, phenotype and endophenotype (e.g. brain changes related to a particular clinical type) may be identified in Tourette syndrome and this is a worthwhile direction for future research.

A wide variety of comorbid psychiatric disorders and/or psychopathology are common, and it seems that the presentation may change over time. Unexpectedly, it appears that uncomplicated Tourette syndrome (without comorbid disorders) may not have the best prognosis. Some comorbidities are common and integral (e.g. OCD, obsessive–compulsive behaviours, ADHD, ASD), whereas some coexistent psychopathologies (e.g. depression) are common but multifactorial in origin, and others (such as personality disorder in adults and bipolar affective disorder) may be due to comorbid conditions (e.g. ADHD, OCD) rather than Tourette syndrome itself.

Treatment should be symptom targeted and, ideally, should also be holistic. This is important as it not only alleviates the suffering but may also improve the outlook in terms of tics, psychopathology and psychosocial functioning. Habit reversal training, exposure response prevention and comprehensive behavioural intervention for tics are gaining momentum in the treatment of tics in Tourette syndrome. Deep brain stimulation is currently the 'quantum leap' in many of our professional lives, but remains a research tool.

References

Alsobrook JP 2nd, Pauls DL (2002) A factor analysis of tic symptoms in Gilles de la Tourette's syndrome. *American Journal of Psychiatry*, **159**, 291–296.

American Psychiatric Association (2013) *Diagnostic and Statistical Manual of Mental Disorders (5th edn) (DSM 5)*. APA.

Bernard BA, Stebbins GT, Siegel S, *et al* (2009) Determinants of quality of life in children with Gilles de la Tourette syndrome. *Movement Disorders*, **24**, 1070–1073.

Burd L, Severud R, Klug MG, *et al* (1999) Prenatal and perinatal risk factors for Tourette disorder. *Journal of Perinatal Medicine*, **27**, 295–302.

Cavanna AE, Schrag A, Morley D, *et al* (2008) The Gilles de la Tourette Syndrome – Quality of Life scale (GTS-QOL): development and validation. *Neurology*, **71**, 1410–1416.

Cavanna AE, Critchley HD, Orth M, *et al* (2011) Dissecting the Gilles de la Tourette spectrum: a factor analytic study on 639 patients. *Journal of Neurology, Neurosurgery and Psychiatry*, **82**, 1320–1323.

Cavanna AE, David K, Orth M, *et al* (1212) Predictors during childhood of future health-related quality of life in adults with Gilles de la Tourette Syndrome. *European Journal of Paediatric Neurology*, **16**, 605–612.

Cavanna AE, Luoni C, Selvini C, *et al* (2013a) The Gilles de la Tourette Syndrome – Quality of Life Scale for children and adolescents (C&A-GTS-QOL): development and validation of the Italian version. *Behavioural Neurology*, **27**, 95–103.

Cavanna AE, Luoni C, Selvini C, *et al* (2013*b*) Disease-specific quality of life in young patients with Tourette syndrome. *Pediatric Neurology*, **48**, 111–114.

Chen K, Budman CL, Diego Herrera L, *et al* (2013) Prevalence and clinical correlates of explosive outbursts in Tourette Syndrome. *Psychiatry Research*, **205**, 269–275.

Chouza C, Romero S, Lorenzo J, *et al* (1982) Clinical trial of tiapride in patients with dyskinesia [article in French]. *La Semaine des Hôpitaux*, **58**, 725–733.

Clarke RA, Lee S, Eapen V (2012) Pathogenetic model for Tourette syndrome delineates overlap with related neurodevelopmental disorders including autism. *Translational Psychiatry*, **2**, e158.

Conelea CA, Woods DW, Zinner SH, *et al* (2011) Exploring the impact of chronic tic disorders on youth: results from the Tourette Syndrome Impact Survey. *Child Psychiatry and Human Development*, **42**, 219–242.

Cooper C, Robertson MM, Livingston G (2003) Psychological morbidity and caregiver burden in parents of children with Tourette's disorder and psychiatric comorbidity. *Journal of the American Academy of Child & Adolescent Psychiatry*, **42**, 1370–1375.

Cordero MI, Sandi C (2007) Stress amplifies memory for social hierarchy. *Frontiers in Neuroscience*, **1**, 175–184.

Cui YH, Zheng Y (2010) [Multiplicity analysis on the risk factors of patients with Tourette syndrome to develop the comorbidity of attention-deficit hyperactivity disorder] [article in Chinese]. *Zhonghua Er Ke Za Zhi [Chinese Journal of Pediatrics]*, **48**, 342–345.

Cui YH, Zheng Y, Yang YP, *et al* (2010) Effectiveness and tolerability of aripiprazole in children and adolescents with Tourette's disorder: a pilot study in China. *Journal of Child and Adolescent Psychopharmacology*, **20**, 291–298.

Cutler D, Murphy T, Gilmour J, *et al* (2009) The quality of life of young people with Tourette syndrome. *Child: Care, Health and Development*, **35**, 496–504.

Deng H, Gao K, Jankovic J (2012) The genetics of Tourette syndrome. *Nature Reviews (Neurology)*, **8**, 203–213.

Eapen V (2012) Neurodevelopmental genes have not read the DSM criteria: Or, have they? *Frontiers in Psychiatry*, **3**, 75.

Eapen V, Pauls DL, Robertson MM (1993) Evidence for autosomal dominant transmission in Tourette's syndrome: United Kingdom cohort study. *British Journal of Psychiatry*, **162**, 593–596.

Eddy CM, Cavanna AE, Gulisano M, *et al* (2011*a*) Clinical correlates of quality of life in Tourette syndrome. *Movement Disorders*, **2**, 735–738.

Eddy CM, Rizzo R, Gulisano M, *et al* (2011*b*) Quality of life in young people with Tourette syndrome: a controlled study. *Journal of Neurology*, **258**, 291–301.

Eddy CM, Cavanna AE, Gulisano M, *et al* (2012) The effects of comorbid obsessive-compulsive disorder and attention-deficit hyperactivity disorder on quality of life in Tourette syndrome. *Journal of Neuropsychiatry and Clinical Neuroscience*, **24**, 458–462.

Eggers C, Rothenberger A, Berghaus U (1988) Clinical and neurobiological findings in children suffering from tic disease following treatment with tiapride. *European Archives of Psychiatry and Neurological Sciences*, **237**, 223–229.

Freeman RD, Fast DK, Burd L, *et al* (2000) An international perspective on Tourette syndrome: selected findings from 3,500 individuals in 22 countries. *Developmental Medicine and Child Neurology*, **42**, 436–447.

Freeman RD, Zinner SH, Muller Vahl KR, *et al* (2009) Coprophenomena in Tourette syndrome. *Developmental Medicine and Child Neurology*, **51**, 218–227.

Gaffney GR, Sieg K, Hellings J (1994) The MOVES: a self-rating scale for Tourette's syndrome. *Journal of Child and Adolescent Psychopharmacology*, **4**, 269–280.

Ganos C, Ogrzal T, Schnitzler A, *et al* (2012*a*) The pathophysiology of echopraxia/echolalia: relevance to Gilles de la Tourette syndrome. *Movement Disorders*, **27**, 1222–1229.

Ganos C, Kahl U, Schunke O, *et al* (2012*b*) Are premonitory urges a prerequisite of tic inhibition in Gilles de la Tourette syndrome? *Journal of Neurology, Neurosurgery and Psychiatry*, **83**, 975–978.

Goetz CG, Tanner CM, Wilson RS, *et al* (1987) A rating scale for Gilles de la Tourette's syndrome: description, reliability, and validity data. *Neurology*, **37**, 1542–1544.

Grados MA, Mathews CA (2008) Latent class analysis of Gilles de la Tourette syndrome using comorbidities: clinical and genetic implications. *Biological Psychiatry*, **64**, 219–225

Haddad ADM, Umoh G, Bhatia, V, *et al* (2009) Adults with Tourette's syndrome with and without attention deficit hyperactivity disorder. *Acta Psychiatrica Scandinavica*, **120**, 299–307.

Hao Y, Tian Q, Lu Y, Chai Y, *et al* (2010) Psychometric properties of the Chinese version of the Pediatric Quality of Life Inventory 4.0 generic core scales. *Quality of Life Research*, **19**, 1229–1233.

Hariz MI, Robertson MM (2010) Deep brain stimulation and the Gilles de la Tourette syndrome. *European Journal of Neuroscience*, **32**, 1128–1134.

Hornsey H, Banerjee S, Zeitlin H, *et al* (2001) The prevalence of Tourette syndrome in 13–14 year olds in mainstream schools. *Journal of Child Psychology and Psychiatry*, **42**, 1035–1039.

Khalifa N, von Knorring AL (2003) Prevalence of tic disorders and Tourette syndrome in a Swedish school population. *Developmental Medicine and Child Neurology*, **45**, 315–319.

Khalifa N, von Knorring AL (2005) Tourette syndrome and other tic disorders in a total population of children: clinical assessment and background. *Acta Paediatrica*, **94**, 1608–1614.

Knight S, Coon H, Johnson M, *et al* (2010) Linkage analysis of Tourette syndrome in a large Utah pedigree. *American Journal of Medical Genetics Part B Neuropsychiatric Genetics*, **153B**, 656–662.

Kurlan R, Daragjati C, Como P, *et al* (1996) Non-obscene complex socially inappropriate behavior in Tourette's syndrome. *Journal of Neuropsychiatry and Clinical Neurosciences*, **8**, 311–317.

Kwak C, Dat Vuong K, Jankovic J (2003) Premonitory sensory phenomena in Tourette's syndrome. *Movement Disorders*, **18**, 1530–1533.

Leckman JF (2003) In search of the pathophysiology of Tourette syndrome. In *Mental and Behavioral Dysfunction in Movement Disorders* (eds MA Bedard, Y Agid, S Chouinard, *et al*), pp. 467– 476. Humana Press.

Leckman JF, Riddle MA, Hardin MT, *et al* (1989) The Yale Global Tic Severity Scale: initial testing of a clinician-rated scale of tic severity. *Journal of the American Academy of Child & Adolescent Psychiatry*, **28**, 566–573.

Leckman JF, Bloch MH, Scahill L, *et al* (2006) Tourette syndrome: the self under seige. *Journal of Child Neurology*, **21**, 642–649.

Lee MY, Chen YC, Wang HS, *et al* (2007) Parenting stress and related factors in parents of children with Tourette syndrome. *Journal of Nursing Research*, **15**, 165–174.

Lees AJ, Robertson M, Trimble MR, *et al* (1984) A clinical study of Gilles de la Tourette syndrome in the United Kingdom. *Journal of Neurology, Neurosurgery and Psychiatry*, 47, 1–8.

Liu J (2011) Early health risk factors for violence: conceptualization, review of the evidence and implications. *Aggression and Violent Behavior*, **16**, 63–73.

Liu ZS, Chen YH, Zhong YQ, *et al* (2011) [A multicenter controlled study on aripiprazole treatment for children with Tourette syndrome in China] [article in Chinese]. *Zhonghua Er Ke Za Zhi [Chinese Journal of Pediatrics]*, **49**, 572–576.

Marquez C, Poirier GL, Cordero MI, *et al* (2013) Peripuberty stress leads to abnormal aggression, altered amygdala and orbitofrontal reactivity and increased prefrontal MAOA gene expression. *Translational Psychiatry*, **3**, e216.

Mathews CA, Waller J, Glidden D, *et al* (2004) Self injurious behaviour in Tourette syndrome: correlates with impulsivity and impulse control. *Journal of Neurology, Neurosurgery and Psychiatry*, 75, 1149–1155.

Mathews CA, Bimson B, Lowe TL, *et al* (2006) Association between maternal smoking and increased symptom severity in Tourette's syndrome. *American Journal of Psychiatry*, **163**, 1066–1073.

McGrath LM, Mustanski B, Metzger A, *et al* (2012) A latent modelling approach to genotype–phenotype relationships, maternal problem behavior clusters, prenatal smoking and MAOA genotype. *Archives of Women's Mental Health*, **15**, 269–282.

McGuire JF, Nyirabahizi E, Kircanski K, *et al* (2013) A cluster analysis of tic symptoms in children and adults with Tourette syndrome: Clinical correlates and treatment outcome. *Psychiatry Research*, **210**, 1198–1204.

Motlagh MG, Katsovich L, Thompson N, *et al* (2010) Severe psychosocial stress and heavy cigarette smoking during pregnancy: an examination of the pre- and perinatal risk factors associated with ADHD and Tourette syndrome. *European Child & Adolescent Psychiatry*, **19**, 755–764.

Neuner I, Nordt C, Schaender F, *et al* (2012) Effectiveness of aripiprazole in the treatment of adult Tourette patients up to 56 months. *Human Psychopharmacology*, **27**, 364–369.

O'Rourke JA, Scharf JM, Yu D, *et al* (2009) The genetics of Tourette syndrome: a review. *Journal of Psychosomatic Research*, **67**, 533–545.

Pappert EJ, Goetz CJ, Loius ED, *et al* (2003) Objective assessments of longitudinal outcome in Gilles de la Tourette's syndrome. *Neurology*, **61**, 936–940.

Pavlov KA, Chistiakov DA, Chekhonin VP (2012) Genetic determinants of aggression and impulsivity in humans. *Journal of Applied Genetics*, **53**, 61–82.

Peterson BS, Leckman JF (1998) The temporal dynamics of tics in Gilles de la Tourette syndrome. *Biological Psychiatry*, **44**, 1337–1348.

Piacentini J, Woods DW, Scahill L, *et al* (2010) Behaviour therapy for children with Tourette disorder: a randomized controlled trial. *JAMA*, **303**, 1929–1937.

Pringsheim T, Lang A, Kurlan R, *et al* (2009a) Understanding disability in Tourette syndrome. *Developmental Medicine and Child Neurology*, **51**, 468–472.

Pringsheim T, Sandor P, Lang A, *et al* (2009b) Prenatal and perinatal morbidity in children with Tourette syndrome and attention-deficit hyperactivity disorder. *Journal of Developmental and Behavioral Pediatrics*, **30**, 115–121.

Rickards, H, Cavanna AE, Worral R (2012) Treatment practices in Tourette syndrome: the European perspective. *European Journal of Paediatric Neurology*, **16**, 361–364.

Rizzo R, Gulisano M, Cali PV, *et al* (2012) Long term clinical course of Tourette syndrome. *Brain Development*, **34**, 667–673.

Robertson MM (2000) Tourette syndrome, associated conditions and the complexities of treatment. *Brain*, **123**, 425–462.

Robertson MM (2003) The heterogeneous psychopathology of Tourette syndrome. In *Mental and Behavioral Dysfunction in Movement Disorders* (eds MA Bedard, Y Agid, S Chouinard, *et al*), pp. 443–466. Humana Press.

Robertson MM (2006a) Attention deficit hyperactivity disorder, tics and Tourette's syndrome: the relationship and treatment implications. A commentary. *European Child and Adolescent Psychiatry*, **15**, 1–11.

Robertson MM (2006b) Tourette syndrome and affective disorders: an update. *Journal of Psychosomatic Research*, **61**, 349–358.

Robertson MM (2008a) The prevalence and epidemiology of Gilles de la Tourette syndrome. Part 1: the epidemiological and prevalence studies. *Journal of Psychosomatic Research*, **65**, 461–472.

Robertson MM (2008b) The prevalence and epidemiology of Gilles de la Tourette syndrome. Part 2: tentative explanations for differing prevalence figures in GTS, including the possible effects of psychopathology, aetiology, cultural differences, and differing phenotypes. *Journal of Psychosomatic Research*, **65**, 473–486.

Robertson MM (2011) Gilles de la Tourette syndrome: the complexities of phenotype and treatment. *British Journal of Hospital Medicine*, **72**, 100–107.

Robertson MM (2012) The Gilles de la Tourette syndrome: the current status. *Archives of Disease in Childhood: Education & Practice*, **97** (5), 166–175.

Robertson M, Cavanna A (2007) The Gilles de la Tourette syndrome: a principal component factor analytic study of a large pedigree. *Psychiatric Genetics*, **17**, 143–152.

Robertson M, Cavanna A (2008) *Tourette Syndrome: The Facts* (2nd edn). Oxford University Press.

Robertson MM, Eapen V (1992) Pharmacologic controversy of CNS stimulants in Gilles de la Tourette's syndrome. *Clinical Neuropharmacology*, **15**, 408–425.

Robertson MM, Eapen V (1996) The National Hospital Interview Schedule for the assessment of Gilles de la Tourette syndrome and related behaviors. *International Journal of Methods in Psychiatric Research*, **6**, 203–226.

Robertson MM, Eapen V (2013) Whither the relationship between etiology and phenotype in Tourette syndrome? In *Tourette Syndrome* (eds D Martino, JF Leckman), pp. 361–394. Oxford University Press.

Robertson MM, Gourdie A (1990) Familial Tourette's syndrome in a large British pedigree: associated psychopathology, severity, and potential for linkage analysis. *British Journal of Psychiatry*, **156**, 515–521.

Robertson MM, Trimble MR (1993) Normal chromosomal findings in Gilles de la Tourette syndrome. *Psychiatric Genetics*, **3**, 95–99.

Robertson MM, Trimble MR, Lees AJ (1988) The psychopathology of the Gilles de la Tourette syndrome: a phenomenological analysis. *British Journal of Psychiatry*, **152**, 383–390.

Robertson MM, Trimble MR, Lees AJ (1989) Self-injurious behaviour and the Gilles de la Tourette syndrome: a clinical study and review of the literature. *Psychological Medicine*, **19**, 611–625.

Robertson MM, Banerjee S, Fox Hiley PJ, *et al* (1997) Personality disorder and psychopathology in Tourette's syndrome: a controlled study. *British Journal of Psychiatry*, **171**, 283–286.

Robertson MM, Banerjee S, Kurlan R, *et al* (1999) The Tourette Diagnostic Confidence Index: development and clinical associations. *Neurology*, **53**, 2108–2112.

Robertson MM, Althoff RR, Hafez A, *et al* (2008) Principal components analysis of a large cohort with Tourette syndrome. *British Journal of Psychiatry*, **193**, 31–36.

Scahill L, Erenberg G, Berlin CM Jr, *et al* (2006) Contemporary assessment and pharmacotherapy of Tourette syndrome. *NeuroRx*, **3**, 192–206.

Scharf JM, Miller LL, Mathews CA, *et al* (2012) Prevalence of Tourette syndrome and chronic tics in the population-based Avon Longitudinal Study of Parents and Children cohort. *Journal of the American Academy of Child & Adolescent Psychiatry*, **51**, 192–201.

State MW (2010) The genetics of child psychiatric disorders: focus on autism and Tourette syndrome. *Neuron*, **68**, 254–269.

Storch EA, Merlo LJ, Lack C, *et al* (2007) Quality of life in youth with Tourette's syndrome and chronic tic disorder. *Journal of Clinical Child and Adolescent Psychology*, **36**, 217–227.

Swedo SE, Leonard HL, Garvey M, *et al* (1998) Pediatric autoimmune neuropsychiatric disorders associated with streptococcal infections: clinical description of the first 50 cases. *American Journal of Psychiatry*, **155**, 264–271.

Timmer M, Cordero MI, Severlings Y, *et al* (2011) Evidence for a role of oxytocin receptors in the long-term establishment of dominance hierarchies. *Neuropsychopharmacology*, **36**, 234–256.

Tourette's Syndrome Study Group (2002) Treatment of ADHD in children with tics: a randomized controlled trial. *Neurology*, **58**, 527–536.

Verdellen C, van de Grient J, Hartmann A, *et al* (2011) European Clinical Guidelines for Tourette Syndrome and other tic disorders. Part III: behavioural and psychosocial interventions. *European Child & Adolescent Psychiatry*, **20**, 197–207.

Verhoeven FE, Booij L, Kruijt AW, *et al* (2012) The effects of MAOA genotype, childhood trauma, and sex, on trait and state-dependent aggression. *Brain and Behavior*, **2**, 806–813.

Walkup JT, Rosenberg LA, Brown J, *et al* (1992) The validity of instruments measuring tic severity in Tourette's syndrome. *Journal of the American Academy of Child & Adolescent Psychiatry*, **31**, 472–477.

Walkup JT, Kahn S, Sehuerholz L (1999) Phenomenology and natural history of tic-related ADHD and learning disability. In *Tourette Syndrome: Developmental Psychopathology and Clinical Care* (eds JS Leckman, DFJ Cohen), pp 63–79. John Wiley & Sons.

Wenzel C, Kleinmann A, Bokemeyer S, *et al* (2012) Aripiprazole for the treatment of Tourette syndrome; a series of 100 patients. *Journal of Clinical Psychopharmacology*, **32**, 548–550.

Woods DW, Piacentini J, Himle MB, *et al* (2005) Premonitory Urge for Tics Scale (PUTS): initial psychometric results and examination of the premonitory urge phenomenon in youths with tic disorders. *Journal of Developmental and Behavioral Pediatrics*, **26**, 397–403.

World Health Organization (1992) *The ICD-10 Classification of Mental and Behavioural Disorders: Clinical Descriptions and Diagnostic Guidelines*. WHO.

Yi MJ, Sun ZY, Ran N, *et al* (2011) [Subjective quality of life in children with Tourette syndrome] [article in Chinese]. *Zhong Guo Dang Dai Er Ke Za Zhi [Chinese Journal of Contemporary Pediatrics]*, **13**, 732–735.

Zhang HY, Liu CY, Wang YQ (2012) [Risk factors for Tourette syndrome] [article in Chinese]. *Zhong Guo Dang Dai Er Ke Za Zhi [Chinese Journal of Contemporary Pediatrics]*, **14**, 426–430.

CHAPTER 18

Sleep disorders

Gregory Stores

Much knowledge about sleep and its disorders has accumulated in recent times, but awareness of these advances among both the general public and professionals remains inadequate. This is especially so regarding sleep disorders in children and adolescents, despite the publication of valuable sources of information relevant to clinical practice such as that by Mindell & Owens (2010).

Before the scientific study of sleep began, important observations were made by some writers. For example, Charles Dickens provided some of the best descriptions of a wide variety of sleep disorders (presumably based on his observations of real people), including some in children and adolescents (Cosnett, 1992). The most notable of these is Joe the Fat Boy in *The Pickwick Papers*, who might well have suffered from obstructive sleep apnoea. Dickens's accounts of this and other sleep disorders preceded those of clinicians many years later.

Although sleep medicine is now a specialty in its own right, all clinicians would benefit from having at least a working knowledge of the field. Many patients seen in both primary and secondary care are likely to have sleep problems, and these can often be treated without recourse to the special sleep centres that are now available for complicated cases. This chapter reviews main aspects of sleep and its disorders, with special emphasis on clinical practice in child and adolescent psychiatry. More detailed accounts are provided elsewhere, both in terms of children's sleep disorders in general (Stores, 2006a) and also sleep disturbance in children and adolescents who have disorders of development (Stores & Wiggs, 2001).

Only selected references to the literature are provided. In places, 'child' or 'children' can be taken to include adolescents.

Links between disturbed sleep and child and adolescent psychiatry

Sleep medicine is a multidisciplinary specialty based on approaches and information from general medicine and paediatrics, adult and child psychiatry, neuropsychiatry, psychology (including developmental aspects) and several other disciplines. Increasingly, advances are being made concerning the neurobiology of sleep, aspects of which are reflected in disorders of sleep and wakefulness (Schwartz & Roth, 2008). Mahowald and colleagues (2011) refer to wakefulness, rapid eye movement (REM) sleep and non-rapid eye movement (NREM) sleep as the 'primary states of being'. These are not necessarily mutually exclusive states and they can occur in various combinations to produce intriguing and surprising clinical consequences in various sleep disorders. In sleepwalking, for example, both adults and children can perform highly complicated acts while still asleep. Failure to recognise this fact easily leads to misinterpretation of the episodes as attention-seeking or otherwise intentional behaviour.

In considering the relationships between sleep problems and psychiatric disorders in children and adolescents, the following points are worthy of note. First, the rate of significant sleep disturbance is increased in children and adolescents with a wide range of psychiatric problems, and not just anxiety states and depression (Ivanenko & Johnson, 2008; Alfano & Gamble, 2009). Conversely, children with inadequate or poor-quality sleep are at increased risk of developing psychological or psychiatric conditions such as attention-deficit hyperactivity disorder (ADHD) behaviour. Second, certain psychotropic medications can disturb sleep. Examples include sleeplessness caused by some antidepressant and stimulant drugs, and daytime sleepiness produced by sedative-hypnotic drugs. Third, some forms of sleep disturbance may be misdiagnosed as psychiatric disorders (Stores, 2007a). For example, pathological sleepiness may be misinterpreted as depression.

Prevalence of sleep disturbance

Overall, a significant sleep disturbance occurs in about 25% of children and adolescents (Owens, 2008). However, prevalence rates well in excess of this are reported in certain high-risk groups, namely, children with an intellectual disability, other neurodevelopmental disorder, psychiatric condition or other chronic paediatric condition. For example, estimated rates are reported to be 50–80% in children with autism spectrum disorders (Richdale & Schreck, 2009) and up to 50% in those diagnosed with ADHD (Corkum et al, 2011).

The lives of such children (and those of their parents) are highly likely to be further complicated by disturbed sleep and its consequences. Children with these high-risk conditions do not have a separate set of underlying sleep disorders compared with other children. The differences lie in the relative pattern of occurrence of the various sleep disorders, the degree of severity and a greater tendency for the sleep disorder to persist if untreated.

The distinction between sleep problems and sleep disorders

It is essential to distinguish between a sleep problem and a sleep disorder. At any age, there are just three basic sleep problems:

- not sleeping well (insomnia or sleeplessness), taking the form of not readily getting to sleep, difficulty staying asleep, or waking early and not returning to sleep
- excessive daytime sleepiness, including sleeping during the day or prolonged overnight sleeping
- behaving in unusual ways, having strange experiences or exhibiting unusual movements at various stages of the sleep process (parasomnias).

Sleep disorder refers to the underlying cause of the sleep problem. The International Classification of Sleep Disorders (ICSD-2) (American Academy of Sleep Medicine, 2005) describes over 80 sleep disorders, many of which occur in children and adolescents. There is some merit in using this system of classification as it is considered to be more diagnostically specific and up to date than the DSM and ICD classifications of sleep disturbance.

Aetiological factors

In children, as in adults, psychological, neurological, respiratory, metabolic, endocrine, genetic, pharmacological and other physical factors may influence sleep. The following examples illustrate the need to consider a wide range of possible explanations for a child's sleep disturbance.

- In very young children, a degree of early brain maturation is required for the biological clock controlling sleep–wake rhythms to develop.
- Parenting practices can profoundly influence young children's sleep patterns: lack of routine, poor limit-setting, and reinforcement by paying too much attention to a child's reluctance to settle to sleep can cause or maintain sleep problems.
- Adolescent sleep difficulties may be caused by a combination of pubertal changes in sleep physiology and altered lifestyle, as well as emotional problems.
- At any age, the possibility of medical causes of sleep problems needs to be considered, including medications the child is taking.

There may be additional considerations concerning children whose development is delayed.

- A child's intellectual limitations or communication problems can interfere with learning good sleep habits, as may parents' mental health and parenting abilities.
- Additional physical and psychiatric conditions associated with the child's condition are likely to contribute to sleep disturbance. This is so in the case, for example, of children diagnosed with ADHD, who may have sleep apnoea and other psychiatric conditions (Konofal et al, 2010), and also those with autism spectrum disorders, where comorbidities can include epilepsy and mood disorders (Richdale & Schreck, 2009). Such comorbidities are common throughout neurodevelopmental disorders. For instance, in Down syndrome, children are prone to

many specific medical problems, including obstructive sleep apnoea, and also various psychiatric conditions (Stores & Stores, 2013).

Continuity of sleep disorders into adulthood

The following examples illustrate this possibility.

- Rhythmic movement disorders such as headbanging usually remit spontaneously by about 3 years of age, and arousal disorders (such as sleepwalking) by puberty. In a minority, both may persist into adulthood.
- Adenotonsillar hypertrophy is the usual cause of obstructive sleep apnoea in children. It is treatable by surgery, but anatomically more complex causes (as in some neurodevelopmental disorders) are more difficult to correct.
- Behavioural insomnia of childhood, largely the result of failure to learn good sleep habits, can continue into adult life if untreated.
- Nightmares usually cease spontaneously by adolescence or adulthood, but if they are part of post-traumatic stress disorder they might persist long term.
- Narcolepsy often begins in childhood or adolescence and can continue well into adult life.
- If untreated, delayed sleep phase syndrome (discussed below) may persist or give rise to potentially long-lasting secondary sleep-disrupting difficulties such as depression, the use of alcohol to combat insomnia, and stimulant drugs to counteract daytime sleepiness.
- Conditioned or learned insomnia results from associating being in bed with being awake and distressed about being unable to sleep. The problem can persist if this negative association is not replaced by positive associations.
- Idiopathic insomnia typically begins in childhood, is resistant to treatment and may well be lifelong.

Developmental aspects of sleep disorders, including differences between children and adults

The literature on sleep disturbance in adults cannot be drawn on freely when considering children and adolescents, as many changes take place before adulthood is reached. There are alterations in sleep physiology, for example, including the gradual reduction of REM sleep, which is particularly abundant in very young children (perhaps because of its importance for early brain development), and the need for daytime naps, which have usually tailed off by 3 years of age. Sleep requirements also gradually lessen throughout childhood until about the time of puberty, when the need for sleep may increase again during the teens.

The pattern of sleep disorders is different from that in adults. Characteristically, childhood sleep disorders are bedtime settling and troublesome night-waking, rhythmic movement disorders, nocturnal enuresis and arousal disorders. Parental behaviour may well be aetiologically relevant to the sleep disorder. Parents' knowledge, attitudes and emotional state often determine whether they see their child's sleep pattern as a problem or not.

Basically, a particular sleep disorder can have different clinical associations in children than in adults. For example, adult obstructive sleep apnoea generally causes sleepiness and reduced activity during the day; but children with this condition (or other sleep disorders causing sleep loss or disruption) can be abnormally active. There may also be differences in significance. Many childhood sleep disorders can be expected to resolve spontaneously in a way that is unusual in adults, and children's sleep disorders are generally less frequently associated with psychiatric illness than in adults. Finally, the need for multidisciplinary involvement in assessment and management of children with disturbed sleep can be greater than in the case of adults. In addition to medical specialties, developmental psychology and child and family psychiatry often have important contributions to make.

Effects on child development of persistently disturbed sleep

There are many potentially serious psychological/psychiatric, social and physical effects of persistently disturbed sleep.

Emotional state and behaviour

'Overtired' children are often irritable and even aggressive. Bedtime can become distressing if associated with upsetting experiences such as night-time fears. Delayed sleep phase syndrome can lead to mood and other emotional changes, both directly because of sleep deprivation and also as a result of the psychosocial consequences of the condition (Gregory & Sadeh, 2012).

Intellectual function and education

Insufficient sleep can cause impaired concentration, memory, decision-making and general ability to learn (Fallone *et al*, 2002). Studies in the USA have suggested that 80% of adolescents obtain less than the average 9 hours of sleep required for satisfactory daytime functioning, 25% obtain less than 6 hours and over 25% fall asleep in class. Also, students whose sleep becomes insufficient generally achieve lower school grades than previously (National Sleep Foundation, 2006).

Physical effects

As the production of growth hormone is closely linked to deep NREM sleep, disruption of this type of sleep may affect physical growth (Smalldone *et al*, 2007). Similarly, obstructive sleep apnoea can impair the depth and quality of sleep, causing failure to thrive in some young children. In addition, persistent sleep loss may be associated with impaired immunity, obesity, hypertension and diabetes.

Family and other social effects

Because of their own loss of sleep, parents (mainly mothers) may become anxious and depressed and unable to cope (sometimes even resorting to an increased use of physical punishment) (Meltzer & Mindell, 2007). Marital relationships can become seriously strained.

Principles of assessment

Screening for sleep disturbance

Routinely, history taking should at least include questions about the items in Box 18.1. If the answers are positive, further details may be obtained using a brief standardised screening questionnaire such as the Children's Sleep Habits Questionnaire, which has versions for school-age children (Owens *et al*, 2000) and toddlers/preschool children (Goodlin-Jones *et al*, 2008). It has been used with typically developing children and others whose development is delayed.

Diagnosis of the sleep disorder

Screening for sleep symptoms simply highlights the possibility of a sleep disorder and does not constitute a diagnosis. Identification of a sleep disorder requires the information listed in Box 18.2.

Box 18.1 Taking a routine history for sleep disturbance

The clinician should ask whether the child:

- has difficulties at bedtime or settling to sleep
- wakes during the night
- has breathing problems while asleep
- shows unusual behaviours, experiences or movements at night
- has difficulty waking up in the morning
- is unusually sleepy or 'overtired' during the day.

Box 18.2 Identification of a sleep disorder

Diagnosis will depend on:

- detailed histories, especially about the sleep problem
- the child's 24 hour sleep–wake pattern, including parenting practices
- the child's developmental history
- family history and circumstances
- physical and behavioural examination
- possibly further assessment in the form of a sleep diary and objective sleep studies such as actigraphy or polysomnography.

It may be necessary to refer the child for assessment at a specialised paediatric service (such as an ear, nose and throat clinic if sleep apnoea is a possibility) or a paediatric sleep disorders service. Sleep centres in the UK can be located through the British Sleep Society's website (http://www.sleepsociety.org.uk/sleep-centre-locator).

General principles of treatment

There are many forms of treatment for sleep disorders. Choice depends on accurate diagnosis of the child's problem. The evidence for the efficacy of these treatments varies (Kuhn & Elliott, 2003) and is often based on a consensus of clinical experience.

Education of parents about the developmental importance of sleep, how to promote good sleep habits from an early age, and also what are realistic expectations at different ages is an important general requirement. An optimistic view of treatment possibilities should be encouraged.

Principles of sleep hygiene help to promote good sleep habits (Jan *et al*, 2008). These might be sufficient in themselves to prevent or treat disturbed sleep, and they are also useful as an accompaniment to more specific treatment for a given sleep disorder. Good sleep hygiene (the details of which vary with the child's age) includes aspects such as those listed in Box 18.3.

Behavioural methods are appropriate, especially (although not only) for insomnia. Pharmacological treatments are suitable in a limited number of circumstances, including when behavioural methods have failed (Hollway & Aman, 2011).

Other treatments include chronotherapy (resetting the biological clock) for sleep–wake cycle disorders, and physical interventions (such as adenotonsillectomy, continuous positive airway pressure and weight reduction for obstructive sleep apnoea). It goes without saying that further assessment and specific treatments may be needed if emotional disturbance is marked in either the child or members of the family.

> **Box 18.3**   Some fundamentals of good sleep hygiene
>
> - Regular daytime and bedtime routines and timing
> - The avoidance of arousing activities and stimulating drinks near bedtime
> - A bedroom conducive to relaxation and sleep, and not associated with entertainment
> - Prevention of negative associations with sleeplessness, such as distress when lying awake in bed unable to sleep

Management of specific sleep disorders

The following summary is organised in terms of the sleep disorders that might underlie the three basic sleep problems mentioned earlier. Child psychiatrists and their teams might usefully incorporate the principles and practices into their approaches to patients with disturbed sleep whatever their primary diagnosis. The importance of screening for sleep problems and, where indicated, accurate diagnosis of the underlying sleep disorder has already been emphasised. Treatment possibilities and issues are considered in detail elsewhere (Kotagal, 2012).

Insomnia

The origins of this type of sleep problem might lie in a failure to encourage good sleep habits at an early age (under 5). Basic guidelines for achieving this are well described, including teaching children to fall asleep alone so that when they wake in the night they will be able to fall asleep again without requiring parents' attention ('self-soothing'), and establishing a consistent 24-hour routine, especially at bedtime.

Problems of resisting going to bed at the required time, and/or waking repeatedly at night and demanding their parents' attention (including coming into their bed), are extensively treated by behavioural methods (such as 'graduated extinction') in typically developing children (Mindell *et al*, 2006). They are also advocated for children with developmental disorders in whom insomnia is particularly common because of medical, psychiatric as well as neurodevelopmental conditions (Richdale & Wiggs, 2005).

In general, behavioural methods are recommended in preference to pharmacological treatment. However, sedative/hypnotic drugs are often used, despite little evidence in support of the practice (Owens & Moturi, 2009).

Melatonin deserves special mention because of its current popularity, mainly as a treatment for sleeplessness. How far it deserves this popularity has yet to be clarified because of the relatively few methodologically sound studies and inconsistent findings (London New Drugs Group, 2008). However, some recent reports (e.g. Lerchl & Reiter, 2012; Gringras *et al*,

2012) provide more convincing evidence that melatonin can be effective, perhaps especially in children with neurodevelopmental disorders, although inconsistency of response from one child to another has yet to be explained. Other important issues concern dosage, short- and long-acting forms of the drug, possible adverse effects and long-term efficacy. Generally, it might be considered appropriate to assess the usefulness of melatonin if behavioural treatments have been adequately tried without success.

In school-age children some of the causes of insomnia in younger children still apply but enquiry might reveal other factors such as night-time fears. These fears are usually transient and require only reassurance and comfort, but in some children they are so intense and persistent as part of an anxiety state, including post-traumatic stress disorder (PTSD), that they need special attention. Other possibilities include worry about daytime matters, conditioned insomnia and the restless legs syndrome.

Early morning waking, where the child wakes very early, does not go back to sleep and is noisy or demands attention, can be very distressing to parents and other members of the family. It can result from bedtime being too early (in which case the time the child goes to sleep should be gradually reset), or it may be part of an anxiety state or depressive disorder.

High rates of insomnia have been consistently reported in adolescents. Implicated factors can be worries, anxiety and depression, or an excess of caffeine-containing drinks, alcohol or nicotine, as well as illicit drug use and withdrawal. Difficulty getting to sleep because of a physiological shift in the sleep phase (as well as daytime sleepiness) is a prominent part of delayed sleep phase syndrome. Instead of recriminations and attempts to set limits, the timing of the sleep phase needs to be reset.

For further details of the clinical management of insomnia in children and adolescents see Mindell & Owens (2010).

Excessive daytime sleepiness

Excessive sleepiness is mainly a problem in older children and adolescents, in whom it has been associated with behavioural and psychiatric problems as well as with educational underperformance and other disadvantages (Carskadon, 2011). Extreme sleepiness will cause a reduction of activity at any age, but lesser degrees in young people may produce irritability, overactivity, restlessness, poor concentration, impulsiveness or aggression. These symptoms can lead to a diagnosis of ADHD without it being realised that the origin of the behaviour was a sleep disorder. Kothare & Kaleyias (2008) have described the diagnostic approach to excessive sleepiness. It is useful to consider the following three main categories of possible causes.

Insufficient sleep

Delayed sleep phase syndrome causes both insomnia and excessive daytime sleepiness. It is said to be common in adolescents. Its main diagnostic features are listed in Box 18.4.

> **Box 18.4** Key diagnostic features of delayed sleep phase syndrome
>
> - Persistently severe difficulty getting to sleep, often staying awake until very late
> - Usually uninterrupted sound sleep once it is achieved
> - Considerable reluctance to get up for school, college or work; school attendance may be sporadic or even discontinued
> - Sleepiness and underfunctioning, especially during the first part of the day, giving way to alertness in the evening and early hours
> - The abnormal sleep pattern is maintained by sleeping in very late when able to do so (e.g. at weekends and during holidays)

Treatment consists of gradually and consistently changing the sleep phase to an appropriate time. Additional measures to achieve or maintain the improved sleep schedule include early-morning exposure to light and possibly the use of melatonin (Gradisar *et al*, 2011).

Disturbed nocturnal sleep

Daytime sleepiness, despite sleep duration at night being within normal limits, suggests that the restorative quality of the sleep is impaired. Poor-quality sleep can be caused by physical illness and psychiatric disorders (such as anxiety or depression) and some of their pharmacological treatments, obstructive sleep apnoea (which occurs in at least 2% of all children, with a much higher prevalence in children with various intellectual disabilities, notably Down syndrome (Stores & Stores, 2013)), and other sleep disorders, such as periodic limb movements in sleep.

Disorders involving an increased tendency to sleep

In some cases, prolonged or otherwise excessive sleep is an intrinsic part of the condition, rather than a consequence of it. Narcolepsy is the prime example, with the classic combination of daytime sleep attacks, overnight sleep disruption, cataplexy, hypnagogic hallucinations and sleep paralysis. Narcolepsy with cataplexy occurs in about 0.1% of the population. Onset is common in childhood and adolescence, when its clinical manifestations can be complex and easily misinterpreted with the correct diagnosis often delayed by many years (Stores, 2006*b*). Narcolepsy can be associated with serious psychosocial difficulties and psychiatric disorders, as might other causes of excessive daytime sleepiness (Stores *et al*, 2006).

Other possibilities (usually involving intermittent episodes of excessive sleepiness) include Kleine–Levin syndrome (classically with the addition of bouts of hyperphagia and hypersexuality, as well as other bizarre behaviour), major depressive disorder, substance misuse, menstruation-related hypersomnia and certain other neurological diseases. Misdiagnosis is a particular risk in Kleine–Levin syndrome (Pike & Stores, 1994).

Parasomnias

More than 20 types of parasomnia are described in ICSD-2 (American Academy of Sleep Medicine, 2005). They can easily be confused with each other if the distinctive features of each are not known, or not carefully described on clinical assessment. Precise diagnosis is important, as different parasomnias may well need contrasting types of treatment. Accurate diagnosis depends principally on a detailed account of the subjective and objective sequence of events from the onset of each episode to its resolution, as well as the circumstances in which it occurs. Audio-visual recordings combined with polysomnography can be helpful if the nature of the episodes remains unclear. Preliminary home video recordings by parents also may reveal features omitted from the descriptions provided in the clinic.

The more dramatic forms of parasomnia seem to be a main cause of diagnostic confusion and imprecision, as well as unnecessary concern about their psychological significance, as many are benign. However, parasomnias may lead to psychological complications if the child is frightened, embarrassed or otherwise upset by the experience, or because of the reactions of other people to the episodes.

As many childhood primary parasomnias remit spontaneously within a few years, children and parents can often be reassured about the future, although protective measures (e.g. in severe headbanging or sleepwalking) may be required in the meantime.

Specific treatment, including medication, is needed in only a minority of cases of primary parasomnia, but is likely to be required for the underlying disorder in the secondary parasomnias.

For more detailed information on parasomnias in children and adolescents see Stores (2007b).

Primary parasomnias

Primary parasomnias are primary sleep phenomena and generally common in children. They include hypnagogic (at sleep onset) and hypnopompic (on waking) hallucinations, which are common and benign but can be frightening and even misdiagnosed as psychosis if associated with sleep paralysis (Stores, 1998). Sleep-related rhythmic movement disorders (such as headbanging) occur in many young children, almost always remitting spontaneously by 3 to 4 years of age. Nocturnal enuresis can usually be classified as a primary parasomnia.

Parents are often distressed to witness confusional arousals, sleepwalking (especially of the agitated type) or sleep terrors, which are forms of 'arousal disorder' common in young children. The degree of agitation and confused behaviour may be extreme, suggesting that the child is suffering in some way. In fact, during an arousal disorder episode the child remains asleep and unaware of the events. Understandable attempts to arouse the child and provide comfort should be discouraged as this may cause real distress.

The term 'nightmare' is sometimes used misleadingly for any form of dramatic parasomnia. True nightmares (frightening dreams), if frequent and associated with intense bedtime fears, may indicate an anxiety disorder and their content may suggest a cause.

Secondary parasomnias

Secondary parasomnias are manifestations of a physical or psychiatric disorder. Examples of the former type are sleep-related epilepsies, including benign centrotemporal (Rolandic) epilepsy (the most common form of childhood epilepsy) and nocturnal frontal lobe epilepsy. As the clinical manifestations of seizures in these two forms of epilepsy can consist of changes in behaviour (which may be dramatic), the conditions are likely to be misdiagnosed as non-epileptic, such as attention-seeking or dissociative states.

Other parasomnias

Other parasomnias that are part of physical or psychiatric disorders include those associated with obstructive sleep apnoea, gastrointestinal reflux, REM sleep behaviour disorder (in many cases), nocturnal panic attacks, nocturnal disturbances in PTSD and dissociative states. Simulated parasomnias, shown by polysomnography to be enacted during wakefulness, sometimes occur in children and adolescents.

Conclusion

In various ways sleep and its disorders can be seen as a central topic in child and adolescent psychiatry (and, indeed, other branches of psychiatry). Therefore, all psychiatrists should be familiar with the principles of modern sleep disorders medicine. The sleep disorders field is advancing rapidly, but the accumulated knowledge is not yet sufficiently represented in professional teaching and training (Peile, 2010). However, in principle, there are now many opportunities for child and adolescent psychiatrists (including those whose work involves the care of children with neurodevelopmental disorders) to contribute as part of their practice to the accurate diagnosis, prevention and successful treatment of sleep disorders to the benefit of their patients and their families.

References

Alfano CA, Gamble AL (2009) The role of sleep in child psychiatric disorders. *Child Youth Care Forum*, **38**, 327–340.
American Academy of Sleep Medicine (2005) *International Classification of Sleep Disorders, 2nd Edition: Diagnostic and Coding Manual*. American Academy of Sleep Medicine.
Carskadon MA (2011) Sleep's effects on cognition and learning in adolescence. *Progress in Brain Research*, **190**, 137–143.

Corkum P, Davidson F, Macpherson M (2011) A framework for the assessment and treatment of sleep problems in children with attention-deficit/hyperactivity disorder. *Pediatric Clinics of North America*, **58**, 667–683.

Cosnett JE (1992) Charles Dickens: observer of sleep and its disorders. *Sleep*, **15**, 264–267.

Fallone G, Owens JA, Deane J (2002) Sleepiness in children and adolescents: clinical implications. *Sleep Medicine Reviews*, **6**, 287–306.

Goodlin-Jones BL, Sitnick SL, Tang K, *et al* (2008) The Children's Sleep Habits Questionnaire in toddlers and preschool children. *Journal of Developmental & Behavioral Pediatrics*, **29**, 82–88.

Gradisar M, Dohnt H, Gardner G, *et al* (2011) A randomised controlled trial of cognitive-behavior therapy plus bright light therapy for adolescent delayed sleep phase disorder. *Sleep*, **34**, 1671–1680.

Gregory AM, Sadeh A (2012) Sleep, emotional and behavioral difficulties in children and adolescents. *Sleep Medicine Reviews*, **16**, 129–136.

Gringras P, Gamble C, Jones AP (2012) Melatonin for children with neurodevelopmental disorders: randomized double masked placebo controlled trial. *BMJ*, **345**, e6664, doi: 10.1136/bmj.e6664.

Hollway JA, Aman MG (2011) Pharmacological treatment of sleep disturbance in developmental disabilities. *Research in Developmental Disabilities*, **32**, 939–962.

Ivanenko A, Johnson K (2008) Sleep disturbances in children with psychiatric disorders. *Seminars in Pediatric Neurology*, **15**, 70–78.

Jan JE, Owens JA, Weiss MD, *et al* (2008) Sleep hygiene for children with neurodevelopmental disorders. *Pediatrics*, **122**, 1343–1350.

Konofal E, Lecendreux M, Cortese S (2010) Sleep and ADHD. *Sleep Medicine*, **11**, 652–658.

Kotagal S (2012) Treatment of dyssomnias and parasomnias in childhood. *Current Treatment Options in Neurology*, **14**, 630–649.

Kothare SV, Kaleyias J (2008) The clinical and laboratory assessment of the sleepy child. *Seminars in Pediatric Neurology*, **15**, 61–69.

Kuhn BR, Elliott AJ (2003) Treatment efficacy in behavioral pediatric sleep medicine. *Journal of Psychosomatic Research*, **54**, 587–597.

Lerchl A, Reiter RJ (2012) Treatment of sleep disorders with melatonin. *BMJ*, **345**, e6968, doi: 10.1136/bmj.e6968.

London New Drugs Group (2008) *APC/DTC Briefing: Melatonin in Paediatric Sleep Disorders*. LNDG.

Mahowald MW, Cramer Bornemann MA, Schenck CH (2011) State dissociation, human behavior, and consciousness. *Current Topics in Medicinal Chemistry*, **11**, 2392–2402.

Meltzer LJ, Mindell JA (2007) Relationship between child sleep disturbances and maternal sleep, mood, and parenting stress: a pilot study. *Journal of Family Psychology*, **21**, 67–73.

Mindell JA, Owens JA (2010) *A Clinical Guide to Pediatric Sleep* (2nd edn). Lippincott Williams and Wilkins.

Mindell JA, Kuhn B, Lewin DS, *et al* (2006) Behavioral treatment of bedtime problems and night wakings in infants and young children. *Sleep*, **29**, 1263–1276.

National Sleep Foundation (2006) *Summary of Findings: 2006 Sleep in America Poll*. National Sleep Foundation.

Owens J (2008) Classification and epidemiology of childhood sleep disorders. *Primary Care*, **35**, 533–546.

Owens JA, Moturi S (2009) Pharmacologic treatment of pediatric insomnia. *Child and Adolescent Psychiatric Clinics of North America*, **18**, 1001–1116.

Owens JA, Spirito A, McGuinn M (2000) The Children's Sleep Habits Questionnaire (CSHQ): psychometric properties of a survey instrument for school-aged children. *Sleep*, **15**, 1043–1051.

Peile E (2010) A commentary on sleep education. In *Sleep, Health and Society: From Aetiology to Public Health* (eds FP Cappuccio, MA Miller, SW Lockley), pp. 412–416. Oxford University Press.

Pike M, Stores G (1994) Kleine–Levin syndrome: a cause of diagnostic confusion. *Archive of Disease in Childhood*, **71**, 355–357.

Richdale AL, Schreck KA (2009) Sleep problems in autism spectrum disorders: prevalence, nature, & possible biosocial aetiologies. *Sleep Medicine Reviews*, **13**, 403–411.

Richdale A, Wiggs L (2005) Behavioral approaches to the treatment of sleep problems in children with developmental disorders: what is the state of the art? *International Journal of Behavioral Consultation and Therapy*, **1**, 165–189.

Schwartz JRL, Roth T (2008) Neurophysiology of sleep and wakefulness: basic science and clinical implications. *Current Neuropharmacology*, **6**, 367–378.

Smalldone A, Honig JC, Byrne MW (2007) Sleeplessness in America: inadequate sleep and relationships to health and well-being of our nation's children. *Pediatrics*, **119** (suppl 1), S29–37.

Stores G (1998) Sleep paralysis and hallucinosis. *Behavioural Neurology*, **11**, 109–112.

Stores G (2006a) Sleep disorders. In *A Clinician's Handbook of Child and Adolescent Psychiatry* (eds C Gillberg, R Harrington, H-C Steinhausen), pp. 304–338. Cambridge University Press.

Stores G (2006b) The protean manifestations of childhood narcolepsy and their misinterpretation. *Developmental Medicine & Child Neurology*, **68**, 307–310.

Stores G (2007a) Clinical diagnosis and misdiagnosis of sleep disorders. *Journal of Neurology, Neurosurgery & Psychiatry*, **8**, 1293–1297.

Stores G (2007b) Parasomnias of childhood and adolescence. *Sleep Medicine Clinics*, **2**, 405–417.

Stores G (2009) Aspects of the parasomnias in children and adolescents. *Archive of Disease in Childhood*, **94**, 63–69.

Stores G, Stores R (2013) Sleep disorders and their clinical significance in children with Down syndrome. *Developmental Medicine & Child Neurology*, **55**, 126–130.

Stores G, Wiggs L (eds) (2001) *Sleep Disturbance in Children and Adolescents with Disorders of Development: Its Significance and Management*. Mac Keith Press.

Stores G, Montgomery P, Wiggs L (2006) The psychosocial problems of children with narcolepsy and those with excessive daytime sleepiness of uncertain origin. *Pediatrics*, **118**, e1116–1123.

CHAPTER 19

Self-harm in adolescents

Alison Wood

The National Institute for Health and Care Excellence (NICE) has defined self-harming behaviour as:

> 'an expression of personal distress, usually made in private, by an individual who hurts him or herself. The nature and meaning of self-harm, however, vary greatly from person to person. In addition, the reason a person harms him or herself may be different on each occasion, and should not be presumed to be the same' (National Institute for Clinical Excellence, 2004: p. 8).

Self-harm can be divided into two broad types: self-injury and self-poisoning. The definition of self-harm is therefore purely behavioural and it includes a spectrum of risk-taking behaviours (Box 19.1). This spectrum includes smoking, tattooing, recreational alcohol and drug misuse, food restriction and promiscuity. Motivation must be appraised separately. Suicidal intent is associated with self-harming behaviour, particularly with self-poisoning, but the behaviour does not in itself predict underlying intent. Suicidal intent must be assessed specifically (see Risk assessment).

This chapter focuses on self-harming behaviours in 12- to 18-year-olds presenting to professionals working in child and adolescent mental health services (CAMHS), from single acts of self-harm posing little medical risk to multiple acts posing serious risk to life. Young people who self-harm form a highly heterogeneous population.

Self-harming behaviour has been the focus of scrutiny from public health, service provision, professional/therapeutic and patient/carer perspectives

---

Box 19.1 Types of self-harm

Self-injury: cutting, swallowing objects, insertion of objects into body, burning, hanging, stabbing, shooting, jumping from heights or in front of vehicles

Self-poisoning: overdosing with medicines, swallowing poisonous substances

Other risk-taking behaviours: smoking, tattooing, recreational drug/substance misuse, over-eating, food restriction, promiscuity

---

over the past decade or so. Although awareness of self-harm has increased, little progress has been made in its evidence-based management by professionals (Hawton *et al*, 2009).

The NICE guideline on longer-term management of self-harm was published in 2012 (National Institute for Health and Clinical Excellence, 2012). This covers young people aged 8 years and over and focuses on the longer-term management (after the first 48 hours) of both single and recurrent episodes of self-harm. The guideline is both an update and a continuation of the 2004 guideline on short-term management (National Institute for Health and Clinical Excellence, 2004), and it informs this chapter.

Epidemiology

In community surveys, around 10% of adolescents report self-harming behaviour. It is estimated that about 25000 adolescents present to hospitals following self-harm each year in England and Wales. These rates are among the highest in Europe. Although self-harm is commonly reported in such surveys, young people presenting to hospitals represent less than 10% of the adolescent population who self-harm.

Most information about self-harm as a medical phenomenon and as a symptom of mental illness is derived from clinical populations, and it is important to question how far this can generalise to the general population. For example, Hawton *et al* (1996) found that almost 70% of young people admitted to hospital following episodes of self-harm (mainly self-poisoning) described previous acts of self-harm which had not been reported. Subsequently, Hawton & Rodham (2006) described their questionnaire survey of 6020 year 11 pupils (15- to 16-year-olds) in the Oxford area. This in-depth study reported that 13.2% of the young people questioned had tried to harm themselves at some point in their lives: 6.9% had done so in the previous year. A total of 15% of adolescents in this survey reported thoughts of suicide and 54% of those reporting self-harm described more than one episode. Only 12.6% ($n = 50$) of those who had engaged in self-harm had presented to hospital. The largest proportion of acts of self-harm, possibly amounting to 80–90%, is therefore invisible to professionals.

Meltzer *et al* (2001) conducted an interview-based study of over 4000 young people aged between 5 and 15 years in Great Britain. They found rates of self-harm of 1.3% for 5- to 10-year-olds and of 5.8% for 11- to 15-year-olds. The behaviour was associated with mental health disorders and psychosocial disadvantage, and parents were largely unaware of it.

As self-harm is common among adolescents, it is important to gain an understanding of the associated features and also of the relationship between self-harming behaviour and completed suicide.

Associated features

Gender

Self-harming behaviour is 2–4 times more common in girls than in boys, a difference found consistently in international studies (Evans *et al*, 2005). This may be related to the higher rates of depression in girls, the greater tendency for boys to externalise and a possible underreporting by boys.

Age

Although studies vary with respect to age ranges reported, in adolescents there is a peak in suicidal thinking and behaviour between the ages of 14 and 18. In England, presentations for both genders are rare under the age of 12, but increase steadily until 16 and remain at this level until the late teens (Hawton *et al*, 2003).

Genetics and neurobiology

Psychiatric disorder, suicidal behaviour and severe aggression all tend to run in families and this may be due to genetic or environmental factors or both. It may be that neurobiological anomalies mediate the heritability of these behaviours. Dysregulation of the serotonin system has been found to be associated with suicidal behaviour and this effect may be mediated by increases in impulsivity or disinhibition (Brent & Mann, 2005). There is a growing body of evidence associating abnormalities in the serotonin system with self-harming behaviour (Asberg & Forslund, 2000).

Ethnicity and international differences

Data in this area are difficult to interpret owing to classifications of ethnicity, sampling and variations in reporting. Self-harm is reported in most minority ethnic groups and may be more prevalent in all minority groups, suggesting that the social experience of being part of a minority may be more important than being of a particular ethnicity (for a comprehensive review see Roberts *et al*, 1997). The Child & Adolescent Self-harm in Europe (CASE) study (Madge *et al*, 2008) is a seven-country comparative community study of over 30 000 15- and 16-year-olds. In four of the seven countries, at least one in ten females had harmed themselves in the previous year. Rates were highest in Australia, England, Belgium and Norway, and lowest in The Netherlands. There are suggestions (the trends did not reach significance) that the prevalence of suicidal phenomena is higher in the USA, Canada and Australia than in Europe and Asia.

Risk factors for adolescent suicidal behaviour

Although self-harming behaviours are very common, their significance as a risk factor for completed suicide needs examination. An inquiry into self-harm in England (Mental Health Foundation, 2006) examined the behaviour from the perspective of young people and their carers. The vast majority of young people who self-harm see it as a means of coping with difficult feelings and circumstances, and regard it as a private experience. The role of professionals is to alleviate suffering where this is indicated, and to assess and manage risk in situations where self-harm poses threats to life from suicidal urges and intent or significant risk to physical health due to the consequences of the behaviour. The remainder of this chapter focuses on the young people who present to services.

The psychological autopsy is an accepted method of investigating mental and psychosocial characteristics of suicides. Research using this approach for adolescents has revealed that the risk factors for completed suicide are the presence of a psychiatric disorder, previous suicide attempt and substance/alcohol misuse (Shaffer *et al*, 1996).

Suicidal behaviour can usually be seen as arising from a complex set of interacting vulnerabilities and situations, with a final trigger. Various models have been proposed of the factors that need to be considered. Sutton (1998), for example, used the idea of the four 'Ms': means, motivation, moment(s) of madness. Hawton & Rodham (2006) found that young people described psychological pain (wanting relief from a terrible state), wanting to die, wanting to punish themselves, and wanting to show how desperate they were feeling as the most common motives driving the self-harming behaviour. For further reading the comprehensive review of suicide and suicidal behaviour by Bridge *et al* (2006) is recommended.

Risk assessment and risk management

The purpose of risk assessment is to identify those at significant risk of suicide and enable risk management strategies and treatment interventions to be put in place. Risk assessment should take place as soon as possible after an incident, when the young person is medically fit and parents or carers are available. The interview should include an assessment of the young person on their own and history from parents/carers. Key areas of enquiry are shown in Box 19.2.

The NICE guidelines (National Institute for Health and Clinical Excellence, 2004, 2012) include a separate section for 8- to 16-year-olds. Recommendations include admission for assessment of all young people presenting to hospital following an overdose. Risk assessment is often conducted on a medical/paediatric ward or in an accident and emergency (A&E) department. If risk of further self-harm is identified, therapy or outreach is recommended for at least 3 months. The Royal College of Psychiatrists (2006) reviewed services for people who self-harm and produced a manual of standards of good practice for A&E staff, ambulance services, mental health teams and primary care practitioners. In addition, a review from the Royal College of Paediatrics and Child Health (2003)

Box 19.2   Risk assessment

- The attempt: detailed description, suicide ideation, lethality, intent/motivation and current intent. Previous suicidal behaviours and triggers.
- Presence of mental health disorder: assess for depression, conduct disorder, eating disorder, anxiety, post-traumatic stress disorder and psychosis. Ask about substance and alcohol misuse. Previous history of mental disorders/treatment. Family–environmental factors: parental psychopathology, family history of suicidal behaviour, family dislocation, experience of loss, family discord, and physical, emotional and sexual abuse.
- Social/educational: not attending education, disaffection, learning difficulties, social isolation, bullying, and social-related difficulties. Marginalisation and 'not fitting in' are important in adolescents, for whom being accepted by a peer group is crucial to healthy development.
- Previous experience of treatment: motivation to change, engagement, assessment of ability to take responsibility for own safety, availability of carers, wider support in accessing treatment.

---

highlights the need for separate services for adolescents, confidentiality, privacy, expertise and continuity of care. Child and adolescent mental health services are responsible for providing care for young people up until their 18th birthday (CAMHS Review Expert Group, 2008).

A number of screening instruments have been developed for the identification of at-risk individuals. These have been comprehensively reviewed by Fox & Hawton (2004) and were reviewed recently by the NICE guideline group (National Institute for Health and Clinical Excellence, 2012). Prospective studies are needed to investigate the predictive validity of assessment instruments, the majority of which have been developed in the USA for use with adults. These instruments may be useful in assessment, but they do not replace clinical interview and have limited value with adolescents.

When assessing risk it is important to engage the young person, family and professionals involved in a shared understanding of the recent self-harm and a formulation of future risk. Where there is ongoing risk and/or a mental health disorder, care should be coordinated and monitored by a named professional.

Self-harming behaviours may represent unmet need or a method of dealing with emotional pain. Professionals should be calm, containing and non-judgemental, and respond to any needs for medical attention.

For adults, therapeutic risk-taking is advocated. This involves a range of approaches in which services share responsibility for risk with patients, supporting them in taking responsibility for their actions. It can include advice regarding self-management of injuries and provision of first aid, as well as harm minimisation. These interventions need to be delivered by appropriately trained and supervised staff. Most patients with longer-term histories of self-harm will have significant personality difficulties and research emphasises the importance of offering longer-term (at least 12 months) interventions (Alwyn *et al*, 2006).

Such approaches are not considered appropriate for adolescents. It should be explained to the young person that, although they find self-harm helpful, it is maladaptive and alternative solutions can and must be found. Key to therapeutic work is a collaborative approach where young people are required to take increasing responsibility for their own behaviour and emotions, and learn methods of managing them. Sometimes a young person will refuse emergency medical treatment or psychological support, and in such situations assessment of capacity is required to decide whether compulsory treatment is indicated. Urgent medical treatment can be provided under common law. Occasionally, when risk is assessed to be very high and the person has a mental illness, detention under section 2 or 3 of the Mental Health Act 1983 is indicated. The Mental Health Act amendments of 2007 place a duty on mental health trusts to provide age-appropriate accommodation for people under 18 who require hospital admission.

General management

Hawton *et al* (1982) classified adolescents who took overdoses into three groups. Although this publication is now 20 years old the approach remains relevant to everyday clinical practice and is helpful to practitioners in structuring district CAMHS treatments:

- group 1, acute: problems identified at the time of the overdose had persisted less than 1 month; no behavioural disturbance
- group 2, chronic: problems identified at the time of the overdose had persisted for 1 month or more; no behavioural disturbance
- group 3, chronic with behavioural disturbance: problems identified at the time of the overdose had persisted for more than 1 month; recent behavioural disturbance (e.g. truanting, stealing, drug-taking, heavy drinking, fighting, in trouble with the police).

The Hawton system was evaluated in a case-note study in West Glamorgan of 50 adolescents (47 of them girls) consecutively referred for psychiatric assessment after taking overdoses (Davies & Ames, 1998). The 50 were among 157 adolescents (81 of whom were admitted) who had presented to A&E with an overdose over the study period. The most frequent diagnoses among the 50 were adjustment disorder (38%), conduct disorder (28%) and depressive episode (20%); no psychiatric disorder was found in 4% (note that the study preceded the 2004 NICE guidelines on self-harm). By the Hawton classification, 12 (24%) were in group 1, 21 (42%) in group 2 and 17 (34%) in group 3. The study concluded that this is a clinically useful classification that can be used to guide discussion of treatment.

Group 1: acute

An appointment with a healthcare professional provides an opportunity to describe current concerns. The young person may find this validating and it can be therapeutic in itself. Brief intervention consists of psychoeducation about risk and problem-solving for the young person and the parents. A crisis plan will be identified, but there will be no continuing involvement with CAMHS.

Group 2: chronic

In chronic self-harm, the behaviour is likely to be a symptom of an underlying problem and to resolve with treatment of that problem. For example, if depression is diagnosed, an evidence-based treatment such as a brief problem-focused intervention may be indicated (National Collaborating Centre for Mental Health, 2005). If the young person is under 16, their parents/carers will also be involved in the treatment programme. Prognosis is good for adolescents who fall into this category.

Group 3: chronic with behavioural disturbance

This group has the poorest prognosis and is the most difficult to treat with conventional approaches. Risk of repetition is likely to be high. The severity of the self-harm and suicidal intent must be assessed. Young people who frequently self-harm but for whom this is clearly a coping method need continuous surveillance and support. Anxiety levels among parents, carers and professionals may be very high. If the individual has expressed suicidal intent, psychiatric admission may be indicated for assessment, but this should be avoided if possible because of the risk of escalation.

The role of the child psychiatrist is to work in partnership with social, paediatric and educational services. A multi agency meeting is essential as soon as possible to engage members of the care team across agencies, and care coordination is crucial. A proportion of these young people will require alternative accommodation or admission to a psychiatric unit. Interventions should be focused on underlying diagnosis. Drug and alcohol use may be problematic and contribute to ongoing risk. Some young people in this group may be showing features of an emerging borderline personality disorder.

Young people presenting with severe self-harming behaviour associated with suicidal intent may evoke complex emotions in staff. The multidisciplinary team can be polarised in views about such patients. Staff need regular clinical supervision to enable them to manage their emotions, because when the young person feels that they cannot control their emotions, it is important that the professionals caring for them can take charge of their own. Managing self-harm in in-patient populations is particularly difficult for staff.

Evidence-based practice

There is a paucity of research evidence available on the benefit of interventions for adolescent self-harm (Box 19.3). A Cochrane review of pharmacological and psychosocial treatments for self-harm (Hawton *et al*, 2009) provides a comprehensive summary of the available interventions, together with the evidence base. Approaches can be based in the in-patient or out-patient setting.

In-patient treatment

In-patient psychiatric assessment is indicated for young people presenting with evidence of a mental illness and who are at high risk of suicide. For treatment to be beneficial, the individual needs to have a placement/home base that the in-patient team can work with, as admission should be goal-directed and discharge planned at the outset. In-patient treatment can be problematic for young people with features of borderline personality disorder. Self-harming behaviour can worsen and discharge is often difficult. In-patient stay should be as brief as possible.

There are no studies evaluating intensive or residential therapeutic placements. However, my own local case-note audit of young people admitted to a Tier 4 service for whom self-harm was the principal reason for referral showed that the outcomes of admission were less negative than the staff perceived them to be. For the 45 in-patient episodes (41% total admissions) that I reviewed, 82% of the patients were female (mean age 14 years), 40% were admitted from paediatric wards, 86% had a diagnosis of depression, and 93% were living at home. Mean length of stay was 62 days. Seventy-five per cent did not engage in serious self-harm (requiring medical intervention) as in-patients and two-thirds were discharged home. Three young people needed to be transferred to a secure facility because the risk they posed to themselves could not be managed in an open unit.

Box 19.3 Interventions for self-harm in adolescents

- In-patient treatment
- Medication
- Family intervention
- Dialectical behaviour therapy
- Developmental group psychotherapy
- Multisystemic therapy

Out-patient treatment

A stepwise approach to care is helpful, based on the premise that there is no evidence firmly in favour of any specific treatment in the absence of mental illness (Box 19.4).

Medication

Medication may have a role in the treatment of an underlying disorder in self-harm. A small placebo-controlled study reported a reduction in self-harming in patients receiving flupentixol (Montgomery *et al*, 1979). However, a review of the use of medication in the management of self-harm (Hawton *et al*, 2009) found no evidence for the benefit of antidepressants for the disorder. Medication is used in clinical practice for symptom relief, but the lack of evidence base for its efficacy in reducing self-harm itself should be noted.

Brief family intervention

A brief home-based family intervention has been assessed as part of a randomised controlled trial (Harrington *et al*, 1998). Following admission for self-poisoning, patients were allocated to routine care or to routine care plus the intervention. The intervention involved two therapists visiting the young person and their family at home on four occasions. Each session focused on an aspect of adolescence and self-harm. The intervention is manualised and a video is available. Results showed a low repeat rate and low rates of psychopathology, with no differences in any primary outcome between the two groups, although the intervention was well received.

Box 19.4   Stepwise approach to self-harm in CAMHS

1   Risk assessment: risk of suicide; presence of mental illness; psychosocial evaluation involving key family/carers

2   Offer specific treatment/review if there is presence of a mental health disorder

3   For young people who repeatedly self-harm and are assessed as low risk, offer consultation by CAMHS and multi-agency problem-focused approach

4   For young people assessed as being at high risk, involvement of CAMHS is appropriate: offer specific interventions (e.g. group therapy, family therapy or cognitive–behavioural therapy); aim to manage in the community if possible; take a long-term view and involve Social Services if indicated; minimise the number of professionals involved; care coordination is essential

5   If there is no response to focused out-patient intervention and the young person is assessed as being at high risk, consider specialist Tier 4 referral for residential assessment/very specialist interventions such as dialectical behaviour therapy

Dialectical behaviour therapy

Dialectical behaviour therapy (DBT) was developed to treat women with borderline personality disorder who repeatedly self-harmed. The approach is based on Linehan's biosocial theory, in which borderline personality disorder is caused by pervasive emotional dysregulation (Linehan, 1993). Self-harm is considered to be a maladaptive solution to overwhelming intensely painful emotions.

Borderline personality disorder in young people can be diagnosed (for symptoms of at least 12 months' duration) using adult criteria, but this is not recommended for children under 16 years of age. The NICE guidelines include a chapter on the treatment and management of the disorder in young people under 18 years of age (National Institute for Health and Clinical Excellence, 2009). The concept of 'emerging borderline personality disorder' has been suggested to describe children under 16 presenting with symptoms or showing vulnerability to the disorder.

Dialectical behaviour therapy is the only empirically supported treatment for adults with multiple mental health problems at risk of suicide. In a 2-year randomised controlled trial, DBT reduced suicidal behaviour, in-patient days and anger ratings compared with treatment as usual (Linehan et al, 2006).

Miller and colleagues have adapted DBT for adolescents at risk of suicide (see Miller et al, 2007). Therapy comprises individual sessions, including 24-hour telephone access and group skills training. The emphasis is on balancing change and acceptance, and improving capabilities and coping. Treatment is intensive and requires therapist and team supervision. The adolescent programme was designed to take place over 12 weeks.

Rathus & Miller (2002) reported a quasi-experimental investigation of their adaptation of DBT for suicidal behaviour in adolescents with features of borderline personality disorder. They compared 29 adolescents who received DBT with 82 adolescents who received a combination of individual supportive psychotherapy and family therapy. The DBT group had fewer hospital admissions and a higher treatment adherence rate. Katz et al (2004) compared outcomes for adolescents on an in-patient unit adopting a DBT approach with those from an in-patient unit run on psychodynamic principles. Fewer self-harm incidents were reported for the DBT unit. Thus, DBT shows promise in this population.

Developmental group therapy

Developmental group therapy (DGT) was developed in the context of a district CAMHS as an intervention for young people presenting with repeated self-harm. It functions as an open long-term group therapy that young people can access in crisis and can continue to attend until they are ready to leave. The focus is on 'growing up despite multiple problems', and therapy attempts to reduce exclusion and social isolation, and combine and enhance other CAMHS treatments. It provides a long-term therapeutic intervention designed to reduce the need for individual therapy.

A randomised controlled trial within a district CAMHS in Manchester, UK, was undertaken to evaluate DGT. Sixty-three young people aged 12–18 were randomised to receive DGT plus treatment as usual or treatment as usual alone. The risk of being a 'multiple repeater' (more than two further episodes of self-harm) was higher in the treatment-as-usual group (32% v. 6%). Fewer episodes of self-harm and a longer time to first repetition were reported in the DGT group (Wood et al, 2001). Following the pilot study, a large multicentre study (Assessment and Treatment in Suicidal Teenagers, ASSIST) was conducted. A total of 366 young people aged between 12 and 18 were recruited from CAMHS across North West England (Green et al, 2011). The addition of DGT did not improve self-harm outcomes for participants who repeatedly self-harmed, nor was there evidence of cost-effectiveness. The outcomes of the cohort, however, were better than clinical expectations, with 40% of the sample reporting no self-harming for the previous month. The sample as a whole received many interventions, including in-patient treatment and alternative accommodation, and some of the participants had been referred to a Tier 4 service with complex and chronic difficulties for which they had had multiple previous treatments. This is the largest treatment study of adolescents to date.

A randomised controlled trial of DGT in Australia, however, showed higher rates of self-harm in the treatment group (Hazell et al, 2009). The methodology was identical to that used for the British studies and collaboration took place with the Manchester study team. The young people recruited had higher levels of cutting at the outset and lower levels of psychiatric morbidity. This serves to illustrate that the risk of 'contagion' of self-harm among young people is high and group interventions must be conducted by experienced practitioners with access to regular supervision.

Multisystemic therapy

Multisystemic therapy was developed in the USA by Henggeler (1999) as an intensive home-based treatment for delinquent youths presenting with repeated risk-taking behaviour. It comprises individual, parent, family and school interventions centred on the young person. Multisystemic therapy is not an alternative to in-patient management, but it can significantly reduce hospital stays. Although it is not focused on self-harm in itself, it shows promise for populations with multiple problems.

Outcomes and continuity into adult life

There are few UK follow-up studies, but outcomes that have been studied include suicide, repeated self-harm and personality disturbance in adult life. Hawton et al (2006) identified, via the Oxford Monitoring System for Attempted Suicide, a cohort of over 11 000 patients aged 15 who self-harmed. Follow-up over a mean period of 11 years found a death rate of

10.2%. All causes of death (e.g. respiratory disease, neurological, circulatory and endocrine disorders) had increased. Suicide/probable suicide accounted for 2.6%. In a subsequent follow-up study of 710 consecutive under-15-year-olds presenting to hospitals in Oxford over a 26-year period, Hawton & Harriss (2008) concluded that self-harm is most often triggered by life events, but is generally of low suicidal intent. Follow-up occurred on average 11 years after first presentation, and long-term risk of suicide was very low (1.1%). Repetition rates vary but are reported as between 6 and 30%, depending on sample selection/size, length of follow-up and location (Hawton *et al*, 1982; NHS Centre for Reviews and Dissemination, 1998).

Harrington *et al* (2006) published their 6-year follow-up of adolescents who had participated in a randomised controlled trial of the brief family intervention mentioned earlier (Harrington *et al*, 1998). The majority of individuals (70%) had stopped self-harming within 3 years of the trial. At 6 years, less than 10% reported frequent self-harm; 50% had used adult mental health services, and among the adults who continued to self-harm, childhood adversity (e.g. sexual abuse) was prevalent.

Andrews & Lewinsohn (1992) and Sadowski & Kelly (1993) describe poor problem-solving, impaired peer relationships and repeated separations in later life for young people who had presented to services following self-harm in adolescence. Psychiatric disorder is very common in adult suicides, but 40% of individuals under the age of 16 who die by suicide do not appear to have had a diagnosable psychiatric disorder. For these young people, intent was low and lethality of means high (Brent *et al*, 1999).

Conclusion

Self-harming behaviour is common among adolescents, and young people who engage in self-harm come into contact with a large number of different professionals. The role of the psychiatrist is to identify and prescribe treatment for those young people presenting with mental health disorders and/or ongoing high risk to self. Part of the role of the psychiatrist or other mental health professional is to work in partnership with other agencies (using collaborative approaches) to ensure that the mental health, social care, physical health and educational needs of the young person within their family system are met.

Further research is needed into long-term outcomes, in particular early identifiers of borderline personality disorders and investigation into which treatments and interventions are most effective. For some young people, involvement of mental health services may be counterproductive, and core parenting problems and unmet social and emotional needs may be obscured by intensive interventions. For the vast majority of young people who self-harm it is a transient adolescent experience. The challenge for professionals is to identify those who are at risk of death and for whom therapeutic intervention could be life-saving.

References

Alwyn N, Blackburn R, Davidson K, *et al* (2006) *Understanding Personality Disorder: A Report by the British Psychological Society*. BPS.

Andrews J, Lewinsohn P (1992) Suicidal attempts among older adolescents: prevalence and co-occurence with psychiatric disorders. *Journal of the American Academy of Child & Adolescent Psychiatry*, **31**, 655–662.

Asberg M & Forslund R (2000) Neurobiological aspects of suicide behaviour. *International Review of Psychiatry*, **12**, 62–74.

Brent DA, Mann JJ (2005) Family genetic studies, suicide and suicidal behaviour. *American Journal of Medical Genetics Part C: Seminars in Medical Genetics*, **133C**, 13–24.

Brent D, Baugher M, Bridge J, *et al* (1999) Age and sex-related risk factors for adolescent suicide. *Journal of the American Academy of Child & Adolescent Psychiatry*, **38**, 1497–1505.

Bridge J, Goldstein T, Brent D (2006) Adolescent suicide and suicidal behaviour. *Journal of Child Psychology and Psychiatry*, **47**, 372–394.

CAMHS Review Expert Group (2008) *Children and Young People in Mind: The Final Report of the National CAMHS Review*. Department of Health.

Davies G, Ames S (1998) Adolescents referred following overdose: support for Hawton's classification and the role of a primary child and adolescent mental health worker. *Psychiatric Bulletin*, **22**, 359–361.

Evans E, Hawton K, Rodham K (2005) In what ways are adolescents who engage in self-harm or experience thoughts of self-harm different in terms of help-seeking, communication and coping strategies? *Journal of Adolescence*, **28**, 573–587.

Fox C, Hawton K (2004) *Deliberate Self-Harm in Adolescence*. Jessica Kingsley.

Green JM, Wood AJ, Kerfoot M, *et al* (2011) Group therapy for adolescents with repeated self harm: randomised controlled trial with economic evaluation. *BMJ*, **342**, d682, doi: 10.1136/bmj.d682.

Harrington R, Kerfoot M, Dyer E, *et al* (1998) Randomised trial of a home-based family intervention for children who have deliberately poisoned themselves. *Journal of the American Academy of Child & Adolescent Psychiatry*, **37**, 512–518.

Harrington R, Pickles A, Aglan A, *et al* (2006) Early adult outcomes of adolescents who deliberately poisoned themselves. *Journal of the American Academy of Child & Adolescent Psychiatry*, **45**, 337–345.

Hawton K, Harriss L (2008) Deliberate self-harm by under-15-years-olds: characteristics, trends and outcome. *Journal of Child Psychology and Psychiatry*, **49**, 441–448.

Hawton K, Rodham K (2006) *By Their Own Young Hand: Deliberate Self-Harm and Suicidal Ideas in Adolescents*. Jessica Kingsley.

Hawton K, Osborne M, O'Grady J, *et al* (1982) Classification of adolescents who take over-doses. *British Journal of Psychiatry*, **140**, 124–131.

Hawton K, Fagg J, Simkin S (1996) Deliberate self-poisoning and self-injury in children and adolescents under 16 years of age in Oxford, 1976–1993. *British Journal of Psychiatry*, **169**, 202–208.

Hawton K, Hall S, Simkin S, *et al* (2003) Deliberate self-harm in adolescents: a study of characteristics and trends in Oxford, 1990–2000. *Journal of Child Psychology and Psychiatry and Allied Disciplines*, **44**, 1191–1198.

Hawton K, Harriss L, Zahl D (2006) Deaths from all causes in a long-term follow-up study of 11,583 deliberate self-harm patients. *Psychological Medicine*, **36**, 397–405.

Hawton K, Townsend E, Arensman E, *et al* (2009) Psychosocial and pharmacological treatments for deliberate self-harm. *Cochrane Database of Systematic Reviews*, **2**, CD001764.

Hazell PL, Martin G, McGill K, *et al* (2009) Group therapy for repeated deliberate self-harm in adolescents: failure of a replication of a randomized trial. *Journal of the American Academy of Child & Adolescent Psychiatry*, **48**, 662–670.

Henggeler S (1999) Multisystemic therapy: an overview of clinical procedures, outcomes, and policy implications. *Child Psychology and Psychiatry Review*, **4**, 2–10.

Katz L, Cox B, Gunasekara S, *et al* (2004) Feasibility of dialectical behaviour therapy for suicidal adolescent in-patients. *Journal of the American Academy of Child & Adolescent Psychiatry*, **43**, 276–282.

Linehan M (1993) *Cognitive Behavioural Therapy for Borderline Personality Disorder*. Guilford Press.

Linehan MM, Comtois KA, Murray AM, *et al* (2006) Two-year randomized trial and follow-up of dialectical behavior therapy vs therapy by experts for suicidal behaviors and borderline personality disorder. *Archives of General Psychiatry*, **63**, 757–766.

Madge N, Hewitt A, Hawton K, *et al* (2008) Deliberate self-harm within an international community sample of young people: comparative findings from the Child & Adolescent Adolescent Self-harm in Europe (CASE) Study. *Journal of Child Psychology and Psychiatry*, **49**, 667–677.

Meltzer H, Harrington R, Goodman R, *et al* (2001) *Children and Adolescents Who Try to Harm, Hurt or Kill Themselves*. Office for National Statistics.

Mental Health Foundation (2006) *Truth Hurts: Report of the National Inquiry into Self-harm among Young People*. Mental Health Foundation.

Miller AL, Rathus JH, Linehan MM (2007) *Dialectical Behavioural Therapy with Suicidal Adolescents*. Guilford Press.

Montgomery SA, Montgomery DB, Jayanthi-Rani S, *et al* (1979) Maintenance therapy in repeat suicidal behaviour: a placebo controlled trial. In *Proceedings of the Tenth International Congress for Suicide Prevention and Crisis Intervention*, pp. 227–229. International Association for Suicide Prevention.

National Collaborating Centre for Mental Health (2005) *Depression in Children and Young People: Identification and Management in Primary, Community and Secondary Care* (Clinical Guideline 28). National Institute for Health and Clinical Excellence.

National Institute for Clinical Excellence (2004) *Self-Harm: Short-Term Treatment and Management: Understanding Nice Guidance – Information for People Who Self-Harm, their Advocates and Carers, and the Public (Including Information for Young People Under 16 Years)*. NICE.

National Institute for Health and Clinical Excellence (2004) *Self-Harm: The Short-Term Physical and Psychological Management and Secondary Prevention of Self-Harm in Primary and Secondary Care* (NICE Clinical Guideline 16). NICE.

National Institute for Health and Clinical Excellence (2009) *Borderline Personality Disorder: Treatment and Management* (NICE Clinical Guideline 78). NICE.

National Institute for Health and Clinical Excellence (2012) *Self-Harm: Longer-Term Management* (NICE Clinical Guideline 133). NICE.

NHS Centre for Reviews and Dissemination (1998) Deliberate self-harm. *Effective Health Care*, **4** (6).

Rathus J, Miller A (2002) Dialectical behavior therapy adapted for suicidal adolescents. *Suicide and Life-Threatening Behavior*, **32**, 146–157.

Roberts RE, Chen YR, Roberts CR (1997) Ethnocultural differences in prevalence of adolescent suicidal behaviors. *Suicide and Life-Threatening Behavior*, **27**, 208–217.

Royal College of Paediatrics and Child Health (2003) *Bridging the Gaps: Health Care for Adolescents*. Royal College of Paediatrics and Child Health.

Royal College of Psychiatrists (2006) *Better Services for People who Self-Harm: Quality Standards for Health Care Professionals*. Royal College of Psychiatrists.

Sadowski C, Kelly M (1993) Social problem-solving in suicidal adolescents. *Journal of Consulting and Clinical Psychology*, **61**, 121–127.

Shaffer D, Gould M, Fisher P, *et al* (1996) Psychiatric diagnosis in child and adolescent suicide. *Archives of General Psychiatry*, **53**, 339–348.

Sutton A (1998) Psychodynamics of self-directed destructive behaviour in adolescence. *Advances in Psychiatric Treatment*, **4**, 31–38.

Wood A, Trainor G, Rothwell J, *et al* (2001) Randomized trial of group therapy for repeated self-harm in adolescents. *Journal of the American Academy of Child & Adolescent Psychiatry*, **40**, 1246–1253.

CHAPTER 20

Adolescent substance misuse: an update on behaviours and treatments

Paul McArdle and Bisharda Angom

Substance misuse emerged as a relatively common behaviour among Westernised young people towards the end of the 20th century. The trend appeared first in English-speaking countries and, at least in the UK, in a context of deteriorating mental health: national cohort studies reveal 'a substantial increase' in emotional and conduct problems in 16-year-olds over a 20-year period (Collishaw et al, 2010). Whether this link with poor mental health is more than coincidental is unclear. However, the substances used may adversely affect maturing cortical white matter, memory, and educational and psychosocial progress during a critical developmental period (Newbury-Birch et al, 2009). In this way they potentially reduce the life chances and perhaps the lifespan (Impinen et al, 2010) of a substantial minority of young users.

Substance misuse is the term used in the UK to refer to patterns of maladaptive use of substances. DSM-5 refers to 'substance use disorder', requiring specification of the substance used and, depending on the number of symptoms, whether the disorder is mild, moderate or severe (American Psychiatric Association, 2013). Although it acknowledges 'a severe state of chronically relapsing compulsive drug taking', DSM-5 has controversially (Drummond 2011) dropped the term 'dependence'. This may be more applicable to young people, among whom, some argue, physiological dependence appears to be uncommon (National Treatment Agency for Substance Misuse, 2010).

The epidemiology of the problem

Much of the available epidemiological data on young people still comes from school surveys. UK school survey data show a reduction in numbers reporting being offered drugs and in the proportion reporting ever having tried them: the latter figure fell from 30% in 2003 to 22% in 2009 (Fuller & Sanchez, 2010). Nevertheless, among the 22% of 15-year-olds reporting any use, at least a third are regular users (10% of all boys surveyed and 6%

of the girls report use on 'more than 10 occasions', indicative of regular use), many or most of whom 'misuse'. About a quarter of all users (5% of the total surveyed), say that they 'need help or treatment'. Although drinking also appears to have declined over the past decade, 1% of girls and 2% of boys drink daily, and of those 15-year-olds who drink, 31% of boys and 29% of girls drink 15 or more units per week. About 5% smoke cigarettes, drink and use drugs. More girls than boys first used drugs 'to forget my problems' (13 v. 9%) but otherwise their patterns of use are now similar. This 'equality' is a major change that has occurred over a generation and, because of their smaller body size, disproportionately risks the health of females.

School-survey data from the USA also show declines in alcohol drinking and cigarette smoking (Johnston et al, 2009; Lopez et al, 2009). However, from a plateau in 2007, cannabis use has again increased. In their report for the National Institute on Drug Abuse, Johnston et al (2009) comment that this followed evidence of reduced perception of risk – not (yet) apparent in the UK data – which they term 'generational forgetting'. This is a process whereby a particular generation's knowledge of the widely recognised adverse consequences of a highly prevalent action fades as that generation is replaced. The survey also shows that the perceived risks of LSD, inhalants and ecstasy (MDMA) among participants had declined appreciably.

The 2011 European School Project on Alcohol and other Drugs (ESPAD) is an international schools survey of 15- to 16-year-olds repeated on five occasions since 1995. The project, which now covers 30 European countries and 100 000 pupils, offers estimates of current trends in substance use (Hibell et al, 2012). In brief, across the continent, substance use has broadly plateaued since 2007, but rates remain higher than in 1995. Initially apparent mainly in the UK and Ireland, binge use of alcohol and lifetime and regular cannabis use spread from west to east and from north to south across the continent. Nevertheless, the UK still has the third highest and Ireland the sixth highest numbers of young people who admitted being drunk in the previous 30 days. Comparing the genders, with the exception of cigarettes (equality), inhalants (girls have caught up with boys in the most recent survey) and tranquillisers (across the duration of the surveys girls have used more than boys), boys consume more substances than girls. The UK is sixth (France is first) in the ranking for use of cannabis during the previous 30 days.

In 2011, cocaine was second only to cannabis as the most tried drug in Europe (European Monitoring Centre for Drugs and Drug Addiction, 2012), although its use is concentrated in a small number of countries (Table 20.1).

Novel psychoactive substances

According to European data, there has been a decline in numbers of injecting drug users presenting to clinical services. However, the European

Table 20.1 European Union countries with lowest and highest prevalences of previous-month cocaine use among 15- to 34-year-olds in 2007

Ranking	Countries	Population prevalence, %
Low-prevalence countries	Romania	0
	Greece, Lithuania, Norway, Poland	0.1
	Czech Republic, Estonia, Hungary	0.2
High-prevalence countries	UK	2.1
	Spain	2.0
	Cyprus	1.3
	Italy	1.1

Source: European Monitoring Centre for Drugs and Drug Addiction (2011).

Monitoring Centre for Drugs and Drug Addiction (2012) now reports new drugs emerging at a rate of almost one a week. These are mainly synthetic cannabinoids (23 substances) and synthetic cathinones (8), but they also include phenethylamines such as amfetamine and methamfetamine, and natural cathinones. This situation is challenging governments' capacity to regulate (Advisory Council on the Misuse of Drugs, 2011). These inexpensively manufactured, unregulated synthetic compounds can circumvent legal controls and have been commonly available over the counter in 'head-shops' or legally from the internet. The molecular structure of cathinone can be altered to produce various compounds, known as cathinones or cathinone derivatives (Fig. 20.1), and analysis suggests that most of the new agents seen in the UK are stimulants, similar in effect to amfetamine (Advisory Council on the Misuse of Drugs, 2010a, 2011).

Noting legislation that would come into effect in December 2009 to control synthetic cannabinoid receptor agonists such as 'Spice', the UK's Advisory Council on the Misuse of Drugs (ACMD) argued for a similar response to other 'legal highs', focusing on the cathinones, of which mephedrone is the class member most commonly appearing in police drug

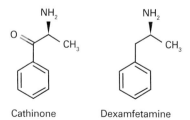

Cathinone   Dexamfetamine

Fig. 20.1 Chemical structures of cathinone and dexamfetamine.

seizures (Iversen, 2009). Owing to their reduced ability to cross the blood–brain barrier, the cathinones may be less potent than amfetamines but they can cause pronounced autonomic effects, tachycardia, hypertension and vasoconstriction leading to blue peripheries, as well as agitation and depression as the stimulant effect wanes. Interestingly, despite the reported marketing of cathinones as plant fertiliser or bath salts, the ACMD stated that they have no recognised efficacy or suitability for such uses.

Since recent UK control of mephedrone, some websites are said to have switched to selling a structurally related compound, naphyrone, a triple monoamine reuptake inhibitor (dopamine, serotonin and noradrenaline). Drugs such as dexamfetamine, which interact selectively with the dopamine transporter, have psychostimulant properties; those such as MDMA (ecstasy) interact selectively with the serotonin transporter and have 'empathogenic' profiles'; and triple reuptake inhibitors such as cocaine combine these properties (Advisory Council on the Misuse of Drugs, 2010b). Consequently, naphyrone may have a cocaine-like profile, while being more potent than cocaine. Sometimes naphyrone is marketed as NRG-1, but test purchases are said to show a markedly inconsistent range of chemicals. The toxic effects are likely to be similar to those of other stimulants. The ACMD warns that naphthyl compounds have been shown to have carcinogenic properties.

What causes substance misuse?

Genetic contribution

Substance misuse is clearly linked with environmental adversities such as family and community breakdown. However, young people who misuse substances commonly exhibit a complex inherited predisposition, of which early use of drugs, alcohol or cigarettes may be a behavioural marker. For instance, data from the Minnesota Twin Family Study (McGue & Iacono, 2008) confirm the long-held view that use of alcohol before the age of 15 is associated with increased risk of later alcohol misuse. Moreover, in a comparison with boys without early alcohol use, early drinking was linked to a range of adverse outcomes: the odds ratio for antisocial personality disorder was 5.8, for drug dependence 3.2, for nicotine dependence 1.7 (and for major depression 1.3). With the exception of a much lower risk for antisocial personality disorder, the pattern of associations was similar for girls. However, the risk of adverse outcomes, including alcohol dependence, associated with early-onset problem behaviour not related to alcohol misuse was sometimes even higher. Compared with young people without early problem behaviour, the risk for lifetime alcohol dependence among early smokers and early drug users was around 7 times higher. The corresponding risk for young people who had been in trouble with the police or had had early sexual intercourse was also considerably higher. McGue & Iacono referred to this array of behaviours as 'disinhibitory psychopathology'.

A population of adopted and non-adopted adolescents (King *et al*, 2009) revealed that young people living with an alcohol-dependent adoptive parent were more likely to drink than those living with a non-drinking adoptive parent, suggesting an environmental effect. However, those with alcohol-dependent biological parents displayed a range of 'disinhibited' behaviours, reflecting what the study's authors argue is the inherited disinhibited predisposition. Figure 20.2 shows that the disinhibition is passed to the biological child of drinking parents; the adopted child of the drinking parent is 'protected' from the disinhibition syndrome.

These datasets support the view that what is transmitted genetically is not a specific predisposition to misuse substances, but a broad behavioural disposition. This disposition is likely to include clinical syndromes such as attention-deficit hyperactivity disorder (ADHD) and conduct disorder, each of which is independently predictive of substance misuse; these risk factors potentially act throughout adolescence (Lynam *et al*, 2009). It appears also to include new forms of disinhibitory psychopathology such as cyberbullying (Sourander *et al*, 2010).

'Self-medication'

Self-treatment may be another contributory factor in substance misuse. Forms of psychopathology such as bipolar disorder and post-traumatic stress disorder (PTSD) are independently associated with higher risk of substance misuse (Goldstein & Bukstein, 2010), perhaps especially among the most vulnerable in society (Bender *et al*, 2010). The effect of depression on risk of substance misuse appears substantially reciprocal, but depression may more often lead to misuse in females (Gallerani *et al*, 2010). Similarly,

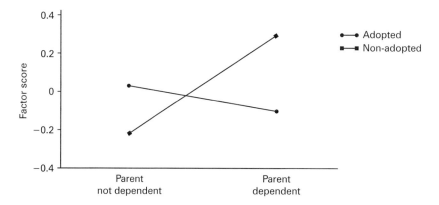

Fig. 20.2 Effect of parental alcohol dependence on standardised disinhibition factor scores in adopted and non-adopted adolescent offspring (after King *et al*, 2009, with permission).

a study of females with PTSD that included older adolescents showed that successful treatment of PTSD predicted reduction in substance use but not *vice versa* (Hien *et al*, 2010). In a large adolescent population study, depression contributed to the uptake of smoking, and continued smoking contributed to 'a dampening or levelling off of depression symptoms'. These findings, perhaps due to the modulating effect of nicotinic acetylcholine receptors on the release of neurotransmitters, suggest that smoking is an 'effective' self-therapy for depression (Audrain-McGovern *et al*, 2009).

Environment

Environmental factors interact with predisposition. For instance, constrained environments (e.g. those characterised by strong family bonds or those in which substances are less available) appear to suppress genetic risk, whereas unconstrained or stressful environments give it freer rein. Indeed, Hicks *et al* (2009) concluded that the greater the environmental stress, the greater the genetic effect. In disorganised environments with easy access to substances, or in which young people are left to their own devices, predispositions are more likely to be fulfilled than in environments where access to substances is limited, a potential gene–environment interaction. Social adversity may not so much 'cause' misuse as permit it.

Pre-existing mental illness

Swendsen *et al* (2010) examined risks posed by a range of mental disorders and the degree to which substance use, misuse and dependence might be eliminated through their treatment. Analysing follow-up data from the US National Comorbidity Survey, and consistent with other longitudinal studies, they argue that risk is linked to affective disorders but that pre-existing behavioural disorders, including ADHD and conduct disorder, are the most powerful antecedents of substance misuse and that their successful early treatment could reduce illicit drug use and dependence by more than 70%. Indeed, early treatment of ADHD appears to reduce risk of later misuse: in a longitudinal case–control study of girls with ADHD, those treated with stimulants were 73% less likely to develop a substance use disorder (Wilens *et al*, 2008).

Intervention

Knowledge concerning the effectiveness of intervention derives mainly from studies of prevention and treatment. However, the body of high-quality randomised controlled trial (RCT) research exclusively concerning young people is relatively limited. Consequently, in the search for useful insights and reflecting the often complex comorbid conditions of those presenting to services, it may be possible cautiously to extrapolate from treatment trials of complex adult psychopathology.

Prevention programmes

Riggs *et al* (2009) presented a long-term follow-up (from 11 to 28 years of age) of a universal intervention in the form of an early-adolescent substance misuse prevention programme. This comprised 10–13 approximately monthly teacher-led sessions of 'resistance skills' and 'social-normative change', a five-session booster 12 months later (at age 13), and a parent programme including interactive sessions about homework and parent–child communication. Significant programme effects emerged at age 15 (2 years after the end of the programme) and appeared to increase until age 17, with differences between the intervention and control groups persisting thereafter. A European study has reported reduced drunkenness and less frequent cannabis use following a teacher-led classroom intervention (Faggiano *et al*, 2010). A parent-only intervention was significant at 12-month outcome, but a pupil-only intervention had no effect on any outcomes (Koning *et al*, 2009). However, compared with no intervention, two sessions of a school-based targeted intervention involving group work with at-risk young people yielded reduced illicit use over the 2-year follow-up (Conrod *et al*, 2010). Perhaps by helping mothers develop a sense of mastery, nurse home visiting of vulnerable mothers during their pregnancy and the first 2 years of their children's lives was linked to reduced affective symptoms and substance misuse in the children 12 years later (Kitzman *et al*, 2010).

These data suggest that altering school curricula to attend to wider aspects of personal development can be effective in enhancing life skills, thus reducing later problem behaviours, and that combined and booster interventions may be important for detecting sustained effects in universal interventions. However, targeted interventions have the advantage of excluding those at low risk and, because of their smaller scale, are likely to be cheaper. What the exact balance of universal and targeted programmes should be remains unclear and is likely to depend on local social and political priorities as much as on science. Prolonged follow-up can detect important delayed or sleeper effects, perhaps reflecting altered developmental trajectories. Any interventions should be evaluated in different cultures. If successful, they may be cost-effective and may benefit whole societies, although reasonable fidelity to the original concept or technology is likely to be important.

Treatment

Opportunistic brief interventions in healthcare settings have shown positive effects on adult drinking. Consistent with this, focusing on adolescents exposed to aggression and substance use, a half-hour therapy in an emergency department reduced reported exposure to violence and aggression at 3-month and alcohol consequences at 6-month follow-up compared with an information brochure control intervention (Walton *et al*, 2010). The precise components of a successful brief intervention for young people are not known, but such a finding shows that even taking a substance history and briefly discussing its findings may be helpful, opening to a wide range of clinicians the possibility of intervening.

In an RCT targeting substance-misusing adolescents with ADHD, individual psychotherapy was linked with significant reduction in substance misuse (Riggs *et al*, 2011). Those additionally treated with long-acting osmotic-release methylphenidate (OROS MPH) over the course of the 4-month trial showed additional benefits. Diversion of the methylphenidate (e.g. selling it on) and interaction with drugs of misuse were not reported, allowing the authors to state that OROS MPH is safe to use in this population. Focusing on opiate-dependent adolescents, Woody *et al* (2008) reported the greater efficacy (as measured by abstinence) of 12 weeks as opposed to 2 weeks of buprenorphine treatment and concluded that a case exists for longer-term maintenance for this group, supplemented by psychosocial interventions.

Adolescent development occurs in 'an ecology of nested systems' (Liddle *et al*, 2009), such as peers, family, schools, recreation and juvenile justice. Within these systems, the relative influence of attachments to family and school versus, for instance, to deviant peers may shape behaviour. Multidimensional family therapy (MDFT) focuses on engagement of the young person and family, targeting adolescent, parental and family interactions as well as extra-familial domains of functioning (Henderson *et al*, 2009).

Henderson *et al* (2010) conducted a secondary analysis of two RCTs comparing MDFT with either cognitive–behavioural therapy (CBT) or enhanced (through support with engagement and transport) treatment as usual. This demonstrated that, for milder forms of misuse, the more intensive MDFT treatment had no greater impact than less intensive CBT (Fig. 20.3). However, statistically significant differences favouring MDFT emerged among those with indicators of more severe substance misuse. Consistent with clinical experience, this important interaction seems to confirm that treatment should be tailored to the severity and complexity of the presenting problems.

Prognosis may be related to aftercare. In an 8-year follow-up of adolescents who had received in-patient treatment for alcohol or drug dependence, Kelly *et al* (2008) showed a relationship between abstinence and attendance at Alcoholics or Narcotics Anonymous meetings. Attending one meeting per week independently predicted abstinence, and most attending three meetings were abstinent. Attendance during the first 6 months after discharge from hospital was associated with abstinence but this effect diminished over the period. Kaminer *et al* (2008) demonstrated reduced relapse rates among young people with alcohol use disorders initially treated as in-patients who were offered aftercare comprising face-to-face contact but not those offered only telephone contact. This

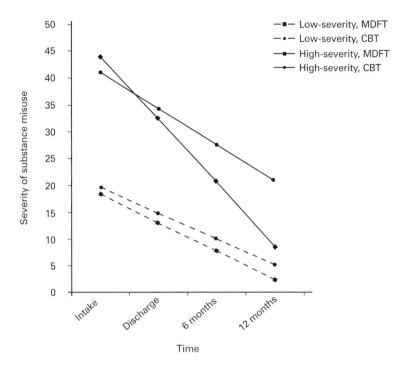

Fig. 20.3 Treatment effect differences for milder and more severe substance misuse. MDFT, multidimensional family therapy; CBT, cognitive–behavioural therapy. After Henderson *et al* (2010), with permission.

underlines the importance for many of a continued relationship with a helping other or others.

Research implications

A review of the 'first 10 years' of the US National Institute on Drug Abuse Clinical Trials Network, which mainly focuses on adult misusers, concluded that the overall efficacy of short-term detoxification was 'poor', so that 'only' 29% had opiate-free urine post-treatment (Wells *et al*, 2010). The review concluded that 'the pooled impact on substance use, especially on maintenance of reduction or abstinence, of all the trials is disappointing'. It noted too the debate in the literature about the degree to which specific psychotherapeutic methods account for variance in outcome, adding that 'care should be taken in simply continuing to test one treatment after another in designs similar to those that have been employed'. The authors concluded that combinations of treatments, and flexible treatment protocols, more focus on subcomponents of treatments such as therapist effects and longer-term follow-up to detect sleeper effects are required.

Treatment for individuals with features of personality disorder

Borderline personality disorder

Many young substance misusers display impulsive aggression, self-harm, interpersonal difficulties, affective distress and mistrust. These are core features of borderline personality disorder, and adults exhibiting them have shown benefits from sustained structured interventions such as dialectical behaviour therapy (DBT) and mentalisation-based treatment (MBT).

In a trial involving adults with borderline personality disorder, 59% of whom reported lifetime comorbid substance use disorders, McMain *et al* (2009) compared DBT with expert general psychiatric management (case management, psychodynamic psychotherapy and medication). The core strategies used in the DBT involved balancing validation of patients' experience with behavioural change to help them develop more effective coping strategies, thereby eliminating behavioural dyscontrol. Over a 12-month period, 25 therapists delivered 30+ sessions to 183 patients, 62% of whom completed treatment. Both treatments were associated with equivalent symptomatic improvement.

In another trial, Bateman & Fonagy (2009) compared MBT with structured clinical management (crisis contact and crisis plans, pharmacotherapy, general psychiatric review and written information about treatment). The aim of MBT, a psychodynamic treatment, was to strengthen patients' capacity to understand their own and others' mental states in attachment contexts, thus enabling them to address their difficulties with affect regulation, impulse control and interpersonal functioning. Of the 134 adult participants, 54% reported a substance use disorder. All were offered 18 months or 140 sessions of treatment, delivered by 11 therapists, and 75% completed at least 70 sessions in the first year. The authors concluded that focusing on psychological functions related to symptoms of borderline personality disorder (e.g. difficulty in reflecting on the mental states of oneself and others) could improve a structured programme providing generic psychological support.

Oldham (2009) commented that 'often the biggest hurdle is to engage the patient in treatment – to establish a partnership that can endure so that any one of the many types of effective treatments can take hold and lead to lasting change'. He speculates that the overarching goal of therapy may be to enable rational control of emotion, to 'teach the cortex to control the amygdala'.

Overall, these studies suggest that a coherent package of interventions, sustained over at least 6 months, involving relatively intensive contact can usefully affect symptoms often considered intractable. Taken with the MDFT data, they may also suggest a dose–response effect, so that complex psychopathology requires more elaborate and sustained interventions.

Antisocial personality disorder

Adult antisocial behaviour has close links with child and adolescent conduct disorder, which are closely entwined with substance misuse. As treatment studies of adolescent conduct disorder are rare (Riggs *et al*, 2011), it is instructive to consider lessons from adult treatment studies.

Frank antisocial behaviour can appear intractable. However, even among those with antisocial personality disorder, observer ratings of change in therapeutic alliance predict behaviour change (Polaschek & Ross, 2010). A Cochrane review of psychological interventions for antisocial or dissocial personality disorder (Gibbon *et al*, 2010) found 6 months of treatment that included contingency management to have a positive effect on attendance at counselling sessions as well as on social functioning and cocaine use (assessed by an addiction severity measure). Twenty-four weeks of CBT was associated with a significant reduction in cocaine-positive urine samples. However, CBT was not associated with change in verbal or physical aggression, compared with treatment as usual (TAU). As both interventions were associated with reduced aggression, high-quality TAU could be an effective intervention. Indeed, as the participants came from mental health and forensic services within the National Health Service (Davidson *et al*, 2009), it is likely that TAU was a reasonably sustained intervention emphasising engagement, general supportive interventions and problem-solving.

National guidance

Until April 2013, the UK National Treatment for Agency Substance Misuse (NTA) had the responsibility for 'improving the availability, capacity and effectiveness' of services for drug misusers in England. This organisation has now been subsumed under NHS England. Data published by the NTA revealed that, of the approximately 24 000 young people aged 16 and below seen in English substance misuse services, only 8% received family interventions (National Treatment Agency for Substance Misuse, 2011). Only 3% were 'referred on'. Most young people in the UK receive a relatively brief intervention that excludes considerations of family relationships or collaboration with other agencies. This work is likely to be short of what could be achieved.

Conclusion

The evidence base suggests that substance-misusing young people, who comprise perhaps 5–10% of the adolescent population, display a constellation of behavioural and emotional difficulties. These phenomena are substantially genetically influenced, so that, in general, even dysfunctional parents should not be 'blamed'. Understanding this can aid

325

Box 20.1   Practice implications

- Relatively simple interventions targeted on emergency department attenders or at-risk pupils identified by questionnaire may reduce substance misuse and related behaviours
- In light of the complex psychopathology that accompanies substance misuse, especially more severe misuse, an effective treatment system should have the capacity to:
  - engage families and improve relationships with parents/carers
  - target the 'ecology': the young person's relationship with leisure, education, work, criminal justice system
  - distance young people from substance-using peers
  - be sustained over at least months
  - offer intensive contact.

---

empathy and family engagement. It is possible to prevent some substance use through school-based programmes (Box 20.1). Existing users may show a measurable response to very brief interventions offered opportunistically. It follows that any health or social care professional encountering a young user should, in a non-judgemental way, take a substance use history and thoughtfully feed back and discuss the findings. However, especially among those below 16, substance use may be a marker of more profound or safeguarding problems that are likely to need extensive assessment or referral. In the UK context, multifaceted interventions, the components of which are becoming apparent, require engagement and the capacity to organise a coalition of services to deliver a coherent and substantial package of intervention probably lasting at least some months. However, this type of response is not universal; treatment needs more closely to follow the emerging evidence base.

References

Advisory Council on the Misuse of Drugs (2010a) *Consideration of the Naphthylpyrovalerone Analogues and Related Compounds*. ACMD.

Advisory Council on the Misuse of Drugs (2010b) *Consideration of the Cathinones*. ACMD.

Advisory Council on the Misuse of Drugs (2011) *Consideration of the Novel Psychoactive Substances ('Legal Highs')*. Home Office.

American Psychiatric Association (2013) *Diagnostic and Statistical Manual of Mental Disorders (5th edn) (DSM-5)*. APA.

Audrain-McGovern J, Rodriguez D, Kassel J (2009) Adolescent smoking and depression evidence for self medication and peer smoking mediation. *Addiction*, **104**, 1743–1756.

Bateman A, Fonagy P (2009) Randomized controlled trial of outpatient mentalization-based treatment versus structured clinical management for borderline personality disorder. *American Journal of Psychiatry*, **166**, 1355–1364.

Bender K, Ferguson K, Thompson S, et al (2010) Factors associated with trauma and posttraumatic stress disorder among homeless youth in three US cities: the importance of transience. *Journal of Traumatic Stress*, **23**, 161–168.

Collishaw, S, Maughan, B, Natarajan, L, et al (2010) Trends in adolescent emotional problems in England: a comparison of two national cohorts twenty years apart. *Journal of Child Psychology and Psychiatry*, **51**, 885–894.

Conrod P, Castellanos-Ryan N, Strang J (2010) Brief, personality-targeted coping skills interventions and survival as a non-drug user over a 2-year period during adolescence. *Archives of General Psychiatry*, **67**, 85–93.

Davidson K, Tyrer P, Tata P, et al (2009) Cognitive behaviour therapy for violent men with antisocial personality disorder in the community: an exploratory randomized controlled trial. *Psychological Medicine*, **39**, 569–577.

Drummond C (2011) The end of the dependence syndrome as we know it? *Addiction*, **106**, 892–894.

European Monitoring Centre for Drugs and Drug Addiction (2011) Cocaine and crack cocaine: prevalence and patterns of use. In *Annual Report 2011: The State of the Drugs Problem in Europe*. EMCDDA.

European Monitoring Centre for Drugs and Drug Addiction (2012) *New drugs detected in the EU at the rate of around one per week, say agencies (News Release No. 2/2012)*. EMCDDA.

Faggiano F, Vigna-Taglianti F, Burkhart G, et al (2010) The effectiveness of a school-based substance abuse prevention program: 18-month follow-up of the EU-Dap cluster randomized controlled trial. *Drug and Alcohol Dependence*, **108**, 56–64.

Fuller E, Sanchez M (eds) (2010) *Smoking, Drinking and Drug Use among Young People in England 2009*. NHS Information Centre for Health and Social Care.

Gallerani C, Garber J, Martin N (2010) The temporal relationship between depression and comorbid psychopathology in adolescents at varied risk for depression. *Journal of Child Psychology and Psychiatry*, **51**, 242–249.

Gibbon S, Duggan C, Stoffers J, et al (2010) Psychological interventions for antisocial personality disorder. *Cochrane Database of Systematic Reviews*, **6**, CD007668.

Goldstein B, Bukstein O (2010) Comorbid substance use disorders among youth with bipolar disorder: opportunities for early identification and prevention. *Journal of Clinical Psychiatry*, **71**, 348–358.

Henderson C, Rowe C, Dakof G, et al (2009) Parenting practices as mediators of treatment effects in an early-intervention trial of multidimensional family therapy. *American Journal of Drug and Alcohol Abuse*, **35**, 220–226.

Henderson C, Dakof G, Greenbaum P, et al (2010) Effectiveness of multidimensional family therapy with higher severity substance-abusing adolescents: report from two randomized controlled trials. *Journal of Consulting and Clinical Psychology*, **78**, 885–897.

Hibell B, Guttormsson U, Ahlström S, et al (2012) *The 2011 ESPAD Report: Substance Use among Students in 36 European Countries*. Swedish Council for Information on Alcohol and other Drugs (CAN).

Hicks B, South S, DiRago A, et al (2009) Environmental adversity and increasing genetic risk for externalizing disorders. *Archives of General Psychiatry*, **66**, 640–648.

Hien D, Jiang H, Campbell A, et al (2010) Do treatment improvements in PTSD severity affect substance use outcomes? A secondary analysis from a randomized clinical trial in NIDA's Clinical Trials Network. *American Journal of Psychiatry*, **167**, 95–101.

Impinen A, Mäkelä P, Karjalainen K, et al (2010) High mortality among people suspected of drunk-driving: an 18-year register-based follow up study. *Drug and Alcohol Dependence*, **110**, 80–84.

Iversen L (2009) *Re: ACMD consideration of mephedrone (and related cathinones) (Letter to the Home Secretary)*. Advisory Council on the Misuse of Drugs.

Johnston LD, O'Malley PM, Bachman JG, et al (2009) *Monitoring the Future. National Results on Adolescent Drug Use: Overview of Key Findings, 2009* (NIH Publication No. 10-7583). National Institute on Drug Abuse.

Kaminer Y, Burleson J, Burke R (2008) Efficacy of outpatient aftercare for adolescents with alcohol use disorders: a randomized controlled study. *Journal of the American Academy of Child & Adolescent Psychiatry*, **47**, 1405–1412.

Kelly J, Brown S, Abrantes A, *et al* (2008) Social recovery model: an 8-year investigation of adolescent 12-step group involvement following inpatient treatment. *Alcoholism: Clinical and Experimental Research*, **32**, 1468–1478.

King S, Keyes M, Malone S, *et al* (2009) Parental alcohol dependence and the transmission of adolescent behavioral disinhibition: a study of adoptive and non-adoptive families. *Addiction*, **104**, 578–586.

Kitzman H, Olds D, Cole R, *et al* (2010) Enduring effects of prenatal and infancy home visiting by nurses on children. *Archives of Pediatrics & Adolescent Medicine*, **164**, 412–418.

Koning I, Vollebergh W, Smit F, *et al* (2009) Preventing heavy alcohol use in adolescents: cluster randomized trial of a parent and student intervention offered separately and simultaneously. *Addiction*, **104**, 1669–1678.

Liddle H, Rowe C, Dakof G, *et al* (2009) Multidimensional family therapy for young adolescent substance abuse: twelve-month outcomes of a randomized controlled trial. *Journal of Consulting and Clinical Psychology*, **77**, 12–25.

Lopez M, Compton W, Volkow ND (2009) Changes in cigarette and illicit drug use among US teenagers. *Archives of Pediatrics & Adolescent Medicine*, **163**, 869–870.

Lynam, D, Charnigo, R, Moffitt, T, *et al* (2009) The stability of psychopathy across adolescence. *Development and Psychopathology*, **21**, 1133–1153.

McGue M, Iacono WG (2008) The adolescent origins of substance use disorders. *International Journal of Methods in Psychiatric Research*, **17 (suppl. 1)**, S30–8.

McMain SF, Links PS, Gnam WH, *et al* (2009) A randomized controlled trial of dialectical behaviour therapy versus structured psychiatric management for borderline personality disorder. *American Journal of Psychiatry*, **166**, 1365–1374.

National Treatment Agency for Substance Misuse (2010) *Substance Misuse among Young People: The Data for 2008–09*. NTA.

National Treatment Agency for Substance Misuse (2011) *Substance Misuse among Young People: 2010–11*. NTA.

Newbury-Birch D, Walker J, Avery L, *et al* (2009) *Impact of Alcohol Consumption on Young People: A Systematic Review of Published Reviews (Research Report DCSF-RR067)*. Department for Children, Schools and Families.

Oldham J (2009) Borderline personality disorder comes of age. *American Journal of Psychiatry*, **166**, 509–511.

Polaschek D, Ross E (2010) Do early therapeutic alliance, motivation and stages of change predict therapy change for high risk, psychopathic, violent prisoners? *Criminal Behaviour and Mental Health*, **20**, 100–111.

Riggs N, Chou C, Pentz M (2009) Preventing growth in amphetamine use: long term effects of the Midwestern Prevention Project (MPP) from early adolescence to early adulthood. *Addiction*, **104**, 1691–1699.

Riggs PD, Winhusen T, Davies RD (2011) Randomized controlled trial of osmotic-release methylphenidate with cognitive-behavioral therapy in adolescents with attention-deficit/hyperactivity disorder and substance use disorders. *Journal of the American Academy of Child & Adolescent Psychiatry*, **50**, 903–914.

Sourander A, Klomek A, Iknone M, *et al* (2010) Psychosocial factors associated with cyber-bullying among adolescents: a population-based study. *Archives of General Psychiatry*, **67**, 720–728.

Swendsen J, Conway K, Degenhardt L, *et al* (2010) Mental disorders as risk factors for substance use, abuse and dependence: results from the 10-year follow up of the National Comorbidity Survey. *Addiction*, **105**, 1117–1128.

Walton M, Chermack S, Shope J, *et al* (2010) Effects of a brief intervention for reducing violence and alcohol misuse among adolescents: a randomized controlled trial. *JAMA*, **304**, 527–535.

Wells E, Saxon A, Calsyn D, *et al* (2010) Study results from the Clinical Trials Network's first 10 years: where do they lead? *Journal of Substance Abuse Treatment*, **38** (suppl. 1), S14–S30.

Wilens T, Adamson J, Monuteaux M, *et al* (2008) Effect of prior stimulant treatment for attention-deficit/hyperactivity disorder on subsequent risk for cigarette smoking and alcohol and drug use disorders in adolescents. *Archives of Pediatrics and Adolescent Medicine*, **162**, 916–921.

Woody GE, Poole SA, Subramaniam G, *et al* (2008) Extended vs short-term buprenorphine-naloxone for treatment of opioid-addicted youth. *JAMA*, **200**, 2003–2011.

CHAPTER 21

Eating disorders

Dasha Nicholls and Elizabeth Barrett

This chapter provides an overview of classification and outcome of eating disorders, before focusing on current evidence-based treatment for the two main disorders of anorexia nervosa and bulimia nervosa. Eating disorders in childhood and adolescence present a serious threat to health and well-being, including medical consequences ranging from growth delay to life-threatening effects of starvation and refeeding (Nicholls *et al*, 2011a). Anorexia nervosa is frequently cited as the third most common chronic illness of adolescence (Lucas *et al*, 1991).

Setting the context: classification and epidemiology

Historically, the eating disorders (for which the majority of literature uses DSM terminology) comprise anorexia nervosa, bulimia nervosa and eating disorders not otherwise specified (EDNOS), with separate classification of feeding disorders with onset before age 6. The point at which the responsibility for food intake changes from parent to child is complex, and includes factors such as the accurate recognition of hunger and satiety, knowledge of food hygiene and handling, sensory integration of texture and smell, as well as an understanding of nutritional needs. Eating disturbance is a common manifestation of emotional issues (anxiety, mood) and a medium through which autonomy and control are negotiated. There are therefore many potential mechanisms through which the feeding to eating transition can be deviated or delayed.

The revised classification of feeding and eating disorders in DSM-5 (American Psychiatric Association, 2013) and that proposed for ICD-11 recognises this continuous process. This will be an important conceptual shift. Key changes recommended for the classification of eating disorders (Uher & Rutter, 2012) can be summarised as follows.

- The merging of feeding and eating disorders into a single grouping with categories applicable across age groups.
- Diagnosis that can be made on the basis of behaviours (e.g. parental report of excessive exercise) that indicate fear of weight gain or other underlying fears or beliefs.
- Broadening the criteria for the diagnosis of anorexia nervosa and removing the requirement for amenorrhoea; extending the

weight criterion to any significant underweight; and extending the cognitive criterion to include developmentally and culturally relevant presentations.

- Reducing the frequency requirement to meet diagnostic thresholds for binge eating and vomiting.
- Including binge eating disorder as a specific category defined by subjective or objective binge eating in the absence of regular compensatory behaviour.
- Introduction of a new term, 'avoidant/restrictive food intake disorder' (ARFID), to classify restricted food intake in children or adults that is not accompanied by psychopathology related to body weight and shape (Bryant-Waugh et al, 2010). This category will replace the current diagnosis of 'feeding disorder of infancy and early childhood'. No age criterion is proposed for ARFID and it may occur through nutritional impairment or by virtue of the psychological impact of a highly restricted diet both on personal development and on family function. Individuals with this disorder are more likely to have other medically unexplained symptoms, or comorbid medical or neuro-developmental disorders.
- 'Other specified feeding and eating disorder' (OSFED) will replace EDNOS for cases of atypical anorexia nervosa, atypical bulimia nervosa, atypical binge eating disorder, purging disorder and night eating syndrome.

An overall aim is to minimise use of the catch-all diagnosis of 'unspecified feeding and eating disorder'.

Research using the new criteria is as yet sparse, but in a recent US study utilising the DSM-5 classification system, Stice et al (2013) followed up adolescent girls and reported that lifetime prevalence by age 20 was 0.8% for anorexia nervosa, 2.6% for bulimia nervosa, 3.0% for binge eating disorder, 2.8% for atypical anorexia nervosa, 4.4% for subthreshold bulimia nervosa, 3.6% for subthreshold binge eating disorder, and 3.4% for purging disorder. This gives a combined prevalence for any eating disorder of 13.1% (5.2% had anorexia nervosa, bulimia nervosa or binge eating disorder; 11.5% had feeding and eating disorders not elsewhere classified (FED-NEC)). Early-onset eating disorders therefore include anorexia nervosa and bulimia nervosa and a range of eating disorder-like presentations, currently termed EDNOS, atypical or unclassifiable. The DSM-5 work group decided, having reviewed the evidence, that obesity did not merit classification as an eating disorder (Marcus & Wildes, 2009).

Outcomes and continuity into adult life

Around 50% of adolescents with anorexia nervosa respond to treatment within 12 months, and 75–80% achieve full or partial remission, regardless of treatment type (Lock et al, 2010). This means, however, that 20–25% will still meet diagnostic criteria for anorexia nervosa after 2 years of treatment (Gowers *et al*, 2007). Factors that have been associated with poorer outcome include admission to psychiatric hospital, eating-related obsessionality, eating disorder-specific psychopathology, binge eating and purging, older age and longer duration of illness (Gowers *et al*, 2007; Le Grange *et al*, 2012). For bulimia nervosa, around 40% abstain from bingeing/purging after treatment, but relapse is common even by 6 months. Those with less severe eating concerns at baseline, lower baseline depression, fewer binge/purge episodes at presentation, and receiving family-based rather than individual treatment are more likely to be in remission at follow-up (Le Grange *et al*, 2008).

Previous studies had suggested that outcome for childhood-onset eating disorders might be worse than for those with onset in adolescence. Data from a national sample of patients under 13 with eating disorders found that most were still in treatment at 1 year, and seven had been hospital in-patients for most of the year (Nicholls *et al*, 2011*b*).

Keel & Brown (2010) reviewed long-term outcome data from 26 studies. They found that most patients with anorexia nervosa achieved remission by 5-year follow-up, those receiving in-patient treatment having a poorer prognosis. In a 10-year outcome study, most (69%) participants met criteria for full recovery, but 51% had developed another Axis I disorder (Herpertz-Dahlmann *et al*, 2001). There was a significant association between psychiatric comorbidity and the outcome of the eating disorder. Recovered patients did not differ significantly from normal controls with regard to psychiatric morbidity and psychosocial functioning. Approximately 30% of patients with bulimia nervosa and related EDNOS remain ill 10–20 years after initial presentation, although symptom remission for binge and purge behaviour is high. Early adolescent bulimia nervosa carries a ninefold increase in risk for late adolescent bulimia nervosa and a twenty-fold increase in risk for adult bulimia nervosa (Kotler *et al*, 2001). Field *et al* (2012) report that girls with binge eating disorder were almost twice as likely as their unaffected peers to become overweight or obese or to develop depressive symptoms.

Therapeutic models

Although some advocate a medical illness model for eating disorders, most adopt a psychological formulation and treatment approach that considers developmental and systemic factors but still acknowledges individual genetic and neurobiological risk. Assumptions about the role of the family in aetiology have undergone an enormous cultural shift away from blaming the parents to recognition of the importance of involving them in treatment and decision-making (Treasure *et al*, 2007; Le Grange *et al*, 2010). Controlled treatment trials in anorexia nervosa for patients under the age of 18 with an illness of less than 3 years' duration showed that family work was more effective at 5-year follow-up than individual therapy alone (Eisler *et al*, 1997). The 'Maudsley model' of family-based treatment (Lock *et al*, 2000) has since gained a considerable evidence base and is the best empirically supported treatment available to young people with anorexia nervosa (Lock *et al*, 2010). It is essentially a structural model, with parents clearly in charge, and with externalisation of the anorexia as a key strategy. This involves conceptualising the illness (often given a name) as an entity provoking the child and family. The child, family and professionals are united in their struggle to disempower and banish the illness. A similar model for family-based treatment of bulimia nervosa has been described (Le Grange & Lock, 2007). No specific family therapy techniques have been described for the treatment of the 'atypical' eating disorders.

If a family-based approach is not possible or the young person does not respond to this approach, combination therapies or individual therapy models may be used. Individual therapy for young people would typically occur in conjunction with parental or family work, as the burden of change should not rest solely on the child. It can take the form of various models of psychotherapy, including adolescent-focused psychotherapy (Fitzpatrick *et al*, 2010), interpersonal psychotherapy and psychodynamic psychotherapy. Parents need to support and respect the confidentiality of the sessions, and the therapist is accountable to the parents for the work being done, usually through periodic reviews or feedback. Behavioural techniques have a role in changing concrete, measurable aspects of behaviour, but have little impact on thoughts, beliefs and feelings. They are not much use in isolation, and at worst can be punitive. Cognitive–behavioural techniques, however, are a mainstay of treatment for bulimia nervosa, and can be adapted for use in anorexia nervosa and ARFID (Gowers & Green, 2009). For some types of ARFID, specific focus on systematic desensitisation using graded hierarchies, and techniques addressing sensory sensitivities may also be necessary.

The 'therapeutic tool box' therefore needs to be varied and flexible, depending on the age, developmental stage and degree of cooperation of the child. For example, it is not helpful to sit in prolonged silence with a child who is unwilling or unable to engage in any communication. For a more detailed account of some of the therapeutic techniques of use in young people with eating disorders, see Watkins (2013) and Troupp (2013).

Comprehensive approach

A multidisciplinary approach is essential. Debate sometimes arises over which to tackle first: the eating behaviour or the emotional symptoms. However, growth failure, pubertal arrest and failure of bone accretion can have significant impact in as little as 6 months and so the multidisciplinary team needs not only to be aware of and identify all these competing problems, but also to find constructive ways to resolve them. Although motivation is an important factor to consider, therapeutic alliance does not predict outcome for anorexia nervosa (Pereira *et al*, 2006), and young people recognise that some things do need to be done or decided against their will. It does matter how they are done, however, and respect and trust are important qualities in healthcare professionals managing young people with eating disorders (Tan *et al*, 2003).

Healthcare setting

As a 2009 Cochrane review outlines, current policy in the UK and elsewhere places emphasis on the provision of mental health services 'in the least restrictive setting, whilst also recognising that some children will require inpatient care' (Shepperd *et al*, 2009). A number of studies have emerged looking at health service context rather than the treatment itself. Of these, the most influential has been the Treatment Outcome for Child and Adolescent Anorexia Nervosa (TOuCAN) trial (Gowers *et al*, 2007). This evaluated the clinical and cost-effectiveness of in-patient treatment compared with two variants of out-patient treatment: general (routine) treatment in child and adolescent mental health services (CAMHS) and a specialist adolescent eating disorders service for young people with anorexia nervosa. This was a population-based, pragmatic randomised controlled trial (RCT) involving 215 young people (aged 12 to 18, mean age 14 years 11 months) and 35 CAMHS teams in England. In addition, the satisfaction of the young people and their carers with these treatments was elicited (Gowers *et al*, 2010). On follow-up at 1, 2 and 5 years, using both standardised and self-report measures, there was significant improvement in all groups at each time point. The number achieving a good outcome was 19% at 1 year, 33% at 2 years and 64% (of those followed up) at 5 years. Analysis demonstrated no difference in efficacy of in-patient compared with out-patient treatment, or specialist compared with generalist treatment at any time point, when baseline characteristics were taken into account. The specialist out-patient programme was the dominant treatment in terms of incremental cost-effectiveness. Of note, the specialist out-patient service used a largely cognitive–behavioural rather than family-based treatment model. Out-patient treatment had a higher probability of being more cost-effective than in-patient care (Byford *et al*, 2007).

Overall, the TOuCAN study provides little support for lengthy in-patient psychiatric treatment on clinical or health economic grounds, and broadly supports existing guidelines on the treatment of anorexia nervosa, such as those published by the National Institute for Health and Care Excellence (NICE). These suggest that out-patient treatments should be offered to the majority, with in-patient treatment offered in rare cases (National Collaborating Centre for Mental Health, 2004). Out-patient care, supported by brief (medical) in-patient management for correction of acute complications, may be a preferable approach. The health economic analysis and patients' and carers' views both support NICE guidelines, which suggest that anorexia nervosa should be managed in specialist services that have experience and expertise in its treatment. Comprehensive general CAMHS might, however, be well placed to manage milder cases.

House *et al* (2012) have taken these issues further, exploring the effect of direct access to specialist services on referral rates, admissions for in-patient treatment and continuity of care. In areas where specialist out-patient services were available, 2–3 times more cases were identified than in areas without such services, and there were significantly lower rates of admission for in-patient treatment and considerably higher consistency of care.

Together these studies support the development of specialist eating disorder services able to provide continuity of care where possible. To our knowledge, there is no research about feeding disorders services.

The most common reasons for hospital admission are listed in Box 21.1. Admission to a paediatric ward for primarily medical reasons tends to work successfully only in the context of continuity of paediatric care and where skilled psychiatric care is also available. Staff need to receive adequate training, and health service managers should address barriers to joint working. Admission to psychiatric units can be for one of two reasons: first, acute admission for management of risks that cannot be addressed in the paediatric setting, for example suicidality, some extreme eating behaviours or need for restraint; and second, because out-patient therapy does not provide sufficiently intensive support for change.

Box 21.1 Reasons for admission to hospital

There are various reasons for admission other than being seriously medically unwell. It is important to clarify and agree the necessity for and the purpose of paediatric admission with the young person, family and team members.

Reasons for admission include:

- need for intravenous fluids to correct electrolyte abnormality
- refeeding for severe malnutrition
- management of physical complications of severe malnutrition and/or associated behaviours, such as electrolyte disturbance secondary to purging
- management of an acute medical illness unrelated to the eating disorder
- respite for parents
- assessment
- assessment and management of self-harm
- initiation of/trial of medication
- management of uncontrolled compensatory behaviours (e.g. excessive exercise, vomiting)
- moving the young person towards taking responsibility for their own eating disorder when a family-based approach is not appropriate or effective and out-patient treatment would not be safe.

Help for parents

Mistrust of professionals and self-blame are common for parents. They may have been told explicitly that they are to blame, or have developed a sense of failure while attempting to overcome their child's difficulties. Clear information, both in the form of general literature and specifically about their own child's difficulties, can help in establishing trust. Additionally, eating disorders occur more often in some families. For example, there is a specific association between some ARFID presentations and maternal eating disorder, particularly food avoidance emotional disorder (FAED) (Watkins *et al*, 2012). It is evident that parenting a child with a feeding or eating disorder is stressful, and many carers report mental health problems. Sometimes, parents develop a rejecting stance to their child or see the eating behaviour as a personal attack (indeed, their child may see it in that way too). Except where there are clear safeguarding concerns, it is unhelpful to the child or parents to conceptualise eating disorders in this way. Helping parents to bear the illness and the rejection that goes with it without rejecting their child is essential.

Medication

The evidence for use of medication in the treatment of childhood-onset eating disorders is limited, and the evidence for effectiveness is weak across the age range. Clinical guidelines (e.g. National Collaborating Centre for Mental Health, 2004) regarding medications are therefore mostly based on consensus views rather than strong research. What evidence there is mainly comes from studies in adults. Medications under consideration for anorexia nervosa are usually atypical antipsychotics, selective serotonin reuptake inhibitors (SSRIs) or micronutrient supplementation. For bulimia nervosa, studies have used SSRIs, other antidepressants and mood stabilisers, with reasonable effects on binge/purge frequency in adults. For binge eating disorder, medications that have been studied include SSRIs, serotonin–noradrenaline reuptake inhibitors (SNRIs), mood stabilisers and anti-obesity medications. Pharmacotherapy for bulimia nervosa and binge eating disorder show moderate effect sizes in adults, but generally low recovery rates. Anorexia nervosa is generally more treatment resistant.

Three RCTs have been conducted to date involving adolescents with anorexia nervosa:

- olanzapine *v.* placebo ($n = 20$): preliminary findings did not support adjunctive olanzapine for underweight adolescent girls with anorexia nervosa (Kafantaris *et al*, 2011)
- risperidone *v.* placebo ($n = 40$): there was no benefit for the addition of risperidone during weight-restoration in adolescents with anorexia nervosa (Hagman *et al*, 2011)

- quetiapine *v.* treatment as usual ($n = 33$): low-dose quetiapine in this open-label RCT resulted in both psychological and physical improvements, with minimal side-effects (Court *et al*, 2010).

Antidepressants should be considered for patients who are clearly suffering from depression or obsessive–compulsive disorder. However, given concerns about the safety of SSRIs in adolescents and children, caution is advised in using this class of medication for anorexia nervosa in this age group (Lock *et al*, 2005*a*). The use of SSRIs is of proven efficacy in adults with bulimia nervosa and should be considered in adolescents (Flament *et al*, 2012). Medication can also be considered as an adjunct to other therapies, particularly when it could enhance the capacity of the child to make use of other therapy. Anxiolytic medication may be a useful adjunct in the treatment of functional dysphagia. Medication should never be used in the absence of other treatments.

Management and treatment: specific disorders

Anorexia nervosa

Responsibility

Anorexia nervosa (for definition see Box 21.2) remains the psychiatric disorder with the highest mortality, and it can create enormous anxiety and conflict in personal and professional relationships. Issues of control and responsibility are central to the treatment of anorexia nervosa. With young people, these are further complicated by the need to determine to what extent they can be considered both competent and to have capacity to make decisions about treatment. Responsibility for recovery can be seen to

---

Box 21.2 Features of anorexia nervosa

- Weight lost or maintenance of a significantly low expected weight for height and age, or failure to make weight gain during a growth period
- Fear of gaining weight or becoming fat, even though underweight
- Weight loss achieved by restriction of food intake and specific avoidance of 'fattening foods' and one or more of the following: self-induced vomiting, self-induced purging, excessive exercise, use of appetite suppressants and/ or diuretics
- Disturbance in the way the person experiences their body weight and shape (body image distortion), undue influence of body weight or shape on self-evaluation, morbid preoccupation with weight and shape

(Adapted from: World Health Organization, 1992; American Psychiatric Association, 1994)

lie with the child, the parents or the professionals. When the professionals take charge, this allows the parents and child to be relieved of the anxiety, but it can also reinforce the parents' sense of failure. Occasionally, it causes the parents to withdraw the young person from treatment if they are not in agreement with the professionals.

For these reasons, parents should be helped to take responsibility for managing the eating disorder, unless the age of the young person, urgency or other imperatives suggest otherwise. This means establishing parental control of food and fluid intake. The young person is encouraged to negotiate the 'how' of food intake, but not the 'whether'. For example, children may like their mother to sit with them during meals, and hold their hand. Alternatively, they may prefer for food not to be discussed at meal times, and any extra calories to be made up in drink form at the end of the day. Whatever approach is taken, it should be applied consistently by the parents, even if the parental couple are no longer living together. Once control of eating is established, other areas where the child can develop or regain control are negotiated. These form the first two stages of the family-based treatment model for anorexia nervosa.

In older adolescents moving towards independence, or when the illness is long-standing, it may be appropriate for more responsibility to lie with the young person, with parents moving to a supportive rather than responsible role. Techniques such as motivational interviewing or using workbooks such as *Hunger for Understanding* (Nesbitt, 2005) can engage young people in the idea of change and recovery.

Physical aspects

Doctors have a central role in both the recognition and management of medically unstable children. Physical aspects of care can be both acute (e.g. medical compromise) and chronic (e.g. impaired growth and development) in nature. Differences in size and body composition put children at greater risk than adults for certain aspects of acute and chronic starvation. Prepubertal children become emaciated more quickly than adults, because of the relative deficiency of body fat, and they also dehydrate more quickly. Hudson *et al* (2012) looked in detail at children under 13 with eating disorders in the context of the British surveillance study, and found that over a third had medical instability at presentation (60% had bradycardia, 54% hypotension, 34% dehydration, 26% hypothermia). Over 50% required admission shortly after diagnosis (73% to a paediatric ward). Of those with medical instability, 41% were not underweight. Peebles *et al* (2010), in a case-note review of 1310 females aged 8–19 years treated for anorexia nervosa, bulimia nervosa or EDNOS, found that the medical severity of those with EDNOS was intermediate on all parameters to that of those with anorexia nervosa or bulimia nervosa, but that those with partial bulimia nervosa or bulimia nervosa had longer QTc intervals and higher rates of additional medical complications at presentation than the other groups.

Both studies provide evidence that anthropological indices alone are poor markers for medical instability, and clinical assessment is essential. The Junior MARSIPAN report (Royal College of Psychiatrists, 2012) outlines parameters for risk assessment in young people, and gives guidance on laboratory tests and indicators of concern.

In terms of chronic sequelae of eating disorders, the most important are the impact on growth, pubertal development and bone health. Distinction should be made between children who are appropriately prepubertal and those in whom the onset of puberty has been delayed. Significant delay is usually defined as more than 2 standard deviations (s.d.) from the mean. Menses are deemed to be delayed if there is failure of onset within 4.5 years of the start of puberty, or by the time the girl has reached the chronological or bone age of 14 years. Onset of anorexia nervosa during puberty will result in pubertal arrest. Tanner staging, pelvic ultrasound appearances, and discrepancy between bone age and chronological age can help in evaluating the degree of pubertal delay. Chronic physical illness or genetic factors resulting in pubertal delay need to be taken into account.

Height and weight should be plotted on standard growth charts for comparison with population norms and parental heights. Previous information about the child's growth will give a more complete picture. The 'growth spurt' in girls occurs at age 12 years (s.d. = 1.8 years); thereafter, growth slows down and stature is only likely to be significantly affected if onset is post-menarcheal. Body mass index (BMI) is not a linear constant in childhood, so BMI needs to be adjusted for the young person's age and gender by use of a BMI chart or by calculating how far the BMI is from the median for age and gender. This can be expressed as a standard deviation score (SDS), or as a percentage of the median BMI:

(BMI/median BMI for age and gender) × 100

(this is one way of calculating weight for height). Clinically, however, rate of weight loss may be more important than percentage BMI alone.

Osteoporosis is an established risk in adults with anorexia nervosa. In younger patients, the problem of bone loss is compounded by failure of bone accretion, especially important as adolescence is a critical time for bone accrual. Other contributing factors include hypogonadism and low oestradiol levels seen in anorexia nervosa. Nutritional rehabilitation remains the treatment of choice for low bone density in childhood. Calcium supplementation can be considered, although it is likely to have limited value in an underweight child. There is no evidence at present that high oestrogen doses given as an oral contraceptive improve bone mineral density and they should not be considered without consulting a growth specialist, because of the risks of stunting from premature epiphyseal fusion. Misra et al (2011) have examined physiological oestrogen replacement in adolescent girls, demonstrating increase in bone density of those receiving cyclic transdermal oestrogen for 18 months compared with placebo.

Feeding via nasogastric tube or other method should be considered for children who are unable to tolerate oral refeeding for physical or emotional reasons. It is essential to try to obtain the parents' and/or young person's consent for this – any young person with capacity can consent, although it is uncommon for them to do so in such a situation. In the absence of either, an appropriate legal framework should be invoked. For a young person under the age of 18 and living at home, the options are to use either the Children Act 1989 or the Mental Health Act 1983 (as amended in 2007). Eating disorders are classified as mental disorders under the Mental Health Act, and feeding forms part of the treatment (i.e. does not require a separate legal mandate). Parental responsibility remains intrinsic to the Children Act, and in some cases it may therefore be preferable to use this legislation rather than the Mental Health Act, which puts professionals effectively *in loco parentis*.

Target weight

Patients with anorexia nervosa make every attempt to pin down professionals to giving them a target weight. The clinician's target is for normal growth and development to be restored. Height will change during recovery, and thus the target weight range will also change. Lai *et al* (1994) found that menses resumed at an average of 96% weight for height, but as for most biological parameters, there is a normal distribution and therefore considerable variation around this. Pelvic ultrasound scan can show whether uterine size and ovarian maturation have progressed (Allan *et al*, 2010), and is therefore a more sensitive marker of return of hypothalamic–pituitary axis function. If pelvic ultrasound is not available, then a target weight range of 95–100% weight for height is recommended. Weight recovery tends to occur at a rate of about 2–3 kg per month. In premenarcheal girls and in boys, progress through puberty is a marker that a healthy weight has been regained. Height velocity in growing children should return to normal (or be greater) on restoration to a healthy weight.

Anorexia nervosa and the brain

The effect of anorexia nervosa on the brain is a subject of much interest, given recent advances in neuroscience: two books devoted to eating disorders and the brain have been published in the past few years (Adan & Kaye, 2011; Lask & Frampton, 2011). Neuropsychological and neuroimaging research is being used to better identify those at risk and design treatment interventions. Chui *et al* (2008) studied brain structure and cognitive function in 66 adolescent girls with relatively long-standing anorexia nervosa compared with healthy controls, and showed that participants with anorexia nervosa who remained at low weight had larger lateral ventricles relative to controls, and those who had amenorrhoea or irregular menses showed significant cognitive deficits in a number of domains. Stedal *et al* (2012) studied the specific neuropsychological profiles of 155 young people with anorexia nervosa in an attempt to better characterise the profile of those at risk and identify patients who might respond to therapies directed at addressing thinking style rather than the primary psychopathology. The participants mainly functioned in the normal range, with particular strengths in verbal fluency and relatively weaker visuospatial memory, set shifting and central coherence.

Central to the research in this area are questions concerning what is primary (i.e. predisposing or risk) and what is secondary to illness and weight loss. Findings have been mixed, depending on the tests performed, the age and duration of illness, and the time to follow-up. Many studies have shown a recovery in performance on weight restoration (for a review, see Jáuregui-Lobera, 2013), although in adults with long-standing anorexia nervosa Tchanturia et al (2004) showed that performance on set-shifting tasks did not show any improvement following retesting after weight recovery. It may be that a problem with set shifting is a prognostic indicator, and is therefore found in treatment-resistant individuals.

Recognition of the role of thinking style and its relationship to anxiety and perfectionism has been the rationale for the development of cognitive remediation therapy (CRT) for anorexia nervosa (Tchanturia et al, 2013a). Trials are ongoing of CRT as an adjunctive treatment and, although it can be difficult to disentangle the effects of weight restoration and improvement in other parameters such as mood (Dahlgren et al, 2013), this is a promising new area for study.

A related area of increasing research is the relationship between 'autistic traits' and anorexia nervosa. Similarities in socioemotional and cognitive domains include difficulties with empathy, set-shifting and global processing. Self-report evidence shows that both adult and adolescent patients (Baron-Cohen et al, 2013; Tchanturia et al, 2013b) have elevated autistic traits relative to controls, particularly in the area of stereotyped and repetitive behaviours (Pooni et al, 2012). Further research is needed in this area to understand the role of autism spectrum traits in the maintenance and treatment response of anorexia nervosa.

Family therapy and parental counselling

Several studies have reported on family interventions for eating disorders (see 'Therapeutic models', above). Family-based treatment (FBT) is the best studied treatment for the management of anorexia nervosa and therefore has the strongest evidence base for effectiveness in adolescents. It appears to be effective for the majority of adolescents with anorexia nervosa (Lock et al, 2010), with the caveat that those with marked obsessional features or rigidity may need to be treated for longer than the standard 6 months (Lock et al, 2005b). It can be delivered in several formats and doses. Preliminary data suggest that FBT can be disseminated by training and manuals in diverse clinical settings (Couturier et al, 2010). Two systematic reviews, however (Gardner & Wilkinson, 2011; Couturier et al, 2013), reported that

FBT was not significantly better or only marginally better than individual treatment at inducing remission. Family therapy and parental counselling have been shown to be equally effective (Eisler *et al*, 2000). A conjoint family approach may be appropriate from the start, particularly for children who are to articulate their views or demonstrate their conflicts with family members. Parental counselling provides support and advice, using a similar theoretical framework to FBT. In addition to affirming that the parents are in charge, parents can explore issues they may be reluctant to discuss in front of their child. Parental self-efficacy is an important predictor of outcomes. Throughout FBT, parents experienced an increase in self-efficacy and adolescents experienced a reduction in symptoms. Maternal and paternal self-efficacy scores also predicted adolescent outcomes throughout treatment (Robinson *et al*, 2013).

Group therapy

Group therapy is an established part of most treatment programmes for adolescents with eating disorders, the focus usually being on the development of self-esteem. Groups for younger children are less well-established. The provision of unstructured time for children to explore peer relationships and to develop freedom of expression can be infinitely more accessible and acceptable to the child than individual therapy, in which a child can feel persecuted and withdraw.

Parents' groups, in both structured (e.g. psychoeducational) and therapeutic/supportive form, can address issues such as coping with rejection, and allow parents to hear from other parents what it can be hard to hear from professionals. Skills-based workshops (Treasure *et al*, 2007) for parents and carers of individuals with eating disorders across the age range have also been shown to reduce expressed emotion.

Individual therapy

The place of individual therapy for older adolescents and those with long-standing illness has long been recognised. In their randomised controlled trial, Lock *et al* (2010) evaluated the relative efficacy of family-based treatment (FBT) and adolescent-focused individual therapy (AFT) for adolescents with anorexia nervosa in producing full remission. At end of treatment, there were no differences in full remission between FBT and AFT, and both led to considerable improvement. However, those treated with AFT were more likely to require hospital admission at some point. Thus, AFT is an alternative treatment option when FBT is not feasible or viable.

Fairburn *et al* (2003) have developed a transdiagnostic cognitive–behavioural approach to eating disorders treatment, and have compared individual and family-based approaches. A 40-week intervention with enhanced cognitive–behavioural therapy (CBT-E) was offered. Participants showed a substantial increase in weight together with a marked decrease in eating disorder psychopathology, which was sustained at 60-week follow-up (Dalle *et al*, 2013).

For younger children, the role of individual therapy and the therapeutic style adopted depend on a number of factors, not least the availability of skilled therapists. The nutritional status of the child, as well as their cognitive and emotional development, are important in assessing suitability. Parental support for the therapy is crucial. The focus of work may be to encourage the child to address issues more directly with their parents by rehearsing with the therapist. Individual work should also be considered if family therapy is proving unsuccessful. In such circumstances, previously undisclosed abuse may emerge. Other specific indications for individual work include treatment for concurrent depression, obsessive–compulsive disorder or specific anxieties, such as fear of swallowing or choking. Here, age-appropriate CBT would be the treatment of choice.

It is clear that there is a need therefore to tailor treatments to the individual and family. Le Grange *et al* (2012) suggest that patients with more severe eating-related psychopathology have better outcomes in a behaviourally targeted family treatment (FBT) than an individually focused approach (AFT).

Bulimia nervosa

Bulimia nervosa is rare in the premenarcheal age group (Nicholls *et al*, 2011*b*). When it does occur (usually around age 13 or 14 and predominantly in girls) the features are fairly similar to those in older adolescents and adults (Box 21.3). However, purging with laxatives and other medications is less common in the younger age group, and secretiveness may be more prominent, since most adolescents continue to be under some sort of

---

Box 21.3 Features of bulimia nervosa

- Persistent preoccupation with eating and recurrent episodes (over a period of months) of binge eating characterised by eating a large amount of food in a short period of time, and a sense of lack of control while eating
- Attempts to counteract the 'fattening' effects of food by compensatory behaviours such as: self-induced vomiting, misuse of purgatives, alternating periods of starvation or excessive exercise, use of drugs such as appetite suppressants, diuretics, thyroid preparations or, in diabetes, misuse of insulin
- Psychopathology consisting of a morbid dread of fatness and setting of a target weight way below what might be considered healthy
- Bulimia nervosa may follow a period of anorexia nervosa, but would only be diagnosed if the patient is no longer significantly underweight

(Adapted from: World Health Organization, 1992; American Psychiatric Association, 1994)

parental surveillance. As in adulthood, comorbid depression is often present, and on the rare occasions that in-patient treatment is indicated, depression is more likely to be the reason than the eating behaviour itself. Research among adolescents with bulimia nervosa has lagged behind that among adults, although there is growing evidence that supports the efficacy of family-based interventions and cognitive–behavioural treatments adapted for use with adolescent populations.

Bulimia nervosa is pervaded by a sense of chaos, and the first role of the clinician is to establish clear structures and boundaries. The adolescent's behaviour may seem to demand constant supervision, accompaniment to the toilet, supervision after meals and monitoring at school. On the other hand, the adolescent may feel that their parents are being intrusive and become more secretive. Individual therapy can provide structure, containment and privacy for the adolescent, while family work can focus on helping parents negotiate boundaries with their offspring. For example, parents may decide that the adolescent eats three meals a day with the rest of the family, but agree not to accompany him or her to the toilet unless requested to do so. Within this framework, adapted for age where appropriate, adolescents can start to address their own issues in relation to food.

Most patients with bulimia nervosa will be of normal weight or overweight. Despite healthy weights, irregular menses is a common feature and may affect bone density. The most serious medical concern is potassium depletion as a result of frequent vomiting. Serum potassium is a poor reflection of the body's potassium stores and clinical judgement may be more valuable in deciding whether purging is occurring at a life-threatening level.

Despite advances in cognitive–behavioural techniques for young people and a strong evidence base for adults, there have been only two RCTs comparing their efficacy with family-based treatment in bulimia nervosa (and none in anorexia nervosa). Le Grange et al (2007) aimed to evaluate the relative efficacy of family-based treatment (FBT) and supportive psychotherapy (SPT) for adolescents with bulimia nervosa. Family-based treatment showed a clinical and statistical advantage over SPT at the end of treatment and at 6-month follow-up. Reduction in core bulimic symptoms was also more immediate for patients receiving FBT. However, when Schmidt et al (2007) compared the efficacy and cost-effectiveness of family therapy and CBT guided self-care in adolescents with bulimia nervosa or EDNOS, they found that CBT guided self-care had the advantage of offering a more rapid reduction of bingeing, lower cost and greater acceptability for the adolescents involved, although there were no differences between the treatments overall at 12 months. This suggests that there may be an element of choice for young people about which treatment they would prefer, and some room for clinician judgement based on the level of support from family/parents that the young person may benefit from during their recovery.

Conclusion

Although the rates of true eating disorders (anorexia nervosa, bulimia nervosa) in the population are relatively stable, the overall incidence of eating disorders in younger children and adolescents may be increasing and the definitions of eating disorders changing. Eating disorders with onset during childhood and early adolescence, while sharing many common features with later-onset disorders, need to be considered separately from the point of view of recognition, consequences and management. In children, atypical disorders are frequently seen. Epidemiological evidence suggests that primary care clinicians need to be made aware of these disorders, as they are currently underreferred, relative to expected rates, to eating disorder services. Efforts to prevent eating disorders should focus on cases of subthreshold severity.

The principle of care is a comprehensive, multidisciplinary approach, with close collaboration with parents. Evidence-based psychological interventions for new-onset anorexia nervosa and bulimia nervosa are available and effective. A family-based model of treatment is advocated in most cases as the first line, with alternative approaches placing responsibility for change on the young person, in the context of development of adolescent autonomy. In-patient treatment is of value both to medically stabilise and to initiate refeeding in acute malnutrition and, less commonly, as a form of intensive therapy. Alternatives to in-patient care are undergoing trials. An evidence-based stepped model of care is currently lacking. The burden on parents/carers and siblings is high, and recovery typically takes 2–5 years for anorexia nervosa. Bulimia nervosa has higher remission rates, but relapse is more common than for anorexia nervosa. Specific treatments for most atypical eating disorders have not been systematically described or evaluated.

References

Adan RAH, Kaye WH (eds) (2011) *Behavioral Neurobiology of Eating Disorders*. Springer.

Allan R, Sharma R, Sangani B, *et al* (2010) Predicting the weight gain required for recovery from anorexia nervosa with pelvic ultrasonography: an evidence-based approach. *European Eating Disorders Review*, **18**, 43–48.

American Psychiatric Association (1994) *Diagnostic and Statistical Manual of Mental Disorders (4th edn) (DSM-IV)*. APA.

American Psychiatric Association (2013) *Diagnostic and Statistical Manual of Mental Disorders (5th edn) (DSM-5)*. APA.

Baron-Cohen S, Jaffa T, Davies S, *et al* (2013) Do girls with anorexia nervosa have elevated autistic traits? *Molecular Autism*, **4** (1), 24.

Bryant-Waugh R, Markham L, Kreipe RE, *et al* (2010) Feeding and eating disorders in childhood. *International Journal of Eating Disorders*, **43**, 98–111.

Byford S, Barrett B, Roberts C, *et al* (2007) Economic evaluation of a randomised controlled trial for anorexia nervosa in adolescents. *British Journal of Psychiatry*, **191**, 436–440.

Chui HT, Christensen BK, Zipursky RB, *et al* (2008) Cognitive function and brain structure in females with a history of adolescent-onset anorexia nervosa. *Pediatrics*, **122**, e426–e437.

Court A, Mulder C, Kerr M, *et al* (2010) Investigating the effectiveness, safety and tolerability of quetiapine in the treatment of anorexia nervosa in young people: a pilot study. *Journal of Psychiatric Research*, **44**, 1027–1034.

Couturier J, Isserlin L, Lock J (2010) Family-based treatment for adolescents with anorexia nervosa: a dissemination study. *Eating Disorders*, **18**, 199–209.

Couturier J, Kimber M, Szatmari, P (2013) Efficacy of family-based treatment for adolescents with eating disorders: A systematic review and meta-analysis. *International Journal of Eating Disorders*, **46**, 3–11.

Dahlgren CL, Lask B, Landrø NI, *et al* (2013) Neuropsychological functioning in adolescents with anorexia nervosa before and after cognitive remediation therapy: a feasibility trial. *International Journal of Eating Disorders*, **46**, 576–581.

Dalle GR, Calugi S, Doll HA, *et al* (2013) Enhanced cognitive behaviour therapy for adolescents with anorexia nervosa: an alternative to family therapy? *Behaviour Research and Therapy*, **51**, R9–R12.

Eisler I, Dare C, Russell GF, *et al* (1997) Family and individual therapy in anorexia nervosa. A 5-year follow-up. *Archives of General Psychiatry*, **54**, 1025–1030.

Eisler I, Dare C, Hodes M, *et al* (2000) Family therapy for adolescent anorexia nervosa: the results of a controlled comparison of two family interventions. *Journal of Child Psychology and Psychiatry*, **41**, 727–736.

Fairburn CG, Cooper Z, Shafran R (2003) Cognitive behaviour therapy for eating disorders: a 'transdiagnostic' theory and treatment. *Behaviour Research and Therapy*, **41**, 509–528.

Field AE, Sonneville KR, Micali N, *et al* (2012) Prospective association of common eating disorders and adverse outcomes. *Pediatrics*, **130**, e289–e295.

Fitzpatrick K, Moye A, Hoste RR, *et al* (2010) Adolescent focused psychotherapy for adolescents with anorexia nervosa. *Journal of Contemporary Psychotherapy*, **40**, 31–39.

Flament MF, Bissada H, Spettigue W (2012) Evidence-based pharmacotherapy of eating disorders. *International Journal of Neuropsychopharmacology*, **15**, 189–207.

Gardner J, Wilkinson P (2011) Is family therapy the most effective treatment for anorexia nervosa? *Psychiatria Danubina*, **23** (suppl. 1), S175–S177.

Gowers S, Green L (2009) *Eating Disorders: Cognitive Behavioural Therapy with Children and Young People*. Taylor & Francis.

Gowers SG, Clark A, Roberts C, *et al* (2007) Clinical effectiveness of treatments for anorexia nervosa in adolescents: randomised controlled trial. *British Journal of Psychiatry*, **191**, 427–435.

Gowers SG, Clark AF, Roberts C, *et al* (2010) A randomised controlled multicentre trial of treatments for adolescent anorexia nervosa including assessment of cost-effectiveness and patient acceptability – the TOuCAN trial. *Health Technology Assessment*, **14**, 1–98.

Hagman J, Gralla J, Sigel E, *et al* (2011) A double-blind, placebo-controlled study of risperidone for the treatment of adolescents and young adults with anorexia nervosa: a pilot study. *Journal of the American Academy of Child & Adolescent Psychiatry*, **50**, 915–924.

Herpertz-Dahlmann B, Muller B, Herpertz S, *et al* (2001) Prospective 10-year follow-up in adolescent anorexia nervosa – course, outcome, psychiatric comorbidity, and psychosocial adaptation. *Journal of Child Psychology and Psychiatry*, **42**, 603–612.

House J, Schmidt U, Craig M, *et al* (2012) Comparison of specialist and nonspecialist care pathways for adolescents with anorexia nervosa and related eating disorders. *International Journal of Eating Disorders*, **45**, 949–956.

Hudson LD, Nicholls DE, Lynn RM, *et al* (2012) Medical instability and growth of children and adolescents with early onset eating disorders. *Archives of Disease in Childhood*, **97**, 779–784.

Jáuregui-Lobera I (2013) Neuropsychology of eating disorders: 1995–2012. *Neuropsychiatric Disease and Treatment*, **9**, 415–430.

Kafantaris V, Leigh E, Hertz S, *et al* (2011) A placebo-controlled pilot study of adjunctive olanzapine for adolescents with anorexia nervosa. *Journal of Child and Adolescent Psychopharmacology*, **21**, 207–212.

Keel PK, Brown TA (2010) Update on course and outcome in eating disorders. *International Journal of Eating Disorders*, **43**, 195–204.

Kotler LA, Cohen P, Davies M, *et al* (2001) Longitudinal relationships between childhood, adolescent, and adult eating disorders. *Journal of the American Academy of Child & Adolescent Psychiatry*, **40**, 1434–1440.

Lai KY, de Bruyn R, Lask B, *et al* (1994) Use of pelvic ultrasound to monitor ovarian and uterine maturity in childhood onset anorexia nervosa. *Archives of Disease in Childhood*, **71**, 228–231.

Lask B, Frampton I (eds) (2011) *Eating Disorders and the Brain*. Wiley-Blackwell.

Le Grange D, Lock J (2007) *Treating Bulimia in Adolescents: A Family-Based Approach*. Guilford Press.

Le Grange D, Crosby RD, Rathouz PJ, *et al* (2007) A randomized controlled comparison of family-based treatment and supportive psychotherapy for adolescent bulimia nervosa. *Archives of General Psychiatry*, **64**, 1049–1056.

Le Grange D, Crosby RD, Lock J (2008) Predictors and moderators of outcome in family-based treatment for adolescent bulimia nervosa. *Journal of the American Academy of Child & Adolescent Psychiatry*, **47**, 464–470.

Le Grange D, Lock J, Loeb K, *et al* (2010) Academy for Eating Disorders position paper: the role of the family in eating disorders. *International Journal of Eating Disorders*, **43**, 1–5.

Le Grange D, Lock J, Agras WS, *et al* (2012) Moderators and mediators of remission in family-based treatment and adolescent focused therapy for anorexia nervosa. *Behaviour Research and Therapy*, **50**, 85–92.

Lock J, Le Grange D, Agras S, *et al* (2000) *Treatment Manual for Anorexia Nervosa*. Guilford Press.

Lock J, Walker LR, Rickert VI, *et al* (2005*a*) Suicidality in adolescents being treated with antidepressant medications and the black box label: position paper of the Society for Adolescent Medicine. *Journal of Adolescent Health*, **36**, 92–93.

Lock J, Agras WS, Bryson S, *et al* (2005*b*) A comparison of short- and long-term family therapy for adolescent anorexia nervosa. *Journal of the American Academy of Child & Adolescent Psychiatry*, **44**, 632–639.

Lock J, Le Grange D, Agras WS, *et al* (2010) Randomized clinical trial comparing family-based treatment with adolescent-focused individual therapy for adolescents with anorexia nervosa. *Archives of General Psychiatry*, **67**, 1025–1032.

Lucas AR, Beard CM, O'Fallon WM, *et al* (1991) Fifty year trends in the incidence of anorexia nervosa in Rochester, Minnesota: a population based study. *American Journal of Psychiatry*, **148**, 917–922.

Marcus MD, Wildes JE (2009) Obesity: is it a mental disorder? *International Journal of Eating Disorders*, **42**, 739–753.

Misra M, Katzman D, Miller KK, *et al* (2011) Physiologic estrogen replacement increases bone density in adolescent girls with anorexia nervosa. *Journal of Bone and Mineral Research*, **26**, 2430–2438.

National Collaborating Centre for Mental Health (2004) *Eating Disorders: Core Interventions in the Treatment and Management of Anorexia Nervosa, Bulimia Nervosa and Related Eating Disorders* (Clinical Guideline 9). National Institute for Clinical Excellence.

Nesbitt S (2005) *Hunger for Understanding: A Workbook for Helping Young People to Understand and Overcome Anorexia Nervosa*. Wiley-Blackwell.

Nicholls D, Hudson L, Mahomed F (2011*a*) Managing anorexia nervosa. *Archives of Disease in Childhood*, **96**, 977–982.

Nicholls DE, Lynn R, Viner RM (2011*b*) Childhood eating disorders: British national surveillance study. *British Journal of Psychiatry*, **198**, 295–301.

Peebles R, Hardy KK, Wilson JL, *et al* (2010) Are diagnostic criteria for eating disorders markers of medical severity? *Pediatrics*, **125**, e1193–e1201.

Pereira T, Lock J, Oggins J (2006) Role of therapeutic alliance in family therapy for adolescent anorexia nervosa. *International Journal of Eating Disorders*, **39**, 677–684.

Pooni J, Ninteman A, Bryant-Waugh R, *et al* (2012) Investigating autism spectrum disorder and autistic traits in early onset eating disorder. *International Journal of Eating Disorders*, **45**, 583–591.

Robinson AL, Strahan E, Girz L, *et al* (2013) 'I know I can help you': parental self-efficacy predicts adolescent outcomes in family-based therapy for eating disorders. *European Eating Disorders Review*, **21**, 108–114.

Royal College of Psychiatrists (2012) *Junior MARSIPAN: Management of Really Sick Patients under 18 with Anorexia Nervosa* (College Report CR168). Royal College of Psychiatrists.

Schmidt U, Lee S, Beecham J, *et al* (2007) A randomized controlled trial of family therapy and cognitive behavior therapy guided self-care for adolescents with bulimia nervosa and related disorders. *American Journal of Psychiatry*, **164**, 591–598.

Shepperd S, Doll H, Gowers S, *et al* (2009) Alternatives to inpatient mental health care for children and young people. *Cochrane Database of Systematic Reviews*, **2**, CD006410.

Stedal K, Rose M, Frampton I, *et al* (2012) The neuropsychological profile of children, adolescents, and young adults with anorexia nervosa. *Archives of Clinical Neuropsychology*, **27**, 329–337.

Stice E, Marti CN, Rohde P (2013) Prevalence, incidence, impairment, and course of the proposed DSM-5 eating disorder diagnoses in an 8-year prospective community study of young women. *Journal of Abnormal Psychology*, **122**, 445–457.

Tan JO, Hope T, Stewart A, *et al* (2003) Control and compulsory treatment in anorexia nervosa: the views of patients and parents. *International Journal of Law and Psychiatry*, **26**, 627–645.

Tchanturia K, Morris RG, Anderluh MB, *et al* (2004) Set shifting in anorexia nervosa: an examination before and after weight gain, in full recovery and relationship to childhood and adult OCPD traits. *Journal of Psychiatric Research*, **38**, 545–552.

Tchanturia K, Lloyd S, Lang K (2013*a*) Cognitive remediation therapy for anorexia nervosa: current evidence and future research directions. *International Journal of Eating Disorders*, **46**, 492–495.

Tchanturia K, Smith E, Weineck F, *et al* (2013*b*) Exploring autistic traits in anorexia: a clinical study. *Molecular Autism*, **4**, 44 [Epub ahead of print].

Treasure J, Smith G, Crane A (2007) *Skills-Based Learning for Caring for a Loved One with an Eating Disorder: The New Maudsley Method*. Routledge.

Troupp C (2013) Individual psychotherapy. In *Eating Disorders in Childhood and Adolescence* (4th edn) (eds B Lask, R Bryant-Waugh), pp. 281–300. Routledge.

Uher R, Rutter M (2012) Classification of feeding and eating disorders: review of evidence and proposals for ICD-11. *World Psychiatry*, **11**, 80–92.

Watkins B (2013) Cognitive behavioural approaches. In *Eating Disorders in Childhood and Adolescence* (4th edn) (eds B. Lask, R. Bryant-Waugh), pp. 258–280. Routledge.

Watkins B, Cooper PJ, Lask B (2012) History of eating disorder in mothers of children with early onset eating disorder or disturbance. *European Eating Disorders Review*, **20**, 121–125.

World Health Organization (1992) *The ICD-10 Classification of Mental and Behavioural Disorders: Clinical Descriptions and Diagnostic Guidelines*. WHO.

CHAPTER 22

Gender dysphoria in young people

Domenico Di Ceglie

The film *Boys Don't Cry* illustrates in a highly dramatised form the problems that the phenomenon of gender dysphoria (gender identity disorder in DSM-IV; American Psychiatric Association, 1994) can create in an extreme situation. The film is based on the true story of a young person, Brandon, with a female body who perceived himself as a male. We are not told when the issue of his male gender identity first appeared, but we see him living in a male role as a teenager trying to conceal from his peers the reality of his female body. The struggles of these concealments are well portrayed, as in the scene when Brandon steals tampons from a shop. He joins in male activities and displays of physical strength as a confirmation of his male role. He is well accepted as a boy within a troubled and troublesome group of young people. He falls passionately in love with a girl, Lana, who accepts him as he is without much questioning, and a close intimate relationship develops, which the peer group seems to accept. The reality of his body is eventually revealed. Lana can accept the new situation, but had she really not known or had she turned a blind eye? Unfortunately, two young men become more and more disturbed by this realisation. It stirs a primitive violence in them, which leads first to Brandon's rape and then to his murder.

How can we make sense of this complex tragedy? I would like to suggest that unbearable identity confusion in the two young attackers, against a social background of strong prejudice and stigma, is what leads to the violence. It is aimed at changing Brandon but eventually destroys him when he does not submit to their views of order on gender and sexual matters. For them, having a female body is inextricably connected with having a female identity. Any digression from this rule is a terrible threat to their fragile sense of identity. Obviously, other factors can be invoked in making sense of their behaviour, but these are beyond the scope of this chapter.

The establishment and maintenance of secrecy regarding gender can have serious psychosocial consequences, as the film shows when Brandon's secret is suddenly revealed. However, people who come into contact with a child or teenager they know to have gender dysphoria often experience a sense of confusion. Breaking a cycle of secrecy by promoting openness and creating the conditions for the tolerance of confusion and uncertainty are important factors in the management of gender dysphoria in children.

349

Before the 1960s, secrecy and confusion dominated the area of atypical gender identity development. The first definition of the term 'gender role' was given by John Money (1955, 1994). Money wanted to differentiate a set of feelings, assertions and behaviours that identified a person as being a boy or a girl, a man or a woman (gender roles), from the contrasting conclusion one could have reached by considering only their gonads.

The term 'gender identity' appeared in the mid-1960s in association with the establishment of a gender identity study group at the University of California. Stoller (1992: p. 78) defines it as:

> 'A complex system of beliefs about oneself: a sense of one's masculinity and femininity. It implies nothing about the origins of that sense (e.g. whether the person is male or female). It has, then, psychological connotations only: one's subjective state.'

The concept of gender identity and role having been formulated, it became possible to make sense of experiences that had until then been ill-defined and poorly understood. Incongruity between the natal sex and the psychological/behavioural manifestations of gender identity indicated the presence of a gender dysphoria. This definition opened the way to conceptualising these experiences as new identities and led to their social recognition, which culminated in the UK in the passing of the Gender Recognition Act 2004. This legislation allows transgender people to change their birth certificate in accordance with their perceived gender. Together with these developments there has been a debate on whether or not this condition should remain in the psychiatric classifications.

Classifications of gender dysphoria in young people

Following the definition of gender identity, in 1980 the category of 'gender identity disorder of childhood' (GIDC) and 'transsexualism' (for adolescents and adults) entered the third edition of the Diagnostic and Statistical Manual of Mental Disorders (DSM-III; American Psychiatric Association, 1980). In the following version, DSM-IV, the two categories were amalgamated into a single diagnosis of 'gender identity disorder', with criteria for children, adolescents and adults (American Psychiatric Association, 1994). The recently published DSM-5 (American Psychiatric Association, 2013) reintroduces two separate categories: 'gender dysphoria in children' and 'gender dysphoria in adolescents and adults', with different criteria sets for each category. The diagnostic criteria are divided into A and B: A refers to the clinical features of gender dysphoria, and B to the associated significant distress or impairment in psychosocial functioning (Box 22.1).

'Gender identity disorder of childhood' was also included in the tenth revision of the International Classification of Diseases (ICD-10; World Health Organization, 1992). This classification is currently being reviewed for ICD-11, which is due out in 2015.

Box 22.1   DSM-5 diagnostic criteria for gender dysphoria

Gender dysphoria in children

A. A marked incongruence between one's experienced/expressed gender and assigned gender, of at least 6 months duration, as manifested by at least 6 of the following (one of which must be criterion A1):

1 a strong desire to be of the other gender or an insistence that he or she is the other gender (or some alternative gender different from one's assigned gender)
2 in boys, a strong preference for cross-dressing or simulating female attire; in girls, a strong preference for wearing only typical masculine clothing and a strong resistance to the wearing of typical feminine clothing
3 a strong preference for cross-gender roles in make-believe or fantasy play
4 a strong preference for the toys, games, or activities typical of the other gender
5 a strong preference for playmates of the other gender
6 in boys, a strong rejection of typically masculine toys, games, and activities and a strong avoidance of rough-and-tumble play; in girls, a strong rejection of typically feminine toys, games, and activities
7 a strong dislike of one's sexual anatomy
8 a strong desire for the primary and/or secondary sex characteristics that match one's experienced gender

B. The condition is associated with clinically significant distress or impairment in social, school, or other important areas of functioning.

Specify if: With a disorder of sex development (e.g., a congenital adrenogenital disorder such as 255.2 [E25.0] congenital adrenal hyperplasia or 259.50 [E34.50] androgen insensitivity syndrome).

Coding note: Code the disorder of sex development as well as gender dysphoria.

Gender dysphoria in adolescents or adults

A. A marked incongruence between one's experienced/expressed gender and assigned gender, of at least 6 months duration, as manifested by at least 2 of the following:

1 a marked incongruence between one's experienced/expressed gender and primary and/or secondary sex characteristics (or, in young adolescents, the anticipated secondary sex characteristics)
2 a strong desire to be rid of one's primary and/or secondary sex characteristics because of a marked incongruence with one's experienced/expressed gender (or, in young adolescents, a desire to prevent the development of the anticipated secondary sex characteristics)
3 a strong desire for the primary and/or secondary sex characteristics of the other gender
4 a strong desire to be of the other gender (or some alternative gender different from one's assigned gender)
5 a strong desire to be treated as the other gender (or some alternative gender different from one's assigned gender)
6 a strong conviction that one has the typical feelings and reactions of the other gender (or some alternative gender different from one's assigned gender)

B. The condition is associated with clinically significant distress or impairment in social, occupational, or other important areas of functioning.

Specify if: With a disorder of sex development (e.g., a congenital adrenogenital disorder such as 255.2 [E25.0] congenital adrenal hyperplasia or 259.50 [E34.50] androgen insensitivity syndrome).

Coding note: Code the disorder of sex development as well as gender dysphoria.

Specify if: Posttransition: The individual has transitioned to full-time living in the desired gender (with or without legalisation of gender change) and has gone undergone (or is preparing to have) at least one cross-sex medical procedure or treatment regimen – namely, regular cross-sex hormone treatment or gender reassignment surgery confirming the desired gender (e.g., penectomy, vaginoplasty in a natal male; mastectomy or phalloplasty in a natal female).

(American Psychiatric Association, 2013: pp. 452–453, with permission)

Although there has been a shift towards the recognition of transgender presentations as an issue of identity within a diversity discourse, rather than as a 'psychiatric condition', the incongruence between self-perception and body during the developmental period and beyond is a distressing problem requiring a combination of psychological, social and physical interventions in young people and adults. This is probably the main reason for retaining the condition in DSM-5 under the new names of 'gender dysphoria in children' and 'gender dysphoria in adolescents or adults'. The use of the word 'dysphoria' (from the Greek: state of unease or mental discomfort) instead of 'disorder' emphasises the distressing nature of the condition for the sufferers (Di Ceglie, 2010), but also ensures that there is no need for the individual to retain the diagnosis once the dysphoria has disappeared through gender reassignment procedures or an evolution of the condition with the disappearance of the incongruence between self-perception and the body.

The following case study illustrates an initial clinical presentation (in this and subsequent case studies, details have been altered to protect the individuals' identity).

Case study 1: James

James was referred to a gender identity clinic at the age of 8.

At the assessment interviews, he said that since the age of 5 he had very much wished he were a girl. He had been secretly dressing up in his mother's clothes. He liked to play with dolls and cuddly toys and fantasised that he was a mother feeding them. He played weddings and liked to be in the role of the bride. At school he wanted to play with girls and avoided rough-and-tumble play or other activities with boys.

His maternal grandmother had looked after him from age 6 months to 5 years, as his mother was away often for her work. The grandmother involved him in many activities, including cooking and tidying up the house. After her sudden death in hospital, James developed the features of gender dysphoria. He could not talk about the loss of his grandmother or even mention her, but he concretely identified with her and persistently wished to continue with all the activities in exactly the same way as he once had with her. Family therapy, focusing on a family tree constructed over many sessions, enabled the narrative of his experiences with his grandmother to be heard and understood and this helped him to mourn her death. The clinical features of his gender dysphoria gradually reduced in intensity and disappeared.

In this case the psychological work not only focused on mourning processes, but it also removed the secrecy about James's gender issues, encouraged his curiosity about its origins and established a link between his atypical gender development and the way he had coped with the loss of his grandmother. Symbol formation was stimulated, so that he could have a mental picture of her and memories of the past, rather than concretely identifying with and becoming her. Increased contact with his father seemed also to play an important role.

Prevalence of gender dysphoria in young people

The prevalence of childhood gender dysphoria in the general population has not yet been definitively established. The studies that have been carried out have used differing criteria, such as single behaviours or identity statements. No large-scale investigation with standardised diagnostic criteria has yet been conducted.

Zuger & Taylor (1969) interviewed the mothers of boys around 7 years of age with regard to the presence of six cross-gender behaviours: a desire to be female; feminine dressing; wearing lipstick; doll play; preference for girl playmates; and aversion to boys' games. The mothers were not asked how long the behaviours had been apparent or when they had started. The study showed that these behaviours were not frequently found in children (73% never engaged in any of them).

Feinblatt & Gold (1976) found that of 193 children referred to a Connecticut child guidance clinic, four boys and three girls (3.6% of the total) were referred primarily because of 'gender-role inappropriate behaviour'.

In the final decades of the 20th century, Zucker reported from epidemiological data that extreme forms of cross-gender behaviour seemed to be uncommon among boys in the general population (Zucker, 1985; Zucker & Bradley, 1995). However, in recent years there has been a large increase in referrals of children and adolescents to specialist gender identity services in Western countries (Fig. 22.1). This is probably due to an increase in social awareness or better recognition of the conditions in these countries.

Long-term follow-up studies

An analysis in 1985 of all long-term follow-up studies of children with gender identity disorder (gender dysphoria) referred to mental health professionals (Zucker, 1985) showed that only a small minority of children had a transsexual outcome, while the majority had a homosexual or bisexual outcome. Green et al's (1987) later follow-up study of boys with features of gender dysphoria mirrored these results. Of 44 males in the original 'feminine boy' group who were re-interviewed in adolescence or

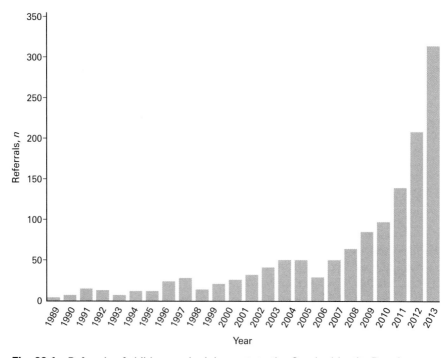

Fig. 22.1 Referrals of children and adolescents to the Gender Identity Development Service at London's Tavistock Centre from the start of the service in 1989 (4 referrals) to 2013 (314 referrals).

young adulthood, three-quarters were homosexual or bisexual. Only one had a transsexual outcome.

More recent studies show that gender dysphoria in prepuberty persists into adolescence and beyond in only 10–30% of individuals (Drummond *et al*, 2008; Wallien & Cohen-Kettenis, 2008). Given the variability of outcomes, some clinicians have defined their approach to the care of children with gender dysphoria as 'watchful waiting'. Factors that may contribute to persistence or desistance are unclear and the subject of current empirical research.

Gender dysphoria in adolescence tends to persist into adulthood in the vast majority of cases (Steensma *et al*, 2011).

Associated psychosocial difficulties

Children with gender identity disorders also present with separation anxiety, depression, and emotional and behavioural difficulties (Coates & Person, 1985). Suicide attempts and self-harming behaviours in adolescence are frequent and in some cases this is how young people with gender identity disorders come to professional attention (Skagerberg *et al*, 2013).

In a survey of the first 124 cases referred to our service, we found that the most common associated features were relationship difficulties with parents or carers (57%), relationship difficulties with peers (52%), depression/misery (42%), family mental health problems (38%), family physical health problems (38%), being the victim of harassment or persecution (33%) and social sensitivity (31%). These data suggest that children with gender identity problems may experience considerable isolation owing to difficulties in their relationships with significant adults and peers. They can also become the victims of persecution, which may contribute to feelings of depression and misery. In this sample, boys appeared to experience more harassment than girls, perhaps because gender non-conformity in boys is less socially acceptable than in girls. The high percentages of mental and physical health problems in the families of children and adolescents referred may indicate that factors such as parental depression or major physical illness could represent a traumatic event for the child, possibly contributing to their gender identity issues. This survey also showed that associated difficulties and case complexity increase during adolescence (Di Ceglie *et al*, 2002).

De Vries *et al* (2010) at the Gender Identity Clinic in Amsterdam found autism spectrum disorders in 7.8% of children and adolescents with gender dysphoria. Jones *et al* (2012) reported elevated scores on the Autism Spectrum Quotient (AQ) in female-to-male transsexuals (transmen).

Explanatory models

No single cause has yet been identified with certainty for the development of gender dysphoria in children and adolescents. Most experts would agree that a combination of biological, psychodynamic/psychological and social factors play a contributory role. The significance of the co-occurrence of gender dysphoria and autism spectrum conditions in some children is the subject of current study. Autistic features may lead to particular styles of thinking, which in some cases contribute to the persistence of gender dysphoria from childhood to adolescence and beyond.

Biological factors include differences in brain anatomy, and genetic and hormonal influences during fetal development and childhood. Taziaux *et al* (2012) found sex differences in the neurokinin B (NKB) system in the infundibular nucleus of the brain. These differences reached significance only in adulthood, and male-to-female transsexuals had a female-typical infundibular NKB system. From their results, the authors suggested that sex steroid hormones in both the perinatal period and during puberty might contribute to the emergence of sex differences in adulthood, and that the gender reversal observed in male-to-female transsexual people may in part reflect an atypical sexual differentiation in the hypothalamus. These data confirm previous findings regarding the difference between sexes in some hypothalamic nuclei, in that male-to-female transsexuals have a configuration of these nuclei similar to those of females (Zhou *et al*, 1995; Kruijver *et al*, 2000). How these differences influence self-perception remains unclear.

Psychodynamic/psychological factors have included attachment problems (Marantz & Coates, 1991), difficulty mourning the loss of an important attachment figure (Bleiberg *et al*, 1986; Di Ceglie, 1998c), consequences of traumatic experiences (Coates *et al*, 1991; Coates & Moore, 1998), maternal depression and particular family constellations (Stoller, 1968). Factors that contribute to the persistence of gender dysphoria from childhood into adolescence and beyond are unclear. On the whole, the interaction between subjective experience, hormonal influences and brain structures is not well understood and requires further study.

For a review of the literature on aetiological factors, see de Vries & Cohen-Kettenis (2012) and Zucker *et al* (2012).

Case study 2: Mark

Mark, aged 16 years, presented with gender dysphoria. He hated his male body intensely. Socially isolated and in despair, he had attempted suicide. Since the age of 3 or 4 he had felt that he was a girl. At the age of 7, his father sexually abused him and this experience confirmed for him that he was a girl as, at that time, he thought that men were sexually attracted only to women. At the time of the referral he felt that his body should be changed immediately, as he could not bear living in a contradictory situation. There was also a real possibility of further suicide attempts.

A structured therapeutic programme, including individual and family sessions, and also consultation with a paediatric endocrinologist made Mark feel that both mind and body had been taken into consideration and helped him to tolerate a transitional phase of uncertainty by containing his feelings of despair. It also supported his hope that the incongruence between his mind and body would eventually be overcome. It was important that network meetings of the professionals involved in his care were held at regular intervals.

Exploration of the young person's expectations, gender identity and roles, body image, self-perception and other people's perception of them is essential preparation for the young person to begin physical (hormonal) interventions and for referral to a gender identity service for adults at the age of 18 for further treatment and perhaps surgical intervention. In Mark's case, this exploration showed a well-established gender dysphoria.

Psychodynamic considerations on the nature of atypical gender identity organisation: continuity and discontinuity

In 1964, Stoller proposed the concept of core gender identity. He saw this as:

'produced by the infant–parent relationship, the child's perception of its external genitalia, and a biologic force, which results from the biologic variables of sex (chromosomes, gonads, hormones, internal accessory reproductive structures and external genitalia)' (Stoller, 1964: p. 453).

Stoller believed that core gender identity is established before the fully developed phallic stage (3–6 years of age), although gender identity continues to develop into adolescence and beyond (1964: p. 453). He further stated that the beliefs comprising the 'mental structure' of core gender identity are the earliest part of gender identity to develop and are relatively permanent after the child reaches 4 or 5 years of age (Stoller, 1992: p. 78).

Further research and clinical experience show that in only 10–30% of children and adolescents with gender dysphoria does the core gender identity have the enduring structural characteristics described by Stoller.

Some years ago, I proposed the concept of atypical gender identity organisation (AGIO) as a clinical entity that can be examined under a number of parameters relevant to clinical management (Di Ceglie, 1998a). These are listed in Box 22.2 and can be explained as follows.

Rigidity–flexibility

This refers to the capacity of an atypical gender identity to remain unchangeable or, alternatively, to be amenable to evolution as the individual develops. Organisations that are more rigid will contribute to the persistence of development of the atypical identity (gender dysphoria), whereas organisations that are more fluid will lead to shifts in gender identity development. As mentioned earlier, only in some prepubertal children (10–30%) will an AGIO possess the unchangeable structural qualities of Stoller's core gender identity. In other words, one could say that there is continuity in the AGIO from childhood to adolescence/adulthood in a small proportion of children and discontinuity in the rest.

Timing of AGIO formation

Atypical organisations that develop very early in the child's life may be more likely to become rigidly structured than organisations that develop later. The early onset of gender dysphoria is in fact one of the criteria for considering early pubertal suppression (see pp. 361–362).

Box 22.2 Clinical features of atypical gender identity organisation (AGIO)

- Rigidity–flexibility
- Timing of formation of the AGIO
- Presence/absence of traumatic events in the child's life in relation to formation of the AGIO
- Position of the AGIO on a continuum from the paranoid-schizoid to the depressive positions

(Di Ceglie, 1998b)

Traumatic events in childhood

In some cases, an AGIO is formed as a psychological coping strategy in relation to a traumatic event in childhood. The earlier the trauma occurs, the more likely it is that the organisation will acquire rigid and unchangeable qualities.

Position on the paranoid-schizoid–depressive continuum

The Klein–Bion model of psychological development posits a continuum from the paranoid-schizoid to the depressive positions. The child's mental state on this continuum when an AGIO is formed is of significance. My hypothesis is that if the AGIO is formed within a mental functioning dominated by paranoid-schizoid processes in response to a traumatic event, it is more likely to become very structured and therefore not amenable to change. Alternatively, if it is formed within a mental functioning of the depressive position, it is likely that the organisation will be amenable to evolution.

Therapeutic exploration may be able to elucidate the characteristics of the organisation and therefore guide management. The following clinical example illustrates this point.

Case study 3: Jennifer

Jennifer was 17 when she presented following three suicide attempts. She was a female-to-male transgender person who presented with depressive episodes and a number of features of borderline personality disorder. She was still living in a female role, maintained her female name and wished to be addressed using a female pronoun. She was uncertain about physical interventions. Her mother, who had died just before Jennifer came to the clinic, had suffered depression after Jennifer's birth, and her father had been physically violent towards his wife during Jennifer's childhood, until they separated. During her psychotherapy sessions, she vividly remembered episodes when her father in fits of temper had kicked her mother, even in the stomach. In one session she admitted, not without a sense of embarrassment and shame, that she had identified with him, an experience that she could not explain. She loved her mother, and her main aim in life was to do something extraordinary that would have made her mother happy. There was no recollection that Jennifer herself had been physically abused by her father, but witnessing violence between her parents had been a traumatic childhood experience.

It is possible to hypothesise that the way Jennifer coped with the fear of damage to her mother, and possibly to herself, was to identify with a male possessing the strength of a masculine body. Once established, this gave her a sense of survival and also of protecting her 'damaged' mother. A female representation of herself had to be strongly avoided, as it was equated in her mind with being weak and damaged.

Another important factor also seemed to play a part. After the birth of two older sisters, her mother had miscarried a baby boy. One year later, Jennifer was born. Jennifer seemed to feel that her mother had expected her to be a boy, and in one session she alluded to her mother having 'psychic qualities', as if she had been part of a magical experience in which she and her mother could read each others' minds. She had probably received, and made her own, her mother's wish that she had been a boy. Her mother probably never consciously expressed this wish, but it remained unconsciously active in the relationship between them.

Two years of psychotherapeutic exploration with this young person allowed the therapist, together with Jennifer, to make this partial reconstruction of her childhood relating to her atypical gender identity development. However, any attempts to explore this understanding further with Jennifer led to continuous interruptions to the therapeutic work, which may have indicated her extreme resistance and fears of having the foundation of her gender identity revisited.

Even if Jennifer retained some of this understanding, it certainly did not alter her gender identity development, that is to say, the sense of who she was. Her AGIO was well established and not amenable to evolution. It formed very early in her life, and traumatic events had played a large part in it. Its formation may have occurred under the dominance of the paranoid-schizoid position.

Towards the end of therapy, Jennifer was able to live in a male role with a male name and his well-being improved. He did not attempt suicide again. He settled in a job and he was more able to establish relationships with other people. One might say that therapy had helped him to cope with his well-established AGIO in a better way, to make the transition to a male role and to give him a sense of hope (an important therapeutic aim, as discussed in the next section). He was eventually referred to an adult service for further treatment.

Management and therapy: the staged approach

The research evidence regarding the management of gender dysphoria in young people is still poor. The Report of the American Psychiatric Association Task Force on Treatment of Gender Identity Disorder states that 'the highest level of evidence available for treatment recommendations for these children can best be characterised as expert opinion' (Byne *et al*, 2012). Our model of management at the Tavistock and Portman NHS Foundation Trust is based on the understanding of atypical gender identity development within a complex paradigm. It has been informed by the fact that the causation of gender dysphoria remains unclear and it is probably multifactorial. It is also influenced by current cultural values and societal attitudes regarding gender identity. Our therapeutic experience has shown that children are very sensitive and feel easily intruded upon by anyone attempting to change who they feel they are and by those who minimise their feelings. Therefore we have developed a model of management in which altering an individual's perceived gender identity is not a primary therapeutic objective. Instead, emphasis is placed on the therapeutic aims listed in Box 22.3.

It is important to add to this list the need to combat the stigma that is often associated with the experience of atypical gender identity and is, at times, internalised by the individual experiencing gender dysphoria. It is also valuable to alleviate the feeling of shame that some children and adolescents and their families experience and to enable individuals to develop skills in handling social interactions and dealing with possible hostility.

The overall aim of therapy is improving the young person's well-being. The aims outlined in Box 22.3 could be achieved through various psychotherapeutic interventions, ranging from individual to family and group therapy. Social and educational interventions are also useful. It is important that these are well coordinated and integrated in a comprehensive management plan agreed with local services (the so-called network model; Di Ceglie, 2013). Some of these aims are more relevant in some cases than in others. The three case studies above give a brief illustration of how these therapeutic objectives could be tackled in clinical work; for a more detailed account see Di Ceglie (1998b).

The recognition and non-judgemental acceptance of the child's gender identity problem, which is not the result of their conscious choice, is important. Without this the child would experience feelings of rejection, and psychological splitting processes might increase to cope with these. Group work for parents of children with gender dysphoria can be very helpful in this respect, as it helps the parents to realise that their experience is not unique and that they are not isolated.

Where an inability to mourn attachment figures has interfered with gender identity development, work enabling mourning to occur may secondarily alter an atypical gender identity development, as shown in case study 1.

Box 22.3 Primary therapeutic aims

- To foster recognition and non-judgemental acceptance of gender identity issues
- To ameliorate associated behavioural, emotional and relationship difficulties (Coates & Person, 1985)
- To break the cycle of secrecy
- To activate interest and curiosity by exploring the impediments to them
- To encourage exploration of the mind–body relationship by promoting close collaboration among professionals in different specialities, including a paediatric endocrinologist
- To allow mourning processes to occur (Bleiberg et al, 1986)
- To enable symbol formation and symbolic thinking (Segal, 1957)
- To promote separation and differentiation
- To enable the child or adolescent and the family to tolerate uncertainty in gender identity development
- To sustain hope

(Di Ceglie, 1998b)

If autistic features coexist with gender dysphoria, psychological interventions aimed at increasing the individual's empathy and symbolic thinking become important (see 'Associated psychosocial difficulties', pp. 354–355). Although this approach has proved useful in clinical work, it needs to be validated by empirical research.

The general approach to the management of gender dysphoria can be best conceptualised as a process involving four stages, in line with the guidance for management originally issued by the Royal College of Psychiatrists (1998) and then further developed in the standards of care published by the World Professional Association for Transgender Health (2011).

Stage 1 The first stage of the process for children and adolescents is a therapeutic exploration, as described above. In adolescents, if the AGIO persists, then physical interventions could be considered if they are requested by the adolescent and the family. There is often pressure for physical intervention because of the high level of distress brought about by the reality of the changing body at puberty. However, the move towards physical intervention should be carefully considered and based on a well-established process of informed consent.

Stage 2 The second stage includes wholly reversible intervention. This involves the use of hypothalamic blockers, which suppress the production of oestrogens or testosterone and produce a state of biological neutrality. In the early stage of pubertal development (Tanner stage 2–3) they induce pubertal suppression. In order that adolescents and parents may make a properly informed decision, it is recommended that young people have some experience of pubertal development (Tanner stage 2–3) before suppression is considered.

Stage 3 When pubertal suppression has been properly assimilated, and while psychological exploration, support and physical monitoring by a paediatric endocrinologist are continued, stage 3 can be considered. This stage includes partially reversible interventions such as hormonal treatment that masculinises or feminises the body.

Stage 4 Finally, stage 4 includes irreversible interventions such as surgical procedures.

In the UK, the Gender Identity Development Service at the Tavistock and Portman NHS Foundation Trust has been offering pubertal suppression within a research protocol since 2011. The treatment, using GnRH at management stages 2/3, is available to children over 12 years of age in whom gender dysphoria persists into adolescence. The protocol was drafted following a wide debate involving young people and their families, professionals and professional organisations such as the British Society for Paediatric Endocrinology and Diabetes (2009). It received ethical approval and has a well-established system for obtaining informed consent from young people and their parents/carers. It adopted eligibility criteria similar to those of the Centre of Expertise on Gender Dysphoria in Amsterdam (Delemarre-van de Waal & Cohen-Kettenis, 2006; de Vries *et al*, 2007).

Children, particularly adolescents, and their families often find the experience of gender dysphoria painful and unbearable, and adolescents are at high risk of suicide attempts. This sense of despair frequently leads to extreme pressure being placed on clinicians to provide immediate solutions through physical intervention. In such cases, a detailed discussion with the adolescent and the family of the treatment as a staged process may relieve the distress by creating space for thinking. This may allow time to explore the issues involved in each stage and gradually reduce the pressure for immediate solutions that have not been properly thought through.

A follow-up study of adolescents with gender dysphoria who were treated with the hypothalamic blockers shows improvement in their psychological functioning during the period of pubertal suppression (de Vries *et al*, 2011).

Conclusion

Gender dysphoria is a complex condition. Clinical practice and research over the past three decades have made it possible to create multidisciplinary models of care that include an integrated programme of psychological, social and physical interventions for children and adolescents suffering from it. As clinical research progresses, new models of care will be developed. Language and nomenclature will also change in line with new cultural and social attitudes.

The relatively recent social and legal recognition of transgender experiences as new identities, protected by equality legislation, has contributed to making the assessment and diagnostic process a temporary phase that lasts only as long as the experience of gender dysphoria persists.

The need remains to combat stigma and raise public awareness about gender identity issues through appropriate social interventions and policies.

In *Boys Don't Cry*, Brandon could not avail himself of the help and support that are now possible. The tragedy portrayed in the film clearly shows the need for making professional services available to all people with gender identity problems and for educating society at large about these unusual life experiences.

References

American Psychiatric Association (1980) *Diagnostic and Statistical Manual of Mental Disorders* (3rd edn) (DSM–III). APA.

American Psychiatric Association (1994) *Diagnostic and Statistical Manual of Mental Disorders* (4th edn) (DSM–IV). APA.

American Psychiatric Association (2013) *Diagnostic and Statistical Manual of Mental Disorders* (5th edn) (DSM-5). APA.

Bleiberg E, Jackson L, Ross JL (1986) Gender identity disorder and object loss. *Journal of the American Academy of Child & Adolescent Psychiatry*, **25**, 58–67.

British Society for Paediatric Endocrinology and Diabetes (2009) *Statement on the Management of Gender Identity Disorder (GID) in Children and Adolescents*. BSPED.

Byne W, Bradley SJ, Coleman E, *et al* (2012) Report of the American Psychiatric Association Task Force on Treatment of Gender Identity Disorder. *Archives of Sexual Behavior*, **41**, 759–796

Coates S, Person ES (1985) Extreme boyhood femininity: isolated behaviour or pervasive disorder? *Journal of the American Academy of Child & Adolescent Psychiatry*, **24**, 702–709.

Coates S, Moore MS (1998) The complexity of early trauma: representation and transformation. In *A Stranger in My Own Body: Atypical Gender Identity Development and Mental Health* (eds D Di Ceglie, D Freedman), pp. 39–62. Karnac.

Coates S, Friedman R, Wolfe S (1991) The aetiology of boyhood gender identity disorder: a model for integrating temperament, development and psychodynamics. *Psychoanalytic Dialogues*, **1**, 481–523.

Delemarre-van de Waal HA, Cohen-Kettenis PT (2006) Clinical management of gender identity disorder in adolescents: a protocol on psychological and paediatric endocrinology aspects. *European Journal of Endocrinology*, **155**, 131–137.

De Vries ALC, Cohen-Kettenis PT (2012) Clinical management of gender dysphoria in children and adolescents: the Dutch approach. *Journal of Homosexuality*, **59**, 301–320.

De Vries ALC, Cohen-Kettenis PT, Delamarre-van de Waal HA (2007) Clinical management of gender dysphoria in adolescents. *Journal of Transgenderism*, **9**, 83–94.

De Vries ALC, Noens ILJ, Cohen-Kettenis PT, *et al* (2010) Autism spectrum disorders in gender dysphoric children and adolescents. *Journal of Autism and Developmental Disorders*, **40**, 930–936.

De Vries ALC, Steensma TD, Doreleijers TAH, *et al* (2011) Puberty suppression in adolescents with gender identity disorder: a prospective follow-up study. *International Society of Sexual Medicine*, **8**, 2276–2283.

Di Ceglie D (1998a) Management and therapeutic aims with children and adolescents with gender identity disorders and their families. In *A Stranger in My Own Body: Atypical Gender Identity Development and Mental Health* (eds D Di Ceglie, D Freedman), pp. 185–197. Karnac.

Di Ceglie D (1998b) Reflections on the nature of the 'atypical gender identity organisation'. In *A Stranger in My Own Body: Atypical Gender Identity Development and Mental Health* (eds D Di Ceglie, D Freedman), pp. 9–25. London: Karnac.

Di Ceglie D (1998c) 'William': working with the family about unresolved mourning and secrecy. In *A Stranger in My Own Body: Atypical Gender Identity Development and Mental Health* (eds D Di Ceglie, D Freedman), pp. 249–259. Karnac.

Di Ceglie D (2010) Gender identity and sexuality: what's in a name? *Diversity in Health and Care*, **7**, 83–86.

Di Ceglie D (2013) The care of the gender dysphoric child. In *Gender Dysphoria and Disorders of Sex Development: Progress in Care and Knowledge* (eds BPC Kreukels, TD Steensma, ALC de Vries), pp. 151–169.

Di Ceglie D, Freedman D, McPherson S, *et al* (2002) Children and adolescents referred to a specialist gender identity development service: clinical features and demographic characteristics. *International Journal of Transgenderism*, **6**(1).

Drummond KD, Bradley SJ, Peterson-Badali M, *et al* (2008) A follow up study of girls with gender identity disorder. *Developmental Psychology*, **44**, 34–45.

Feinblatt JA, Gold AR (1976) Sex roles and the psychiatric referral process. *Sex Roles*, **2**, 109–122.

Green R, Roberts CW, Williams K, *et al* (1987) Specific cross-gender behaviour in boyhood and later homosexual orientation. *British Journal of Psychiatry*, **151**, 84–88.

Jones RM, Wheelwright S, Farrell K, *et al* (2012) Brief report: female-to-male transsexual people and autistic traits. *Journal of Autism and Developmental Disorder*, **42**, 301–306.

Kruijver FP, Zhou JN, Pool CW, *et al* (2000) Mate-to-female transsexuals have female neuron numbers in a limbic nucleus. *Journal of Clinical Endocrinology & Metabolism*, **85**, 2034–2041.

Marantz S, Coates S (1991) Mothers of boys with gender identity disorders: a comparison to normal controls. *Journal of the American Academy of Child & Adolescent Psychiatry*, **30**, 136–143.

Money J (1955) Hermaphroditism, gender and precocity in hyperadrenocorticism: psychological findings. *Bulletin of Johns Hopkins Hospital*, **96**, 253–264.

Money J (1994) The concept of gender identity disorder in childhood and adolescence after 39 years. *Journal of Sex and Marital Therapy*, **20**, 163–177.

Royal College of Psychiatrists (1998) *Gender Identity Disorders in Children and Adolescents – Guidance for Management* (Council Report CR63). Royal College of Psychiatrists.

Segal H (1957) Notes on symbol formation. *International Journal of Psychoanalysis*, **38**, 391–397.

Skagerberg E, Parkinson R, Carmichael P (2013) Self-harming thoughts and behaviours in a group of children and adolescents with gender dysphoria. *International Journal of Transgenderism*, **14**, 86–92.

Steensma TD, Biemond R, Boer FD, *et al* (2011) Desisting and persisting gender dysphoria after childhood: a qualitative follow-up study. *Clinical Child Psychology and Psychiatry*, **16**, 499–516.

Stoller R (1964) The hermaphroditic identity of hermaphrodites. *Journal of Nervous and Mental Disease*, **139**, 453–457.

Stoller R (1968) Male childhood transsexualism. *Journal of the American Academy of Child & Adolescent Psychiatry*, **7**, 193–201.

Stoller R (1992) Gender identity development and prognosis: a summary. In *New Approaches to Mental Health from Birth to Adolescence* (eds C Chiland, JG Young), pp. 78–87. Yale University Press.

Taziaux M, Swaab DF, Bakker J (2012) Sex differences in the neurokinin B system in the human infundibular nucleus. *Journal of Clinical Endocrinology and Metabolism*, **97**, E2210–2220.

Wallien MSC, Cohen-Kettenis PT (2008) Psychosexual outcome of gender dysphoric children. *Journal of the American Academy of Child & Adolescent Psychiatry*, **47**, 1413–1423.

World Health Organization (1992) *The ICD-10 Classification of Mental and Behavioural Disorders: Clinical Descriptions and Diagnostic Guidelines*. WHO.

World Professional Association for Transgender Health (2011) *Standards of Care for the Health of Transsexual, Transgender, and Gender Nonconforming People* (7th version). WPATH.

Zhou JN, Hofman MA, Gooren LJ, *et al* (1995) A sex difference in the human brain and its relation to transsexuality. *Nature*, **378**, 68–70.

Zucker KJ (1985) Cross-gender identified children. In *Gender Dysphoria* (ed. B Steiner), pp. 75–174. Plenum Press.

Zucker KJ, Bradley SJ (1995) *Gender Identity Disorder and Psychosexual Problems in Children and Adolescents*. Plenum Press.

Zucker KJ, Wood H, Singh D, *et al* (2012) A developmental, biopsychosocial model for the treatment of children with gender identity disorder. *Journal of Homosexuality*, **59**, 369–397.

Zuger B, Taylor P (1969) Effeminate behavior present in boys from early childhood. II Comparison with similar symptoms in non-effeminate boys. *Pediatrics*, **44**, 375–380.

CHAPTER 23

The psychiatry of children aged 0–4

David Foreman

Our understanding of the mental health of infancy and early childhood (0–4 years of age) is undergoing a transformation. Traditional psychodynamic developmental accounts are transforming into operationalised, ethological accounts of cognitive processes and adult–child interaction. Intrauterine and early-life development are being increasingly implicated in the aetiology of both child and adult mental illness, while psychological trauma and adversity in this period are being associated with physical as well as mental ill health. The concept of developmentally specific psychiatric syndromes, which underpinned diagnosis for these children, is being eroded. In treatment, there has been increasing recognition of the economic advantages of early intervention, and primary care has engaged extensively with parent training, with good effect. However, in the UK secondary care activity with 0- to 4-year-old children declined by 16.9% between 2006 and 2009, and an unpublished survey conducted by the Royal College of Psychiatrists in 2012 found that 28% of UK child psychiatrists believed that general child and adolescent mental health services (CAMHS) were not appropriate for the problems this group present. This chapter therefore presents an overview of the psychiatry of this age range, with the intention of improving awareness of the importance of mental health in children under 5, exploring the ways in which child psychiatrists may currently contribute, and indicating likely future directions for mental healthcare. A developmental psychopathology approach will be taken, to allow consideration of this group in terms of both current psychopathology and risk (and resilience) factors affecting later health difficulties.

Diagnosis and epidemiology

Diagnosis

The frequency of disorders in 0- to 4-year-olds cannot be determined without an agreed way to detect and classify them, and unfortunately diagnoses in this age range have been contentious. The traditional approach has been to emphasise differing developmental trajectories and adult–child (especially parent–child) relationships across broad behavioural domains, leading to differing forms of classification from those used in other population segments. In classic infant psychiatry, five domains were proposed as defining developmentally specific syndromes:

- pervasive developmental disorders
- reactive attachment disorders of infancy
- eating disorders of infancy
- sleep disorders
- disorders in behavioural organisation.

The first of these has now been extended into the category of autism spectrum disorders and is recognised as a lifespan diagnosis. Reactive attachment disorders have been shown to have a close developmental relationship with a range of similar behavioural, dissociative and affect regulation problems in young adulthood, while eating and sleep problems also extend well outside infancy and so cannot be considered developmentally bound as originally thought. The last domain refers to temperamental problems sufficiently severe to trigger referral; once again, these now can be understood to refer to behavioural styles traceable from early childhood into adult life.

Findings such as these have undermined the validity of defining separate diagnostic classification systems for infants and young children, which were struggling to cope with poor reliability, especially with their proposed developmentally specific syndromes (Egger & Emde, 2011). A recent study used latent class analysis to compare diagnoses made under the best-developed developmentally specific diagnostic system, DC: 0-3R, with the two then current conventional systems, DSM-IV-TR and ICD-10: it found that the three systems identified similar latent classes, although the DSM and ICD coded them differently (Möricke *et al*, 2013). This is also consistent with the extension of dimensional diagnostic approaches into the 0–4 age range. Broad internalising and externalising dimensions have been found for the Child Behavior Checklist (CBCL) for ages 18 months to 5 years (Mothander & Grette Moe, 2008) and the Strengths and Difficulties Questionnaire (SDQ) for 2- to 3-year-olds (Delobel-Ayoub *et al*, 2006), both of which have similar dimensional structures throughout their age ranges.

The evidence thus supports a conceptual shift from qualitatively distinct, developmentally specific syndromes to a developmentally modulated expression of psychopathological processes, which are qualitatively similar across the lifespan. This carries implications for assessment, as the developmental differences between children of different ages then become primarily confounding factors in making accurate diagnoses, rather than markers for different groups of syndromes. This view does not exclude the idea that the onset of disorders may be developmentally related: this seems likely, for example, for depression and schizophrenia, though there is little evidence for such influences on remission. The shift described has led to practical progress, as assessment tools based on its assumptions have proved to have similar reliability to those already existing for older children, with a similar degree of syndrome resolution (Sterba *et al*, 2007). It is therefore now both reasonable and possible to describe the epidemiology of psychiatric disorders in 0- to 4-year-olds in terms of the disorders used across the rest of the age range.

Epidemiology

One effect of these diagnostic concerns has been that, to date, there have only been nine prevalence studies of diagnosis of children aged 0–4. Table 23.1 (page 368) summarises their findings.

Five studies were published since 2009, reflecting the epidemiological advantage of the newly changed paradigm. All the studies in Table 23.1 made use of versions of DSM as their diagnostic schema. It can be seen that the reported prevalence rates closely resemble the patterns found in older children: the range is similar, and the sensitivity to population and instrument choice suggested by the wide variations reported is also found more generally. It therefore seems likely that disorders present similarly, and with similar degrees of impairment, in children aged 0–4 as they do in older children and teenagers. The recent decline in UK CAMHS activity with 0- to 4-year-olds is therefore worrying, as it occurred during a period of increased investment and interest in CAMHS, and rising reported prevalence rates of child psychiatric disorders worldwide (Twenge, 2011).

Clinical assessment of 0- to 4-year-olds in secondary care

In primary care, there are now well-established tools that may be used, or adapted, for the assessment of children with mental health problems, as fine-grained diagnosis is not usually required. However, in secondary care more diagnostic precision is needed, and we have already seen that adequately reliable and valid diagnostic systems have only recently been established for children aged 0–4. In the UK, the lack of confidence this is likely to engender is combined with both low levels of service activity and limited training opportunities. The Royal College of Psychiatrists' survey found that 93% of non-specialist UK child psychiatrists saw not more than four 0- to 4-year-olds a month, and this was true even for 73% of those who reported working in a service that specialised in this age range; unsurprisingly, comments that they were inadequately trained to see this group were common. These concerns were entirely justified under the paradigm of developmentally specific psychopathology, where assessments stress detailed interpretation of (possibly videotaped) parent–child interaction, and the use of instruments to assess individual differences in attachment and temperament that quantify risk and resilience factors, rather than assisting conventional diagnoses. However, the reformulation of early diagnosis described above suggests that child psychiatrists' existing skills, appropriately supported by diagnostically oriented structured assessment tools, will enable effective diagnosis in secondary care. Table 23.2 (pages

Table 23.1 Epidemiology of psychiatric disorders in preschool children

Study	Overall prevalence	Emotional diagnoses	Behavioural diagnoses	Comments
Earls, 1982	14% severe	9%	5%	Local sample of 100 children
Lavigne et al, 1996	21.6% probable, 9.1% severe	<1% for any individual disorder (CBCL identified 3.7%)	16.7% for ODD	Two-stage sample (3860/510) from primary care paediatricians
Keenan et al, 1997	26.4% (definite)	14.9% (definite)	14.9% (definite)	104 low-income families from support programme
Egger et al, 2006	16.2%	10.5%	9%	Two-stage (1191/307) primary care paediatric clinic sample
Lavigne et al, 2009	Not given	0.6–2.1% anxiety, depending on assessment tool; <1% depressive disorders	8.3% ODD (severe); 8.8% ADHD (severe)	Single-stage (796) school and paediatric clinic sample
Bufferd et al, 2011	27.4% (22.5% without specific phobia)	20.3%	10.2%	Area sample (541 interviewed, 815 eligible)
Gleason et al, 2011	8.8%	5.4%	1.4%	Paediatric sample of 1003 children assessed in a two-stage, severity-stratified design
Wichstrøm et al, 2012	12.1% (rate without encopresis 7.1%)	3.3%	3.5%	City-wide sample covering all births over 2 years (3456), severity-stratified sample of 995 assessed
Gudmundsson et al, 2013	10.1% (rate with encopresis and enuresis 18%)	5.7% anxiety; depression percentage not reported (only 1 case was found)	2.8% ODD; 3.8% ADHD	339 sampled at routine check-up, two-stage design, 4–6 age range

ADHD, attention-deficit hyperactivity disorder; CBCL, Child Behavior Checklist; ODD, oppositional defiant disorder.

370–371) provides a list of instruments suitable for this. Although there is an overlap between preschool and autism assessment, the latter is not the focus here, and a comprehensive review of instruments for autism spectrum disorders is available elsewhere (Falkmer *et al*, 2013).

Table 23.2 shows the wide range of valid and reliable assessment tools appropriate for children aged 0–4 that are now available. The validation study of the Schedule for Affective Disorders and Schizophrenia for school-age children (Kiddie-), Present and Lifetime (K-SADS-PL) is especially encouraging, as it supports the view that existing adult instruments may be readily adapted for use in younger age ranges, which follows from the claim that the psychiatric disorders to be identified are not developmentally bound syndromes. Clinicians thus can make detailed, standardised assessments, or use instruments to forewarn or support their clinical impressions and judgements. Either technique supports diagnostic accuracy. Although it measures a risk/resilience factor rather than providing a diagnosis, the Attachment Q-Sort is included in the table because attachment-related difficulties load on different dimensions from conventional psychopathology (Minnis *et al*, 2007), and so could be missed without a specific measure.

Child psychiatry and early intervention

The first strand of the case for early intervention is, in some ways, a return to the roots of psychobiological child guidance as prevention of psychiatric disorders across the lifespan, as described in Chapter 1. There has been an increasing body of evidence consistent with developmental psycho-biological concepts, such as psychobiological developmental pathways to physical and mental difficulties. For example, postnatal depression is associated with children's sleep difficulties, poor weight gain and increased minor physical problems at 9 months, impaired cognition at 16 months, impaired growth as well as behaviour problems at age 2, and increased negative parenting behaviours, which persist, predicting increased behavioural and emotional problems by age 7. Extreme prematurity, a physical perinatal stressor, is associated with subsequent impaired cognition (including executive function) and attention and internalising (though not externalising) behavioural problems (Aarnoudse-Moens *et al*, 2009). However, there is little impact on family functioning in the long term, despite some restriction in opportunities for mothers, even in the presence of enduring neurodisability (Saigal *et al*, 2010). Environmental toxins and recreational drugs are increasingly found to adversely affect the developing fetus, contributing to the risk for subsequent mental health problems. Recreational drugs are more associated with attentional problems, whereas environmental toxins have a general effect on brain development. Early chronic psychosocial trauma, stress and economic disadvantage have also been associated with subsequent neoplastic, gastrointestinal, cardiovascular and immunological illness, possibly via

Table 23.2 Instruments useful in the assessment of children aged 0–4

Instrument	Description	Comments
3Di	Computerised interview for the diagnosis of autism together with likely confounders and comorbidities, including wide diagnostic range in long form; provides ICD diagnoses	Flexible, semi-structured parental interview that also collects school information: many items salient to infants or very young children; some items may also be used as observation points with the child; has long and short form; only the autism diagnosis has published validation
ADI-R/ADOS	Parental interview (ADI-R) and observation schedule (ADOS) for diagnosis of autism	Currently best-validated tool for autism diagnosis; covers much narrower range of diagnoses than long version of 3Di; separate tools, designed to work together
ASEBA	Combination of questionnaires and semi-structured interviews to obtain multi-informant, dimensional assessments with population-based cut-offs	An extension of the well-known CBCL to cover the whole lifespan from 18 months onwards; though distinct, symptom profiles derived from its dimensions have been mapped to common DSM diagnoses
Attachment Q-Sort	Set of cards with descriptors of infant (1 year and over) behaviour, to be sorted by either observer or parent	Best-validated alternative to Ainsworth's Strange Situation, which is not usually appropriate in clinical setting; observer sorting has better validity than maternal sorting; structuring the observational setting may be used to shorten observation time (90 minutes minimum); like the Strange Situation, does not diagnose attachment disorder
CHAT/ M-CHAT[a]	Brief screening tool to detect autism from 18 months; there are associated observer ratings (original CHAT), brief telephone and observational structured interviews	Significant level of false positives obtained from parent-only responses can be reduced by using the additional associated assessments; is one of a number of alternative screening tools available, but was designed to work with the youngest children in whom symptoms could be meaningfully discriminated
DAWBA	Web-based combined structured and semi-structured multi-informant interview for ICD and DSM diagnoses	Validation on 2- to 4-year-olds complete but unpublished (report viewed by author); may underdetect autism
DISCO	Comprehensive clinical assessment for autism spectrum disorders and associated problems said to cover the full age range	Published validation from around 2–3 years onwards, across whole range of autism spectrum; validation includes intellectual disability, may have advantages for this group; collects data on wide range of symptoms, allows diagnosis of other psychiatric disorders also

continued

Table 23.2 *(continued)*

ECI-4	Parent- and teacher-completed rating scale for DSM-IV diagnoses, optimised for age 3–6 years	Items closely matched to DSM-IV criteria, has good convergent validity with other instruments
K-SADS-PL	Semi-structured interview and examination developed for school-age children; provides DSM-IV diagnoses	Has more items dealing with psychotic phenomena than either 3Di or DAWBA
NBAS	Observer-rated scale covering both neurological and behavioural domains of neonatal assessment from birth to 2 months; the scale is to produce a profile, rather than be summative	Although designed as a scale, in clinical use it is recommended both to structure clinical assessment and feed back recommendations to parents on how to respond to baby; has predictive validity, but construct validity and reliability hard to interpret given variability in neonates
PAPA	Standardised psychiatric assessment providing DSM-IV diagnoses	Probably the most extensively validated general diagnostic instrument for DSM diagnoses
PAS-R	30-item checklist for parents of children aged 3–5 years	No obsessive–compulsive items (owing to problems in measurement in this age range), but best-validated scale for preschool anxiety available
PFC	Brief parent-report checklist for identification of depression in 3- to 5-year-old children	The only depression-specific questionnaire of its type
SDQ	Multi-informant screening questionnaire for emotional, behavioural and hyperkinetic disorders and burden from 3 years upwards	Web-based scoring system available; also incorporated as part of the DAWBA

a. *The M-CHAT was preferred to the Social Communication Questionnaire (SCQ) as there was some evidence the latter works less well in younger age ranges, requiring cut-off adjustment (Wiggins et al, 2007).

3Di, Developmental, Dimensional and Diagnostic Interview (Skuse et al, 2004); ADI-R, Autism Diagnostic Interview – Revised (Rutter et al, 2003); ADOS, Autism Diagnostic Observation Schedule (Lord et al, 2002); ASEBA, Achenbach System of Empirically Based Assessment (Achenbach, 2009); Attachment Q-Sort (Waters, no date); CHAT/M-CHAT, (Modified) Checklist for Autism in Toddlers (Kleinman et al, 2008); DAWBA, Development and Well-Being Assessment (Goodman et al, 2000; Posserud et al, 2010); DISCO, Diagnostic Interview for Social and Communication Disorders (Maljaars et al, 2012); ECI-4, Early Childhood Inventory for DSM-IV diagnoses (Bufferd et al, 2011); K-SADS-PL, Schedule for Affective Disorders and Schizophrenia for school-age children (Kiddie-), Present and Lifetime (Birmaher et al, 2009); NBAS, Neonatal Behavioral Assessment Scale (Canals et al, 2011); PAPA, Preschool Age Psychiatric Assessment (Egger et al, 2006); PAS-R, Preschool Anxiety Scale – Revised (Edwards et al, 2010); PFC, Preschool Feelings Checklist (Luby et al, 2012); SDQ, Strengths and Difficulties Questionnaire (Ezpe eta et al, 2013).

long-term immunological activation of macrophages or monocytes and subsequent hypersensitivity (Ford, 2010; Miller *et al*, 2011).

Among disorders more apparent in teens and adults, vulnerability to depression has been associated with the interaction between serotonin transporter gene polymorphisms and early psychological trauma, possibly mediated by impaired coupling between the amygdala and anterior cingulate cortex, as well as such trauma leading to hypothalamic–pituitary–adrenal (HPA) axis and oestrogenic dysregulation; the former is associated with impaired stress management, the latter potentially affects caregiving in subsequent generations. Chronic stress affects both the HPA axis and brain-derived neurotrophic factor (BDNF), leading to reduced hippocampal size and neuronal complexity, especially in the periventricular nuclei (Ansorge *et al*, 2007). Our understanding of schizophrenia is also now neurodevelopmental, with obstetric complications and childhood or adolescent psychosocial stress both contributing to its eventual expression in genetically vulnerable people. Obstetric complications, in particular hypoxia, lead to more severe illness with earlier onset, and a greater likelihood for conversion of prodromal symptoms to the full syndrome. They have also been associated with ventricular enlargement (crucial evidence for the 'over-pruning hypothesis' of excessive brain apoptosis in schizophrenia) and unusual movements at age 4, which both predicted incidence of schizophrenia. Brain-derived neurotrophic factor is implicated here as well: Brain-derived neurotrophic factor is implicated here as well: among individuals who begin life with obstetric complications, those who develop schizophrenia have lower than normal levels of this neuroprotective hormone, rather than the higher than normal levels in those who do not (Karlsgodt *et al*, 2012). Early trauma also mediates this effect, possibly via inflammatory processes (Dennison *et al*, 2012).

Developmental psychopathology has thus proved to be essential to our understanding of the major disorders treated in adult psychiatry, as well as those most prevalent in childhood and adolescence, and it highlights many potential areas for early intervention. The overall picture seems to be that similar stressors and risk factors (physical and psychological trauma and adversity early in life) produce a range of adverse results, the profile of which depends on the interaction between the insult and the individual's genotype, with families being more resilient to the sequelae of physical stressors than psychological or economic ones.

In the second strand of research supporting early intervention, Heckman (2008) developed an economic model based on developmental psycho-pathological findings, which suggested that the benefits across the lifespan of the ratio of early to later intervention in childhood followed a positive curvilinear relationship, i.e., early intervention was disproportionally beneficial compared with later. Data collection problems make this model difficult to test, but Knapp and colleagues have undertaken long-term (6-year) economic reviews of 15 early intervention strategies, with supportive results (Knapp *et al*, 2011). For example, they found that early intervention for conduct disorder (which typically has a childhood onset) had a 20% greater return on investment than early detection of psychosis (which typically begins in adolescence), but even early intervention for conduct disorder has only 10% of the return on investment from prevention of conduct disorder through social and emotional learning programmes. Although these latter were evaluated in school, at 10 years, around 74% of conduct disorders are likely to have begun before then (Meltzer *et al*, 2000) and social education programmes may be successfully adapted for preschool children. It therefore seems likely that the economic benefits of social and emotional learning programmes will be greater if used with preschool children. An interesting counterexample is Knapp *et al*'s (2011) review of postnatal depression: they were not able to confirm any return on investment in the deployment of health visitors, although their model was restricted to the mothers and did not include the children. However, other economic studies have obtained more positive results for such postnatal interventions (McDaid & Park, 2011).

The third strand supporting early intervention refers to cross-sectional, rather than longitudinal, findings. For adult and child health problems, the mean population score is closely related to the number of individuals with extreme values, i.e. the prevalence of relevant cases in the population (Goodman & Goodman, 2011). Therefore, whole-population interventions that reduce mean scores will also reduce associated case prevalences, so effective interventions may offer significant benefit in reducing case-load even if applied to at-risk or whole populations, rather than restricting them to diagnosed patients. From the previous paragraph, it follows that smaller, or even absent cross-sectional effect sizes may be accepted if the intent of an intervention is to reduce disability across the lifespan, given the potential offset in costs. An example where these principles could be applied is in preschool social education (Hamre *et al*, 2012). Although prosocial behaviour in the preschoolers studied was significantly improved, there was no detectable change in the rate of behaviour disorders. However, this was because the base rate was so low in the study population that such change was hard to detect. The results suggested that the intervention would still be valuable in reducing the risk of future behavioural disorders, given their close negative association with prosocial behaviour.

A case can thus be made for child psychiatrists to involve themselves with 0- to 4-year-olds at the population level, as well as treating individual children, i.e. to engage with the public mental health of this age range. External observers consider that the UK (with The Netherlands) already leads the USA in this, and some of this work is undertaken as consultation-liaison to primary care teams and agencies (Embry, 2011). In the UK, such teams can provide, jointly, around one potential worker for every 30 children with a diagnosable psychiatric disorder, and there is an appetite for appropriate training supported by management. In the USA, home-based treatment by such professionals has been shown to be feasible and effective for preschoolers (Lowell *et al*, 2011) and, in general, interventions in this age group produce enduring benefit, which may be enhanced for mental health problems if provided in toddlerhood (Nores & Barnett, 2010). Despite this, and the theoretical account given above, a recent meta-analytic review found no prevention studies for depression covering the preschool age range (Merry *et al*, 2012), though a randomised controlled trial for prevention of anxiety disorders in preschoolers is in progress (Bayer *et al*, 2011).

Treatment

Physical treatments

Although these most frequently refer to psychopharmacology, it is important to remember that other physical treatments may be worthy of research in this age group. Electroconvulsive therapy (ECT) has been used for children, though not preschoolers, and its more acceptable – though possibly less effective – cousin transcranial magnetic stimulation (TMS) has also been trialled with adolescents for depression, with good results (Walter *et al*, 2010). Conversely, vagus nerve stimulation (VNS) has been used extensively with children from less than 2 years of age to 18 for the treatment of epilepsy, and its antidepressant effect has been noted as well as its cognitive benefits (Klinkenberg *et al*, 2013). Given our improved capacity for detecting mood disorders in this age group, and the currently worrying risk–benefit profile for antidepressants in juveniles, research is needed into applicable alternatives to medication. For example, TMS does not require general anaesthetic, does not require administration for months or years, is effective and has fewer side-effects than antidepressants, although it can cause transient discomfort, particularly in its repetitive form. Less controversially, exercise therapy is beneficial for children, including preschoolers, with intellectual disabilities and possibly for ADHD across the ability range (Berwid & Halperin, 2012). However, there have been no trials of exercise therapy for either ADHD in preschoolers without developmental delays, or for emotional disorders in any ability range, despite promising studies showing attenuating depression and anxiety in adults. Despite claims to the contrary, there is also no evidence for the successful use of coordination training (such as the Dore programme) to treat ADHD, dyslexia or Asperger syndrome (Bishop, 2007). Although developed by psychologists, biofeedback is a physical treatment, as it focuses on direct modification of aspects of physical function rather than behaviour. Biofeedback of electroencephalographic recordings (sometimes called neurofeedback) probably improves symptoms of ADHD (Lofthouse *et al*, 2012), though its effect on autism is less clear. However, all studies have been on school-aged children or adults.

Clearly, some of these physical treatments are highly invasive, and should be reserved for very rare and severe cases. However, there appears to have been insufficient research conducted in preschool children even for physical treatments such as exercise or neurofeedback.

In the 1990s, prescribing rates for psychotropic medication in pre-schoolers in the USA were reported at between 3 and 9 per 1000, possibly inflated by some prescriptions for parents not covered by Medicaid, and most prescriptions were for stimulants. A randomised controlled trial found that, while efficacious, stimulant medication in this group showed smaller effect sizes than for older children, a different side-effect profile and a greater withdrawal rate (Wigal *et al*, 2006): the researchers recommended a 'start low and go slow' policy in this age group. A later US review identified prescriptions of antipsychotics to privately insured preschoolers rising from 0.78/1000 in 1999–2000 to 1.54/1000 in 2007, with less than half receiving psychological treatment, a mental health assessment or a visit from a psychiatrist (Olfson *et al*, 2010). The associated diagnoses were either ADHD or disruptive behaviour disorders: durations of treatment were lengthy and polypharmacy common. Introduction of a pre-approval system reduced the rate of requests, but a higher proportion of those continuing to submit were not child psychiatrists (Constantine *et al*, 2012). Antipsychotics have only weak efficacy for ADHD and the core symptoms of autistic disorders, but carry similarly significant metabolic and neurological risks in this age range. Second-generation antipsychotics are effective for disruptive behaviour disorders, but in this age range parenting programmes are also effective, as discussed in the next section, and have better side-effect profiles. There is little information available on medication for emotional disorders in 0- to 4-year-olds.

Thus, although some children aged 0–4 may benefit from psycho-pharmacology, and drugs effective in older children are effective in this age range also, the evidence suggests that its use in this age range carries a less favourable balance of benefits and harms than in older children, as well as having less supporting evidence, and so more caution is advised.

Psychological and social treatments

The treatment of ADHD illustrates how approaches for older children might have to be modified for those of preschool age. It is frequently forgotten that, even for school-age children, well-designed psychological treatments for ADHD have an effect, albeit less than medication, and with little evidence of additive benefit. With preschool children, the picture is different. Greenhill *et al* (2006) report an effect size for methylphenidate of 0.55 (probability of replication: 0.95) following behavioural treatment. The Incredible Years parenting programme has been reported to have an effect size of 0.73 (probability of replication: 0.96) for immediate effect on ADHD symptoms, which was maintained at 18-month follow-up (Jones *et al*, 2008). A parenting intervention specifically designed to target ADHD symptoms achieved an effect size of 0.79 (probability of replication: 0.99), maintained at 15 weeks. However, the programme could not be implemented effectively by newly trained staff outside the envelope of specialist care (Sonuga-Barke *et al*, 2004). The success of this approach using specialist delivery may have been replicated (Thompson *et al*, 2009), though the very high effect sizes reported could reflect the combination of a high drop-out rate and failure to analyse using intention to treat.

High levels of heterogeneity between studies and variable study quality have also characterised early interventions for autism, although effect sizes at least as large as for drug treatment have been reported, and some trends are evident. A recent set of guidelines based on a systematic review concluded that children with autism spectrum disorders require a minimum of 25 hours a week of behaviourally focused programmes, possibly including a developmental component. The studies on which this was based reported outcomes in the preschool period (Maglione *et al*, 2012). Not only does there seem to be a dose–response relationship between time taken and effectiveness, but a large study in preschoolers using a focused parent-training approach achieved only small effect sizes on an intervention lasting 6.5 hours a week, of which 2.5 hours were unsupported homework, despite otherwise good design (Green *et al*, 2010). Despite the large initial outlay required, the return on investment for such intensive treatments, estimated by cost-offset modelling and assuming intervention at 3 years of age, is around 11 to 1 (Peters-Scheffer *et al*, 2012) by 65 years, consistent with Heckman's model discussed above, and is equivalent to an annualised return of about 16%. It seems unlikely that treatments of the intensity and specificity required could be delivered outside specialist settings.

The implication of the admittedly sparse literature is that psychological treatment of preschoolers with significant autistic or hyperkinetic symptoms is to be preferred to drug treatment where possible, and is best delivered from specialist centres, rather than primary care. However, it seems likely that this will require significant reconfiguration of current secondary care services. In the UK at present it takes, on average, 500 days for a referral for ADHD to lead to treatment, which is clearly far too long for a preschool intervention, while the implementation of intensive treatment for autism will require quite different resourcing from that offered by the typical current CAMHS team (Foreman, 2010). Resolving these issues will require skilled clinical leadership.

Conclusion

Understanding of psychiatric diagnosis, epidemiology and treatment options for children aged 0–4 has changed greatly in the past 10 years, and the current disengagement that UK child psychiatry has with this age range is no longer warranted. Conventional diagnostic systems are appropriate for this age range, provided it is understood that development may affect symptom expression, while convincing evidence for developmentally specific syndromes is lacking. This has allowed the development of instruments that demonstrate that the epidemiology of psychiatric disorders in 0- to 4-year-olds includes similar types and rates of disorder as in older children, with comparable disability. Two strands for intervention seem to hold particular promise for the future: engaging with the public mental health of this age range for both primary and secondary prevention; and psychological treatment of preschool autism and ADHD in secondary care. Both offer cost-effective treatment and prevention opportunities, but will require changes in service configuration, including appropriate child psychiatric engagement.

Public mental health is a newly emerging concept, but for young children, the Integrated Management of Childhood Illness (IMCI) strategy has proved effective and affordable in countries much poorer than the UK (Rakha *et al*, 2013). Developed by the World Health Organization and UNICEF, IMCI targets a relatively small number of common illnesses with high morbidity and mortality by using simple, specific detection tools and treatments administered by primary care personnel. As this chapter has shown, similar tools and interventions are now available for the small number of conditions contributing to the burden of mental disorder in this age group, so the IMCI approach, which would situate appropriately trained and experienced child psychiatrists working in a teaching and consultative role with dedicated primary care staff, could well offer considerable dividends.

There is now also good understanding of psychological treatments for preschool children in secondary care; the major difficulties are establishing appropriate infrastructure to ensure sustained, high-quality delivery. Although the benefits of such interventions seem clear, there have been no studies of the economics driving the decisions that enable or disable infrastructure in this field, and disinvestment is currently occurring despite the opposing weight of academic and political opinion. Interdisciplinary research involving child psychiatrists, academic managers and health economists is likely to be needed if such services are to be successfully established.

References

Aarnoudse-Moens CSH, Weisglas-Kuperus N, van Goudoever JB, *et al* (2009) Meta-analysis of neurobehavioral outcomes in very preterm and/or very low birth weight children. *Pediatrics*, **124**, 717–728.

Achenbach TM (2009) *Achenbach System of Empirically Based Assessment (ASEBA): Development, Findings, Theory, and Applications*. University of Vermont Research Center of Children, Youth and Families.

Ansorge MS, Hen R, Gingrich JA (2007) Neurodevelopmental origins of depressive disorders. *Current Opinion in Pharmacology*, **7**, 8–17.

Bayer JK, Rapee RM, Hiscock H, *et al* (2011) The Cool Little Kids randomised controlled trial: population-level early prevention for anxiety disorders. *BMC Public Health*, **11**, 11.

Berwid OG, Halperin JM (2012) Emerging support for a role of exercise in attention-deficit/hyperactivity disorder intervention planning. *Current Psychiatry Reports*, **14**, 543–551.

Birmaher B, Ehmann M, Axelson DA, *et al* (2009) Schedule for affective disorders and schizophrenia for school-age children (K-SADS-PL) for the assessment of preschool children: a preliminary psychometric study. *Journal of Psychiatric Research*, **43**, 680–686.

Bishop DV (2007) Curing dyslexia and attention-deficit hyperactivity disorder by training motor co-ordination: miracle or myth? *Journal of Paediatrics and Child Health*, **43**, 653–655.

Bufferd SJ, Dougherty LR, Carlson GA, *et al* (2011) Parent-reported mental health in preschoolers: findings using a diagnostic interview. *Comprehensive Psychiatry*, **52**, 359–369.

Canals J, Hernández-Martínez C, Esparó G, *et al* (2011) Neonatal Behavioral Assessment Scale as a predictor of cognitive development and IQ in full-term infants: a 6-year longitudinal study. *Acta Paediatrica*, **100**, 1331–1337.

Constantine R, Bengtson MA, Murphy T, *et al* (2012) Impact of the Florida Medicaid Prior-Authorization Program on use of antipsychotics by children under age six. *Psychiatric Services*, **63**, 1257–1260.

Delobel-Ayoub M, Kaminski M, Marret S, *et al* (2006) Behavioral outcome at 3 years of age in very preterm infants: the EPIPAGE study. *Pediatrics*, **117**, 1996–2005.

Dennison U, McKernan D, Cryan J, *et al* (2012) Schizophrenia patients with a history of childhood trauma have a pro-inflammatory phenotype. *Psychological Medicine*, **42**, 1865–1871.

Earls F (1982) Application of DSM-III in an epidemiological study of preschool children. *American Journal of Psychiatry*, **139**, 242–243.

Edwards SL, Rapee RM, Kennedy SJ, *et al* (2010) The assessment of anxiety symptoms in preschool-aged children: the revised Preschool Anxiety Scale. *Journal of Clinical Child & Adolescent Psychology*, **39**, 400–409.

Egger HL, Emde RN (2011) Developmentally sensitive diagnostic criteria for mental health disorders in early childhood: the Diagnostic and Statistical Manual of Mental Disorders–IV, the Research Diagnostic Criteria–Preschool Age, and the Diagnostic Classification of Mental Health and Developmental Disorders of Infancy and Early Childhood–Revised. *American Psychologist*, **66**, 95–106.

Egger HL, Erkanli A, Keeler G, *et al* (2006) Test–retest reliability of the Preschool Age Psychiatric Assessment (PAPA). *Journal of the American Academy of Child & Adolescent Psychiatry*, **45**, 538–549.

Embry DD (2011) Behavioral vaccines and evidence-based kernels: nonpharmaceutical approaches for the prevention of mental, emotional and behavioral disorders. *Psychiatric Clinics of North America*, **34**, 1–34.

Ezpeleta L, Granero R, de la Osa N, *et al* (2013) Psychometric properties of the Strengths and Difficulties Questionnaire (3–4) in 3-year-old preschoolers. *Comprehensive Psychiatry*, **54**, 282–291.

Falkmer T, Anderson K, Falkmer M, *et al* (2013) Diagnostic procedures in autism spectrum disorders: a systematic literature review. *European Child & Adolescent Psychiatry*, **22**, 329–340.

Ford JD (2010) Complex adult sequelae of early life exposure to psychological trauma. In *The Impact of Early Life Trauma on Health and Disease: The Hidden Epidemic* (eds R A Lanius, E Vermetten, C Pain), pp. 69–76. Cambridge University Press.

Foreman DM (2010) The impact of governmental guidance on the time taken to receive a prescription for medication for ADHD in England. *Child and Adolescent Mental Health*, **15**, 12–17.

Gleason MM, Zamfirescu A, Egger HL, *et al* (2011) Epidemiology of psychiatric disorders in very young children in a Romanian pediatric setting. *European Child & Adolescent Psychiatry*, **20**, 527–535.

Goodman A, Goodman R (2011) Population mean scores predict child mental disorder rates: validating SDQ prevalence estimators in Britain. *Journal of Child Psychology and Psychiatry*, **52**, 100–108.

Goodman R, Ford T, Richards H, *et al* (2000) The Development and Well-Being Assessment: description and initial validation of an integrated assessment of child and adolescent psychopathology. *Journal of Child Psychology and Psychiatry*, **41**, 645–655.

Green J, Charman T, McConachie H, *et al* (2010) Parent-mediated communication-focused treatment in children with autism (PACT): a randomised controlled trial. *Lancet*, **375**, 2152–2160.

Greenhill L, Kollins S, Abikoff H, *et al* (2006) Efficacy and safety of immediate-release methylphenidate treatment for preschoolers with ADHD. *Journal of the American Academy of Child & Adolescent Psychiatry*, **45**, 1284–1293.

Gudmundsson OO, Magnusson P, Saemundsen E, *et al* (2013) Psychiatric disorders in an urban sample of preschool children. *Child and Adolescent Mental Health*, **18**, 210–217.

Hamre BK, Pianta RC, Mashburn AJ, *et al* (2012) Promoting young children's social competence through the preschool PATHS curriculum and MyTeachingPartner professional development resources. *Early Education and Development*, **23**, 809–832.

Heckman JJ (2008) Schools, skills, and synapses. *Economic Inquiry*, **46**, 289–324.

Jones K, Daley D, Hutchings J, *et al* (2008) Efficacy of the Incredible Years Programme as an early intervention for children with conduct problems and ADHD: long-term follow-up. *Child: Care, Health and Development*, 34, 380–390.

Karlsgodt KH, Ellman LM, Sun D, *et al* (2012) The neurodevelopmental hypothesis of schizophrenia. In *Schizophrenia: The Final Frontier. A Festschrift for Robin M. Murray* (eds AS David, S Kapur, P McGuffin), pp. 3–18. Psychology Press.

Keenan K, Shaw D, Walsh B, *et al* (1997) DSM-III-R disorders in preschool children from low-income families. *Journal of the American Academy of Child & Adolescent Psychiatry*, **36**, 620–627.

Kleinman JM, Robins DL, Ventola PE, *et al* (2008) The modified checklist for autism in toddlers: a follow-up study investigating the early detection of autism spectrum disorders. *Journal of Autism and Developmental Disorders*, **38**, 827–839.

Klinkenberg S, van den Bosch CN, Majoie H, *et al* (2013) Behavioural and cognitive effects during vagus nerve stimulation in children with intractable epilepsy: a randomized controlled trial. *European Journal of Paediatric Neurology*, **17**, 82-90.

Knapp M, McDaid D, Parsonage M (2011) *Mental Health Promotion and Mental Illness Prevention: The Economic Case*. Department of Health.

Lavigne JV, Gibbons RD, Christoffel KK, *et al* (1996) Prevalence rates and correlates of psychiatric disorders among preschool children. *Journal of the American Academy of Child & Adolescent Psychiatry*, **35**, 204–214.

Lavigne JV, LeBailly SA, Hopkins J, *et al* (2009) The prevalence of ADHD, ODD, depression, and anxiety in a community sample of 4-year-olds. *Journal of Clinical Child & Adolescent Psychology*, **38**, 315–328.

Lofthouse N, Arnold LE, Hersch S, *et al* (2012) A review of neurofeedback treatment for pediatric ADHD. *Journal of Attention Disorders*, **16**, 351–372.

Lord C, Rutter M, DiLavore P, *et al* (2002) *Autism Diagnostic Observation Schedule: ADOS*. Western Psychological Services.

Lowell DI, Carter AS, Godoy L, *et al* (2011) A randomized controlled trial of Child FIRST: a comprehensive home-based intervention translating research into early childhood practice. *Child Development*, **82**, 193–208.

Luby J, Lenze S, Tillman R (2012) A novel early intervention for preschool depression: findings from a pilot randomized controlled trial. *Journal of Child Psychology & Psychiatry*, **53**, 313–322.

Maglione MA, Gans D, Das L, *et al* (2012) Nonmedical interventions for children with ASD: recommended guidelines and further research needs. *Pediatrics*, **130** (suppl 2), S169–S178.

Maljaars J, Noens I, Scholte E, van Berckelaer-Onnes I (2012) Evaluation of the criterion and convergent validity of the Diagnostic Interview for Social and Communication Disorders in young and low-functioning children. *Autism*, **16**, 487–497.

McDaid D, Park AL (2011) Investing in mental health and well-being: findings from the DataPrev project. *Health Promotion International*, **26** (suppl 1), i108–i139.

Meltzer H, Gatward R, Goodman R, *et al* (2000) *Mental Health of Children and Adolescents in Great Britain*. TSO (The Stationery Office).

Merry SN, Hetrick SE, Cox GR, *et al* (2012) Cochrane Review: Psychological and educational interventions for preventing depression in children and adolescents. *Evidence-Based Child Health: A Cochrane Review Journal*, **7**, 1409–1685.

Miller GE, Chen E, Parker KJ (2011) Psychological stress in childhood and susceptibility to the chronic diseases of aging: moving toward a model of behavioral and biological mechanisms. *Psychological Bulletin*, **137**, 959–997.

Minnis H, Reekie J, Young D, *et al* (2007) Genetic, environmental and gender influences on attachment disorder behaviours. *British Journal of Psychiatry*, **190**, 490–495.

Möricke E, Lappenschaar GAM, Swinkels SH, *et al* (2013) Latent class analysis reveals five homogeneous behavioural and developmental profiles in a large Dutch population sample of infants aged 14–15 months. *European Child & Adolescent Psychiatry*, **22**, 103–115.

Mothander PR, Grette Moe R (2008) Infant Mental Health assessment: the use of DC 0-3 in an outpatient child psychiatric clinic in Scandinavia. *Scandinavian Journal of Psychology*, **49**, 259–267.

Nores M, Barnett WS (2010) Benefits of early childhood interventions across the world: (under) investing in the very young. *Economics of Education Review*,**29**, 271–282.

Olfson M, Crystal S, Huang C, *et al* (2010) Trends in antipsychotic drug use by very young, privately insured children. *Journal of the American Academy of Child & Adolescent Psychiatry*, **49**, 13–23.

Peters-Scheffer N, Didden R, Korzilius H, *et al* (2012) Cost comparison of early intensive behavioral intervention and treatment as usual for children with autism spectrum disorder in the Netherlands. *Research in Developmental Disabilities*, **33**, 1763–1772.

Posserud M, Lundervold AJ, Lie SA, *et al* (2010) The prevalence of autism spectrum disorders: impact of diagnostic instrument and non-response bias. *Social Psychiatry and Psychiatric Epidemiology*, **45**, 319–327.

Rakha MA, Abdelmoneim AM, Farhoud S, *et al* (2013) Does implementation of the IMCI strategy have an impact on child mortality? A retrospective analysis of routine data from Egypt. *BMJ Open*, **3** (1), doi: 10.1136/bmjopen-2012-001852.

Rutter M, Le Couteur A, Lord C (2003) *Autism Diagnostic Interview, Revised*. Western Psychological Services.

Saigal S, Pinelli J, Streiner DL, *et al* (2010) Impact of extreme prematurity on family functioning and maternal health 20 years later. *Pediatrics*, **126**, e81–e88.

Skuse D, Warrington R, Bishop D, *et al* (2004) The Developmental, Dimensional and Diagnostic Interview (3di): a novel computerized assessment for autism spectrum disorders. *Journal of the American Academy of Child & Adolescent Psychiatry*, **43**, 548–558.

Sonuga-Barke EJS, Thompson M, Daley D, *et al* (2004) Parent training for attention deficit/hyperactivity disorder: is it as effective when delivered as routine rather than as specialist care? *British Journal of Clinical Psychology*, **43**, 449–457.

Sterba S, Egger HL, Angold A (2007) Diagnostic specificity and nonspecificity in the dimensions of preschool psychopathology. *Journal of Child Psychology and Psychiatry*, **48**, 1005–1013.

Thompson MJ, Laver-Bradbury C, Ayres M, *et al* (2009) A small-scale randomized controlled trial of the revised new forest parenting programme for preschoolers with attention deficit hyperactivity disorder. *European Child & Adolescent Psychiatry*, **18**, 605–616.

Twenge JM (2011) Generational differences in mental health: are children and adolescents suffering more, or less? *American Journal of Orthopsychiatry*, **81**, 469–472.

Walter G, Rey JM, Ghaziuddin N, *et al* (2010) Electroconvulsive therapy, transcranial magnetic stimulation, and vagus nerve stimulation. In *Pediatric Psychopharmacology: Principles and Practice* (2nd edn) (eds A Martin, L Scahill, CJ Kratochvil), pp. 363–375. Oxford University Press.

Waters E (no date) *Assessing Secure Base Behavior and Attachment Security Using the Q-Sort Method.* Stony Brook University (http://www.psychology.sunysb.edu/attachment/measures/content/aqs_method.html). Accessed 23 Jan 2014.

Wichstrøm L, Berg-Nielsen TS, Angold A, *et al* (2012) Prevalence of psychiatric disorders in preschoolers. *Journal of Child Psychology and Psychiatry*, **53**, 695–705.

Wigal T, Greenhill L, Chuang S, *et al* (2006) Safety and tolerability of methylphenidate in preschool children with ADHD. *Journal of the American Academy of Child & Adolescent Psychiatry*, **45**, 1294–1303.

Wiggins LD, Bakeman R, Adamson LB, *et al* (2007) The utility of the social communication questionnaire in screening for autism in children referred for early intervention. *Focus on Autism and Other Developmental Disabilities*, **22**, 33–38.

Index

Compiled by Linda English

abdominal pain 190, 191, 193, 195, 201, 209, 210, 214–215
Abraham, Karl 6
ADAPT (Adolescent Depression Anti-depressant and Psychotherapy Trial) 101, 132, 134, 137
adenotonsillar hypertrophy 290
ADHD *see* attention-deficit hyperactivity disorder
adjustment disorders 187, 193, 196, 201, 209, 214, 306
Adler, Alfred 5–6
adolescent psychiatry, history of 6
adolescents
  management of personality disorder 36–38
  self-harm *see* self-harm in adolescents
  substance misuse 315–329
adult life, continuity into 8
  anxiety disorders 94, 178–179
  ASD 112–113, 228
  eating disorders 331–332
  infancy and early childhood 366
  schizophrenia 246, 257, 258
  self-harm in adolescents 311–312
  sleep disorders 290–291
  somatising 214–215
  Tourette syndrome 280
affective disorders: pharmacology 100–103, 121–122
  see also individual disorders
affect regulation 28–29
  dorsal system 28–29, 35
  identification of emotional significance 28
  negative affect 32, 35
  personality disorders 26–40
  right prefrontal cortex 30
  role of attachment relationships 29–31
  self-regulation 30, 31
  STEPPS 37
  ventral system 28, 29
affects
  definition and formation 26–27

externalisation 30, 32, 34
  functions 27–28
  negative 27–28, 31, 32, 33, 35
  production 28–31
  see also affect regulation
agoraphobia 169, 171
alcohol misuse 34, 318, 319, 321–322
alexithymia 46, 192–193
alpha-2 agonists 81, 85, 121
amantadine 116, 121
amfetamine 79–80
amygdala 28, 35, 60, 172–173, 190, 324, 372
anorexia nervosa 330–343, 345
  autistic traits 341
  brain 340–341
  Children Act 1989 340
  cognitive remediation therapy 341
  family therapy 341–342
  group therapy 342
  individual therapy 342–343
  Mental Health Act 1983 340
  parental counselling 341–342
  physical aspects 338–340
  responsibility 337–338
  target weight 340
anterior cingulate gyrus 28, 34
antidepressants
  ASD 115, 117
  bipolar disorder 140–143, 144
  depression 100–102, 129–137
  personality disorders 36
  Tourette syndrome 276
  see also individual drugs; selective serotonin reuptake inhibitors; tricyclic antidepressants
antipsychotics
  adverse effects 105–107, 118, 143–144, 255–256
  anorexia nervosa 336–337
  antisocial behaviour 69–70
  ASD 89, 115, 117–118, 119–120, 121, 123
  bipolar disorder 102, 139–140

ECG abnormalities 83–84
personality disorders 36
preschoolers 375
psychotic depression 137
schizophrenia 104–107, 255–256
Tourette syndrome 83–85, 86, 276, 279
see also individual drugs
antisocial behaviour, management of 57–73
aetiology 59–60
assessment 60–64
bullying 63, 65
callous-unemotional traits 60, 67
child therapies 67–68
comorbid problems 64–65
contributions from other informants 63–64
developmental history 60–61
early-onset 60, 61
emotional problems 65
family history 61–62
group therapy 67–68
guidelines 66
hyperactivity 64, 69
individual interview 62–63
intellectual disabilities 64–65
intervention principles 65–66
parental discipline 59, 60, 61
parent management training 66–67
pharmacology 64, 69–70
poor regulation of anger 60
reading problems 64, 66
school interventions 68–69
antisocial personality disorder 34, 35, 38, 57, 318, 325
anxiety disorders 165–182
aetiology 171–174
ASD 122, 225
assessment 169–171
CBT and psychological therapy 94, 96–97, 98, 150–151, 174–177
clinical features 167–169
developmental stages 166–167
epidemiology 167
evolutionary basis 165–166
family environment 173–174
generalised anxiety disorder 150–151, 168, 171, 172, 173, 174, 177, 178, 238
genetics 171–172
interventions 174–177
life events 174
medical disorders and drugs 170
neuroimaging and neuropsychology 172–173
NICE guidance 175, 177
parent–child interactions 173–174

pharmacology 94–98, 100–101, 177–178
ADHD 97–98
ASD 122
benzodiazepines and tricyclic anti-depressants 94–95
Child/Adolescent Anxiety Multimodal Study 96
and psychological treatment 94, 96–97, 98
SSRIs 95–96
pregnancy 174
prevention in preschoolers 374
prognosis 178–179
respiratory dysregulation 174
somatising 190, 191, 196–197, 205
temperament 171
aripiprazole
ASD 86, 87, 89, 115, 119, 123
bipolar disorder 102, 103, 140, 143, 144
schizophrenia 105
Tourette syndrome 84–85
arousal disorders 297–298
arylsulfatase-A 255
ASD *see* autism spectrum disorder
Association for University Teachers of Psychiatry 6
asylums 2, 3
atomoxetine
ADHD 79–80, 236, 243
ADHD with anxiety disorders 98
ASD 121
ASD with ADHD 88, 89
Tourette syndrome with ADHD 85, 279
attachment 5
antisocial behaviour 61
caregiving and care-eliciting 29
CBT and 161–162
disinhibited attachment disorder 237–238
dissociation 45
fabrication of illness 16, 17, 20
insecure 31, 38, 44–46
moral defence 45–46
personality disorders and disorganisation of 26–40
PTSD and borderline personality disorder 41–56
reactive attachment disorders of infancy 366, 369
reflective functioning or mentalisation 44
right hemisphere involvement 30, 44
role of relationships in affect regulation 29
secure 29–30, 36, 44, 46, 51, 52
traumatic 45–46
Attachment Q-Sort 369

attention-deficit hyperactivity disorder
(ADHD) 231–244
assessment 234–237
ADHD-RS-IV 239, 243
before clinical contact 234
CADDRA ADHD Checklist 234, 239
Conners 3 234, 235, 237
constructional toys 236
digit span recall 236
first appointment 234–236
further information 237
interview with older child/teenager 236
interview with parents 235
observation and physical examination
of child 236
SNAP-IV-C 235, 237
Strengths and Difficulties
Questionnaire (SDQ) 234
tests 239
Weiss Impairment Scales 239
comorbidity 238
differential diagnosis 237–238
ASD 238
bipolar disorder 238
disinhibited attachment disorder
237–238
disruptive behaviour disorders 237
generalised anxiety disorder 238
simple misbehaviour 237
formulation 239
hyperactivity 232, 233
impairment 239
impulsiveness 232, 233
inattention 231, 233
National Attention Deficit Disorder
Information and Support Service
(ADDISS) 241
neurobiology 233–234
NICE guidelines 76, 80, 123, 151,
237–238, 239–240, 241–242, 243, 244
pharmacology 74–82, 241–243, 375
adverse effects 82
with anxiety disorders 97–98
with antisocial behaviour 69–70
with ASD 87–89
with bipolar affective disorder 102, 144
with OCD 99
with Tourette syndrome 82, 84, 85–86
continued monitoring needed 75
evidence-based treatment and MTA
study 75–76
non-stimulant medications 80–81
stimulant medications 74, 76–80, 81,
88, 89, 236, 241–243, 320, 375

prognosis 244
sleep problems 288, 289
substance misuse 319, 320, 322
treatment
assessing progress 243–244
CBT 151, 161
general principles 239–243
Multimodal Treatment of Attention
Deficit Hyperactivity Disorder (MTA)
study 75–76, 98
parental handling 240–241
pharmacology see above
preschoolers 374, 375–376, 377
psychoeducation 240
Autism Act 2009 112
autism spectrum disorder (ASD)
ADHD differential diagnosis 238
antisocial behaviour 64–65, 69–70, 87
anxiety disorders 167, 168
childhood schizophrenia 246
gender dysphoria 355, 361
infancy and early childhood 366, 369,
374, 375, 376, 377
pharmacology 86–89, 112–128
antidepressants 115, 117
antipsychotics 89, 115, 117–118,
119–120, 121, 123
for anxiety disorders 122
clinical implications 122–123
for comorbid psychiatric symptoms
118–122
for core symptoms 113–118
diagnostic overshadowing 118
diet 115
glutamate-active medication 115–116
for hyperactivity, impulsivity and
inattention 87–89, 119, 120–121, 123
immune function 115
for irritability, aggression and antisocial
behaviour 87, 119–121, 123
management 113
medication management 113
minimum effective dose 123
for mood disorders 120, 121–122
NICE guidance 112, 118, 119, 120
off-label use 113
opiate antagonists 120
for self-injury 119–121, 123
for sleep problems 119
for social deficits 113–116
for stereotypies and repetitive
behaviours 89, 116–118
psychological treatments 218–230
applied behavioural analysis 219, 221

behavioural interventions 219–220, 226
CBT 225–226
communication-based programmes
    221–222
discrete trial training 219
EarlyBird programme 222
Early Intensive Behavioural Inter-
    vention (EIBI) 219–220, 225, 227
Early Start Denver Model (ESDM) 220,
    226
evaluation of treatment outcomes 227
functional communication training 221
future directions 227–228
general educational programmes
    224–225
how to determine what works 226–227
improvement of parent–child
    interactions 222
improvement of social reciprocity 222
joint attention and symbolic play
    programmes 223, 226
Learning Experiences and Alternative
    Program for Preschoolers and their
    Parents (LEAP) 225, 227
More Than Words programme 222
parent training in behavioural
    techniques 220
Picture Exchange Communication
    System (PECS) 221–222, 226–227
pivotal response training 219, 226
Preschool Autism Communication Trial
    (PACT) 222
Research Autism website 218
Responsive Education and Prelinguistic
    Milieu Teaching (RPMT) technique
    222, 226–227
signing and picture systems 221–222
social and emotional competence/
    understanding programmes 223–224
social stories 224
Teaching and Education of Autistic and
    Related Communication-Handicapped
    Children (TEACCH) programme
    224–225
theory of mind programmes 223
schizophrenia and 246, 254
sleep problems 119, 288, 289
Tourette syndrome 265, 269, 272
autonomic nervous system 29–30
avoidant personality disorder 34

behavioural therapy
ASD 219–220, 226

sleep disorders 293, 294
somatising 209
benzodiazepines 94–95, 140, 178, 210
bereavement 14
binge eating disorder 331, 332, 336
biofeedback 374
bipolar disorder 129
additional treatment strategies 144–145
ASD 122
CBT 151
comorbid ADHD 102, 144
differential diagnosis ADHD 238
evidence base 139–140
longer-term management 103
NICE guidelines 102, 103, 138–139,
    140–143, 144
pharmacology 102–103, 137–145
principles of prescribing 143
substance misuse 319
Blacker, C. P. 6
body dysmorphic disorder 196
borderline personality disorder 33, 36, 37
as complex PTSD 41, 42, 43, 48–49
dialectical behaviour therapy 21, 37, 49,
    310, 324
emerging 310
as emotional regulation disorder 37, 43, 310
fabrication of illness 16, 18, 21
PTSD and attachment 41–56
self-harm 35, 307, 308, 310
substance misuse 324
Bowlby, John 4–5
brain-derived neurotrophic factor 372
Broca's speech area 45
bulimia nervosa 330, 331, 336, 337, 338,
    343–344
buspirone 95, 122, 178

CAMHS see child and adolescent mental
    health services
cannabis 248
carbamazepine 143, 144
cathinones 317–318
CBT see cognitive–behavioural therapy
child abuse
corpus callosum 49
fabrication of illness 10–25
of parents 14, 16–17
personality disorders 31
psychobiology 46
PTSD 46, 51, 54
somatising 193, 197–198, 212
see also neglect; sexual abuse

child and adolescent mental health services
(CAMHS) 7
    infancy and early childhood 365, 367, 376
    self-harm 301, 305, 306, 310.311
    somatising 202–203, 204–205, 212–213
Child Behaviour Checklist 366
child guidance clinics 1, 3–5, 6–7
child labour 3
child poverty 7
child psychiatrists: future 7–8
child psychiatry
    early intervention 369–374
    history 1–9
children aged 0–4 see infancy and early
    childhood
Children's Somatization Inventory 205
chronic fatigue syndrome (neurasthenia)
    196–197
    Chalder Fatigue Self-report scale 205
    classification 184–186
    epidemiology 187, 188, 201
    factors associated 191, 192
    outcome 215
    treatment 209, 211
cigarette smoking 320
citalopram 100, 117, 132–133, 135, 136, 210
clomipramine 87, 89, 98, 117, 119, 276
clonidine
    ADHD 81, 243
    ASD 87, 88–89, 119, 121
    Tourette syndrome 85–86, 276, 279
clozapine 106, 107, 119
cocaine 318
cognitive analytic therapy (CAT) 49
cognitive–behavioural therapy (CBT) 150–164
    ADHD 151, 161
    anxiety disorders 96, 150–151, 174–177
    ASD 225–226
    attachment behaviours 161–162
    Beckian cognitive model 153
    collaborative development of case
        formulation 154–156
    computerised 176–177
    concepts and processes fundamental to
        152–154
    conditional assumptions 154
    core beliefs 153
    depression 101, 131, 134, 137, 150–151
    developmental factors 161–162
    eating disorders 333, 344
    evidence base 150–151
    family 151, 157, 158, 160, 161, 177, 209, 211
    incorporating systemic and developmental
        perspectives 151–152
    insights from other psychotherapies
        161–162
    OCD 99, 100, 150–151
    PTSD 48, 51, 150–151
    schizophrenia 256–257
    Socratic questioning 150, 156
    somatisation 209, 211
    systemic formulation 156–161
    use of systemic formulation in practice
        158–161
    vignettes 154–155, 159–161
Commonwealth Fund 4
community services: history 6–7
conduct disorder 7–8, 150–151, 178, 237,
    306, 319, 320, 372–373
    see also antisocial behaviour, management
        of conversion disorder see dissociative
        disorders
Coping Power Program 68
corpus callosum 49
cortisol levels 47, 48
D-cycloserine 116

Dawson, W. S. 4, 7–8
delayed sleep phase syndrome 290, 291,
    295–296
delinquency: history 1, 2, 3, 4–5, 7
dependent personality disorder 34
depression
    additional treatment strategies 137
    adolescent personality disorder 36–37
    ASD 121–122
    comorbid with anxiety 167, 172
    NICE guidelines 100, 132–133, 134–135,
        136, 151
    in parents and fabrication of illness 16
    pharmacology 100–102, 129–137
    postnatal 369, 373
    predictors of response 135
    principles of prescribing 134–135
    psychotic 137, 253–255
    self-harm 131–132, 303, 306
    somatising 190, 191, 196–197, 205
    specialised clinical care 133–134
    substance misuse 319, 320
    suicidality 100–101, 129, 131–132, 134,
        137
    Tourette syndrome 272
dexamfetamine 79–80, 241–242, 318
Diagnostic Classification of Mental Health
    and Developmental Disorders of Infancy
    and Early Childhood-Revised (DC: 0-3R)
    366

Diagnostic and Statistical Manual of Mental
Disorders (DSM)
diagnostic hierarchy concept 120
DSM-III 246, 350
DSM-IV 76, 102, 350
DSM-IV-TR 366
DSM-5
ADHD 86, 87, 231, 239
antisocial behaviour 57
anxiety disorders 165, 168, 169
ASD 120
bipolar disorder 102, 129, 138
eating disorders 330, 331
gender dysphoria 350, 352
personality disorders 32
PTSD 41, 42
somatising 184–187, 195, 215
substance misuse 315
Tourette syndrome 274
dialectical behaviour therapy (DBT) 21, 37,
49, 310, 324
disruptive mood regulation disorder 102,
129
dissociation 45, 49, 50, 193
dissociative (conversion) disorders 184–187,
188, 194, 201, 205, 209, 214
Dissociative Experiences Scale 49
divalproex 120, 122, 139
Down syndrome 290, 296
DSM see Diagnostic and Statistical Manual of
Mental Disorders
Dundee Difficult Times of Day Scale
(D-DTODS) 78
dyspraxia 236

early intervention in psychosis (EIP) teams
258
East London Child Guidance Clinic 4
eating disorders 330–348
ARFID 331, 333, 336
classification 330–331
comprehensive approach 333–334
dissociative disorders 205
EDNOS 330, 331
epidemiology 330–331
healthcare setting 334–335
help for parents 336
of infancy 366
management and treatment for specific
disorders 337–344
Maudsley model of family-based
treatment 333
OSFED 331

outcomes and continuity into adulthood
331–332
personality disorders 36–37
pharmacology 336–337
reasons for hospital admission 335
therapeutic models 332–333
Treatment Outcome for Child and
Adolescent Anorexia Nervosa
(TOuCAN) trial 334
electroconvulsive therapy 374
emotions see affects
epilepsy 16, 298, 374
escitalopram 100, 117, 130, 132–133, 135,
136
ethanol 34
excessive daytime sleepiness 289, 295–296
exercise therapy 374–375
eye-movement desensitisation and
reprocessing (EMDR) 48, 49, 51, 52

fabrication and induction of illness 10–25
assessment of adult(s) 19–21
assessment of child 18–19
bereavement 14
childhood abuse of parents 14
definitions 10
epidemiology 10–11
healthcare professionals 10, 11, 13, 16
impact on children 13
investigation 17–18
management 21
manifestations of abnormal caregiving
11–13
marital and family difficulties 14
motivation and triggers 16–17
parent and child permanently separated
21–22
psychopathology of fabricators 15 16
reunification of parent and child is
planned 22
role of psychiatrist 17–22
social and demographic characteristics of
perpetrators 13–15
treatment for parents 21–22
factitious disorders 15–16, 187, 197–198,
201, 212, 214
see also fabrication and induction of
illness
family therapy
CBT 151, 158, 160, 161, 177, 209, 211
eating disorders 332–333, 341–342
schizophrenia 256, 257
self-harm 309

somatising 210
substance misuse 322
famine, effects on fetus 5
fenfluramine 113
fight/flight response 28, 29–30, 31, 32–33, 35, 45
fluoxetine
  anxiety disorders 95, 177
  ASD 117
  depression 100, 101, 130, 131, 132, 134–135, 137
  OCD 98
flupentixol 309
flutamide 85
fluvoxamine 95, 98, 117, 122, 177
Franco-Prussian war 2
freezing 31, 44, 45
Freud, Anna 5, 6
Freud, Sigmund 6

gender dysphoria 349–364
  ASD 355, 361
  associated psychological difficulties 354–355
  atypical gender identity organisation (AGIO) 357–358
  Boys Don't Cry (film) 349, 362
  case studies 352–353, 356, 358–359
  classifications 350–352
  core gender identity 356–357
  'dysphoria' rather than 'disorder' 352
  explanatory models 355–356
  gender identity 350
  Gender Recognition Act 2004 350
  gender role 350
  hypothalamic blockers 361, 362
  inability to mourn attachment figures 352–353, 360
  long-term follow-up studies 353–354
  position on paranoid-schizoid–depressive continuum 358
  prevalence 353
  rigidity–flexibility 357
  secrecy 349–350
  staged approach 359–362
  traumatic events in childhood 358
  'watchful waiting' 354
generalised anxiety disorder 150–151, 168, 171, 172, 173, 174, 177, 178, 238
genogram 61, 157
group A beta-haemolytic streptococcal (GABHS) infections 266–267
guanfacine 81, 85, 121

Habit Clinic 3
haloperidol 83, 84, 89, 105, 106, 119, 255, 276
Hampstead War Nurseries 5
headaches 190, 193, 201, 204, 211
Health and Social Care Act 2012 2
Healy, William 3
history of child psychiatry 1–9
histrionic personality disorder 33
homeostasis 27, 28
hyperkinetic disorder 64, 76, 119, 120–121, 231
  see also attention-deficit hyperactivity disorder (ADHD)
hypnagogic hallucinations 297
hypnopompic hallucinations 297
hypochondriacal disorder 195–196
hypothalamic–pituitary–adrenal axis 372
hypothalamus 355–356, 361, 362
hypothalamus–periaqueductal grey matter system 35

ICD see International Classification of Diseases and Health Related Problems
infancy and early childhood 365–381
  behavioural organisation disorders 366
  child psychiatry and early intervention 369–374
  clinical assessment in secondary care 367–369
  developmentally specific syndromes 366, 376–377
  diagnosis 365–367
  early trauma and stress 369–372
  eating disorders of infancy 366
  environmental toxins 369
  epidemiology 367
  pervasive developmental disorders 366
  pharmacology 375
  physical treatments 374–375
  postnatal depression 369, 373
  psychological and social treatments 375–376
  public mental health 373–374, 377
  reactive attachment disorders of infancy 366
  recreational drugs during pregnancy 369
  sleep disorders 366
in-patient services, history 6, 7
insomnia 289, 293
  behavioural 290
  conditioned or learned 290
  idiopathic 290
  management 294–295

insula 28, 34
Integrated Management of Childhood Illness
    (IMCI) strategy 377
International Classification of Diseases and
    Health Related Problems (ICD)
    ICD-9 246
    ICD-10
        ADHD 76, 120, 231, 232
        antisocial behaviour 57
        anxiety disorders 165, 167, 168
        ASD 120
        bipolar disorder 138
        gender dysphoria 350
        infancy and early childhood 366
        personality disorders 32, 34
        PTSD 41, 42
        somatising 184–187, 195
        Tourette syndrome 274
    ICD-11 168, 193, 215, 330
International Classification of Sleep
    Disorders (ICSD-2) 289, 297
International Personality Disorder
    Examination (IPDE) 21

Kanner, Leo 4, 6
Kayser–Fleischer ring 255
Klein–Levin syndrome 296
Klein, Melanie 6

lamotrigine 139, 143, 144
lisdexamfetamine 80, 242
lithium 102–103, 122, 139, 140, 143

manic episodes 102–103, 253–254
Mapother, Edward 1–2
mass hysteria/mass sociogenic illness 194
Maudsley Hospital 1–2, 4, 6, 7, 8, 51
measles, mumps and rubella (MMR) vaccine
    115
medication see pharmacology
melatonin 209, 243, 294–295, 296
memantine 116
mentalisation-based therapy (MBT) 21, 324
metachromatic leukodystrophy 254–255
methylphenidate
    ADHD 76–78, 80, 97–98, 241–242, 279,
        322, 375
    ASD 88, 89, 120–121, 123, 124
    preschoolers 375
migration, effects of 1, 3
Miller, Emmanuel 4

mood stabilisers
    antisocial behaviour 69, 70
    ASD 120, 121
    bipolar affective disorder 102
    personality disorders 36
multidimensional family therapy (MDFT)
    322
multisystemic therapy 38
mutism, trauma-induced 45

naltrexone 120
naphyrone 318
narcissistic personality disorder 34
narcolepsy 290, 296
narrative exposure therapy 51
nature v. nurture conflict 2
neglect 13, 15, 30, 31, 44, 46, 193
neurexins 116
neurofeedback 374–375
nightmares 290, 298
nocturnal enuresis 297
noradrenaline 29–30
0–4, children aged see infancy and early
    childhood

obsessive–compulsive disorder (OCD)
    anxiety 165
    ASD 116, 119
    CBT 99, 100, 150–151
    comorbid with Tourette syndrome 82, 84,
        99, 262, 269, 276, 280
    duration of treatment and response rates
        99
    non-response 99–100
    pharmacology 98–101
obsessive–compulsive personality disorder
    34, 99
obstructive sleep apnoea 287, 290, 291,
    292, 293, 296, 298
OCD see obsessive–compulsive disorder
olanzapine
    bipolar disorder 102, 103, 140, 143, 144
    eating disorders 336
    schizophrenia 105–106, 255
    Tourette syndrome 84, 86
oppositional defiant disorder 57, 69, 98,
    193, 237

paediatric autoimmune neuropsychiatric
    disorders associated with streptococcal
    infections (PANDAS) 266

paediatrics, term first used 2
pain disorders (persistent somatoform pain
    disorders) 187, 188, 194–195, 196, 205
panic disorder 169, 171, 172, 174, 178, 205
paranoid personality disorder 32–33
parasomnias 289, 297–298
parasympathetic system 30, 46
Parental Bonding Instrument (PBI) 20
parents
    ADHD 240–241
    eating disorders 336, 337–338, 341–342
    infancy and early childhood 365–366,
        375–376
    parent–child interactions and anxiety
        disorders 173–174
    sleep disorders 289, 291, 292, 293
    somatisation 191, 192–193
    Tourette syndrome 262–265
    training in behavioural techniques in ASD
        220
    training programmes in antisocial
behaviour 65
    see also fabrication and induction of illness
paroxetine 95–96, 98, 100, 135, 136
paroxysmal non-epileptic events 194,
    205–206, 211–212
pentoxifylline 87, 115
personality disorders
    affect regulation 26–40
    Cluster A 32–33, 35
    Cluster B 33–34, 35
    Cluster C 34, 35
    disorganisation of attachment 26–40
    management in adolescence 36–38
    in parents and fabrication of illness 16,
        20–21
    polypharmacy 36
    self-harm 31, 35, 307, 308, 310
    self-preservative behaviour 31–32
    substance misuse 34–35, 36, 324–325
    therapeutic communities 36
    Tourette syndrome 272, 273
    treatment 35–36, 37–38
    violence 35
    see also individual types
pervasive withdrawal (pervasive refusal
    syndrome) 187, 197
pharmacology 74–149
    ADHD 74–82, 241–243
    antisocial behaviour 69–70
    anxiety disorders 94–98, 177–178
    ASD 86–89, 112–128
    bipolar disorder 102–103, 137–145
    depression 100–102, 129–137

eating disorders 336–337
infancy and early childhood 375
OCD 98–100
research in paediatric psycho-
    pharmacology 74
schizophrenia 103–107, 255–256
self-harm 309
somatising 210
Tourette syndrome 82–86, 275–279
phobias, specific or simple 168–169, 171,
    172, 174, 178
pimozide 83, 84
post-traumatic stress disorder (PTSD)
    anxiety 165
    assessment of adults with complex PTSD
        50–51
    attachment and borderline personality
        disorder 41–56
    child abuse 46, 51, 54
    complex PTSD and borderline personality
        disorder 41, 42, 43, 48–49
    cultural issues 50–51
    development of attachment behaviour
        43–46
    dissociation 45, 49, 50
    EMDR 49
    group therapy 53
    need for phase-oriented treatment 51–53
    personality integration and rehabilitation
        52–53
    in pregnant women 47
    psychobiology of neglect and abuse 46
    rape 50–51
    remembering, reprocessing and grieving
        52
    as sensitisation disorder of attachment
        system 47–48
    shame 46, 49, 50
    sleep disorders 298
    social support 41–42
    somatic symptoms 49, 205
    stabilisation 52
    substance misuse 319–320
    termination of therapy 52–53
    transgenerational transmission of
        vulnerability 48
    treatment of complex PTSD 48–53
    vignettes 45, 51
    Yalom's therapeutic factors 53
postwar period 5–6
prefrontal cortex 28, 30, 34, 35, 233,
    248–249
prematurity, extreme 369
problem-solving skills training 68

pseudologia fantastica 17
psychoanalysis 5–6
psychological therapies
    antisocial behaviour 67–68
    anxiety disorders 96–97, 107, 175–177
    ASD *see* autism spectrum disorder,
psychological treatments
    bipolar disorder 145
    depression 133–134
    schizophrenia 256–257
    self-harm 309–311
    see also cognitive–behavioural therapy
psychopathy 35, 38
psychostimulants *see* stimulants
PTSD *see* post-traumatic stress disorder

quetiapine 102, 103, 105, 119, 139, 140, 144, 337

reading delay 64, 66
reflex sympathetic dystrophy 196
Relationship Scales Questionnaire (RSQ) 20
relaxation training 211
rhythmic movement sleep disorders 290, 297
right hemisphere 30, 44, 46
risperidone
    ASD 87, 89, 115, 117–118, 119, 123, 124
    bipolar disorder 102, 103, 139, 140, 144
    eating disorders 336
    schizophrenia 105–106, 255
    Tourette syndrome 84, 86, 279
Royal College of Psychiatrists 2
Rutter, Michael 8

St Ebba's Hospital 6
Schedule for Affective Disorders and Schizophrenia for School-Age Children (K-SADS-PL) 369
schizoid personality disorder 33
schizophrenia 246–261
    aetiology and risk factors 247–248
    affective psychosis and 253–254
    ASD and 246, 254
    'atypical' psychosis and 253–254
    cannabis 248
    CBT 256–257
    childhood schizophrenia 246
    clinical assessment 251–252
    clinical characteristics 251

clinical phases 249–251
    course and outcome 257–258
    cytogenetic abnormalities 247–248, 252
    developmental issues in assessment 252–253
    diagnosis 251–255
    differential diagnosis 253–255
    effects of famine during pregnancy 5
    epidemiology 246–247
    evidence base for antipsychotics 105–106
    family interventions 256, 257
    gender ratio 247
    genetics 247–248
    hallucinations 252–253
    identification of 'at risk' young people 250
    investigations and monitoring 252, 256
    neurobiology 248–249, 372
    neurodegenerative disorders and 254–255
    NICE guidelines 106–107, 257, 258
    obstetric complications 372
    organisation of treatment services 258
    pharmacology 103–107, 116, 255–256
    premorbid psychopathology 249–250
    premorbid social and developmental impairments 249
    prodromal symptoms and onset of psychosis 250–251
    prognostic factors 257
    schizoaffective psychosis and 253–254
    structural brain abnormalities 248–249
    treatments 106–107, 255–257
schizotypal personality disorder 33, 38, 247, 251
secretin 113
selective serotonin reuptake inhibitors (SSRIs)
    adverse effects 135
    anxiety disorders 95–97, 177
    ASD 115, 116, 117, 119, 122, 123, 124
    Committee on Safety of Medicines (CSM) report 129, 130, 131, 136
    depression 100–102, 129–137
    eating disorders 336, 337
    long-term safety 96
    OCD 98, 99, 100
    Tourette syndrome 276
    see also individual drugs
self-harm in adolescents 301–314
    age 303
    brief family intervention 309
    developmental group therapy 310–311
    dialectical behaviour therapy 310
    emotions of staff 307–308

epidemiology 302
ethnicity and international differences
303
evidence-based practice 308–311
four 'Ms' model 304
gender 303
gender dysphoria 354
general management 306–308
genetics 303
groups 1 to 3 306–308
in-patient treatment 308
Mental Health Act 1983 306
multisystemic therapy 311
neurobiology 303
NICE guidelines 301, 302, 304, 305
outcomes and continuity to adulthood
311–312
out-patient treatment 309–311
personality disorders 31, 35, 307, 308,
310
pharmacology 131–132, 309
risk assessment and risk management
304–306
risk of 'contagion' 311
risk factors for suicidal behaviour
303–304
self-injury 301
self-poisoning 301, 309
serotonin system 303
stepwise approach to care 309
self-identity 30, 44
separation anxiety disorder 165, 167, 171,
172, 174, 177, 178
serotonergic proteins: allele length 26
serotonin transporter gene 135, 172, 190,
272–273, 372
sertraline
anxiety disorders 95, 96, 177
ASD 117
depression 100, 132, 133, 136
OCD 98
Tourette syndrome 279
services: model of four-tiered provision 7
sexual abuse
antisocial behaviour 65
of parents in fabrication of illness 14
personality disorders 31
PTSD 45, 46
sleep disorders 287–300
aetiological factors 289–290
assessment 292–293
British Sleep Society's website 293
Children's Sleep Habits Questionnaire
292

continuity into adulthood 290
developmental aspects 290–291
diagnosis 292–293
distinction between problems and
disorders 288–289
effects on child development 291–292
emotional state and behaviour effects 291
family and social effects 292
infancy and early childhood 366
intellectual function and education effects
291
links with child psychiatry 287–288
management of specific disorders
294–298
medication causing 288
physical effects 292
prevalence of sleep disturbance 288
screening 292
treatment principles 293
sleep hygiene 209, 293
sleepwalking 288, 297
social anxiety disorder 168, 178
social phobia 168, 171, 174, 177, 178
Somatic Symptom Checklist 205
somatising 183–217
aetiology 188–193
appropriate clinician to manage 201–203
assessment 203–205
biopsychosocial approach 203, 204, 213
CAMHS referral not accepted by family
212–214
child protection 214
classification 184–187
clinical presentations 193–198
comorbid psychiatric conditions 203,
205–206, 210
cultural factors 190–191, 208
depressive and anxiety disorders 190,
191, 196–197, 203, 205, 214
education and school liaison 210–211
epidemiological studies 187–188
factors associated with physical symptoms
191
genetics 190
girls 188, 194, 195, 196, 197
illness behaviour 183, 189–190, 192–193,
195, 209
management 206–214
outcomes and continuities 214–215
pharmacology 210
pubertal status 188
questionnaires and interview schedules
205
rehabilitation 211

sick role 192
specific treatments 208–212
treatment principles 206–208
treatment setting 206
treatment in severely disturbed families 212
somatoform disorders 194–195, 201, 209
in parents and fabrication of illness 15–16, 17, 18
SSRIs *see* selective serotonin reuptake inhibitors
STEPPS (Systems Training for Emotional Predictability and Problem Solving) 37
stimulants
ADHD 74, 76–80, 81, 97–98, 236, 241–243, 279, 320, 375
antisocial behaviour 69
ASD 88, 89, 120–121
bipolar disorder 144
misuse 317
preschoolers 375
Tourette syndrome 279
Strengths and Difficulties Questionnaire (SDQ) 64, 234, 366
Structured Clinical Interview for DSM-IV Axis II Personality Disorders (SCID-II) 20–21
substance misuse
adolescents 315–329
aetiology 318–320
disinhibitory psychopathology 318–319
environment 320
epidemiology 315–316
genetics 318–319
medication in ADHD 80
national guidance 325
personality disorders 34–35, 36, 324–325
pre-existing mental illness 320
pregnancy 369
prevention programmes 321
psychoactive substances 316–318
PTSD 46, 50
research 323
schizophrenia 248, 250
self-medication 319–320
treatment 321–325
suicidality
depression 100–101, 129, 131–132, 134, 137
gender dysphoria 354, 362
personality disorders 31
psychological autopsy 304
PTSD 50
risk factors for behaviour 303–304

self-harm and 131–132, 301, 302, 303–304, 308, 312
SSRIs 129, 131–132, 177
sulpiride 83, 84
supraorbital area 44, 52
sympathetic system 30, 31, 46

tardive dyskinesia 144
Tavistock Clinic for Functional Nerve Cases 4
tetrabenazine 276
Texas guidelines 132, 136
therapeutic communities 36
tic disorders
ADHD 236
ASD 119
OCD 99
pharmacology 83–85
Tourette syndrome 83–85, 267, 268–269
Tourette syndrome 262–286
aetiology 266–267
aggression and behavioural difficulties 272–273
androgen exposure 267
assessment 274–275
behavioural interventions 276
botulinum toxin injection 275–279
clinical features 267–269
coexistent psychopathology 272
comorbidity 269–272, 280–281
ADHD 82, 84, 85–86, 262, 267, 269, 273, 279
ASD 265, 269, 272
obsessive–compulsive behaviours 262, 265, 269, 272, 276
OCD 82, 84, 99, 262, 269, 276, 280
continuity into adulthood 280
coprolalia 268
echo phenomena 267–268
epidemiology 265
GABHS infections 266–267
genetics 266, 272–273
Gilles de la Tourette Syndrome–Quality of Life scale (GTS-QOL) 262
management and treatment 275–279
monoamine oxidase A (MAOA) gene 272–273
neuroimmunological theories 266–267
PANDAS 266
parents 262–265
pharmacology 82–86, 276–279
comorbid ADHD symptoms 82, 84, 85–86
for tics 83–85

quality of life 262
  scales 275
  smoking during pregnancy 267
  tics 83–85, 267, 268–269
  types 269, 274
transcranial magnetic stimulation 374
trauma-focused cognitive–behavioural
  therapy 48
Treatment for Adolescents with Depression
  Study (TADS) 101, 131, 137
tricyclic antidepressants 94–95, 100, 116
  see also clomipramine
Triple P-Positive Parenting Program 67

UNICEF report 2007 7
USA: history of child psychiatry 1, 3

vagus nerve stimulation 374
valproate 103, 143, 144

valproic acid 87, 89
vancomycin 115
velocardiofacial syndrome (22q11DS)
  247–248, 252
venlafaxine 95, 96, 100, 101, 117, 130, 135,
  136
ventral striatum 28, 34
violence
  instrumental 35
  personality disorders 35
  PTSD 46, 50
  reactive 35

war, effects of 2, 5
well-being of children 7
Wilson's disease 254, 255, 275

ziprasidone 84, 102, 119

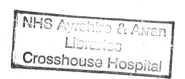